RN to BSN

Review and Challenge Tests

RN to BSN

Review and Challenge Tests

Diane M. Billings, RN, EdD
Professor of Nursing
Indiana University School of Nursing
at Indianapolis

Pamela R. Jeffries, RN, MSN
Assistant Professor of Nursing
Indiana University School of Nursing
at Indianapolis

Carol H. Kammer, RN, EdD
Formerly Associate Professor of Nursing
Indiana University School of Nursing
at Indianapolis and Kokomo

11 Contributors

J.B. LIPPINCOTT COMPANY Philadelphia
Grand Rapids   New York   St. Louis   San Francisco
London   Sydney   Tokyo

Acquisitions Editor: Nancy L. Mullins
Coordinating Editorial Assistant: Ellen Campbell
Manuscript Editor: Diana Merritt
Indexer: Helene Taylor Associates
Design Coordinator: Caren Erlichman
Designer: Susan Blaker
Cover Design: Kevin Curry
Production Manager: Carol A. Florence
Production Coordinator: Barney Fernandes
Compositor: TAPSCO, Inc.
Text Printer/Binder: R.R. Donnelly & Sons Company, Inc.
Cover Printer: New England Book Components

Copyright © 1989 by J.B. Lippincott Company.

All rights reserved. No part of this book may be used or reproduced in any manner whatsoever without permission except for brief quotations embodied in critical articles and reviews. Printed in the United States of America. For information write J.B. Lippincott Company, East Washington Square, Philadelphia, Pennsylvania 19105.

3 5 6 4 2

Library of Congress Cataloging-in-Publication Data

RN to BSN : review and challenge tests.

  Includes bibliographies and index.
    1. Nursing—Examinations, questions, etc. 2. Nursing—Outlines, syllabi, etc. I. Billings, Diane McGovern. II. Jeffries, Pamela R. III. Kammer, Carol Highsmith, [date]   . [DNLM: 1. Nursing—examination questions. 2. Nursing—outlines. WY 18 R6275]
RT55.R63 1989   610.73'076   89–2422
ISBN 0-397-54718-8

The authors and publisher have exerted every effort to ensure that drug selection and dosage set forth in this text are in accord with current recommendations and practice at the time of publication. However, in view of ongoing research, changes in government regulations, and the constant flow of information relating to drug therapy and drug reactions, the reader is urged to check the package insert for each drug for any change in indications and dosage and for added warnings and precautions. This is particularly important when the recommended agent is a new or infrequently employed drug.

Any procedure or practice described in this book should be applied by the health-care practitioner under appropriate supervision in accordance with professional standards of care used with regard to the unique circumstances that apply in each practice situation. Care has been taken to confirm the accuracy of information presented and to describe generally accepted practices. However, the authors, editors and publisher cannot accept any responsibility for errors or omissions or for consequences from application of the information in this book and make no warranty, express or implied, with respect to the contents of the book.

Contributors

Diane M. Billings, RN, EdD
Professor
Indiana University School of Nursing at Indianapolis
Editor; author, Chapter 2, *Study Skills and Test-Taking Strategies*

Marguerite Casey, RN, MSN
Assistant Professor
Indiana University School of Nursing at Indianapolis
Author, Chapter 4, *The Nurse as Communicator*; test item writer

Marsha Dowell, RN, MSN
Assistant Professor
University of Virginia School of Nursing
Charlottesville, Virginia
Author, Chapter 7, *Nursing Care of the Client with Impairment in Sensorimotor Function*, and Chapter 8, *Nursing Care of the Client with Dysfunction of the Genitourinary and Reproductive Systems*; test item writer; audiotape presenter

Pamela R. Jeffries, RN, MSN
Assistant Professor
Indiana University School of Nursing at Indianapolis
Editor; author, Chapter 3, *The Nursing Process*; audiotape presenter

Carol H. Kammer, RN, EdD
Formerly Associate Professor
Indiana University School of Nursing at Indianapolis and Kokomo
Editor; author, Chapter 1, *Introduction to RN Mobility*

Julie Lamothe, RN, MSN, CPNP
Lecturer
Indiana University School of Nursing at Indianapolis
Author, Chapter 13, *Nursing Care of the Infant*, and Chapter 14, *Nursing Care of the Toddler and Preschooler*; test item writer; audiotape presenter

Kathy Jo Morrical, RN, MSN
Assistant Professor
Indiana University School of Nursing at Kokomo
Author, Chapter 5, *Nursing Care of the Client Who Has a Deficiency in the Delivery of Oxygen to the Cells*; test item writer; audiotape presenter

Ann Nice, RN, MSN, OCN
Assistant Professor
Indiana University School of Nursing at Indianapolis
Author, Chapter 6, *Nursing Care of the Client Who Has a Problem with Digestion,*

Metabolism, Elimination, and Providing Nutrients to the Cells; test item writer; audiotape script developer

Virginia Richardson, RN, MSN, CPNP
Assistant Professor
Indiana University School of Nursing at Indianapolis
Author, Chapter 15, *Nursing Care of the School-age Child,* and Chapter 16, *Nursing Care of the Adolescent;* test item writer; audiotape presenter

Mary Van Allen, RN, MSN
Assistant Professor
Indiana University School of Nursing at Indianapolis
Author, Unit III, *Care of the Client During Childbearing;* test item writer; audiotape presenter

Ruth Woodham, RN, MSN
Psychiatric Nurse Therapist
St. Vincent Stress Center
Indianapolis, Indiana
Formerly Assistant Professor
Indiana University School of Nursing at Indianapolis
Author, Unit V, *Care of the Client with a Mental Health Problem;* test item writer; audiotape presenter

Preface

Registered nurse (RN) students, once considered the nontraditional consumers of nursing education, have become a major sector of the nursing student population, representing more than 30% of total baccalaureate and higher degree nursing students. When RN students enter BSN or MSN programs, they are usually required to demonstrate their previously acquired nursing knowledge by taking standardized or teacher-made validation examinations in order to receive advanced placement standing. *RN to BSN: Review and Challenge Tests* is written especially for RN students to use in independent review for validation or challenge examinations given by schools of nursing to evaluate and award credit for previous learning. However, it can also be used for self-assessment and remedial study of a troublesome topic area.

The book is organized in six units. Unit I contains introductory chapters designed to orient students to typical processes used by schools of nursing to award advanced placement credit for previous learning. Specific examination preparation skills (such as how to develop a study plan) and test-taking strategies are included to help students individualize their review. In addition, a chapter on nursing process and a chapter on communication skills serve as foundation content for subsequent units. Units II through V are organized according to the four main clinical areas of nursing:

Care of the Adult Client
Care of the Client During Childbearing
Care of the Child
Care of the Client with a Mental Health Problem

Separation of units according to the traditional nursing content areas enables review and testing over individual units.

The audiotapes that accompany this book are a unique learning feature. The tapes were developed by chapter authors to enhance the written content and personalize the learning process. The content matches written chapters and is presented in a conversational style. Two 90-minute tapes cover all four units. Listening to audiotapes helps break the monotony of reading outline reviews and affords students flexibility in learning. For example, students may listen and learn while driving or doing household tasks.

The testing portion of the book (Unit VI) contains one practice examination for each of the four units listed above, as well as answers with rationales and a diagnostic grid for each test, to help learners identify areas needing additional study. Practice tests included in this book are typical of teacher-made and standardized tests. Answers are coded according to the nursing content area(s) being tested:

Health status
Nursing actions/interventions
Drugs/pharmacology
Nutrition
Communication skills

Answers are also coded according to the nursing process area(s) being tested:

Assessment
Analysis/nursing diagnosis
Planning
Implementation/intervention
Evaluation

The diagnostic grid uses these codes to help students identify patterns of incorrect responses. Students can then plan subsequent study based on knowing their areas of strength and weakness. See the instructions accompanying the Practice Tests for further information about using the grids.

It is suggested that Unit I be read first because it provides orientation and foundation for subsequent chapters. Units II through V may be reviewed in any sequence. For example, a student may focus the initial review on Unit IV, Care of the Child. One study plan might include reading the chapters in that unit, listening to the audiotape of that unit, and taking Practice Test 3. The diagnostic grid accompanying Test 3 could then be used to determine readiness for taking validation examinations in that area. If review is needed beyond the scope of the chapters in Unit IV, the student may choose to read one or more of the suggested texts listed in the bibliography for Unit IV. The student may then progress through the remaining units as needed, at his or her own pace.

Special features of this book include:

- The introductory section describes the RN-to-BSN and RN-to-MSN process as well as types, administration, and scoring of validation examinations.
- An entire chapter is devoted to specific study skills and test-taking strategies.
- A review of nursing process, including information on nursing diagnosis, is included.
- A special chapter focuses on communication and interpersonal skills.
- Content review is organized in an easy-to-read outline format covering traditional areas of nursing content tested on both standardized and teacher-made validation examinations.
- The testing section contains 566 multiple choice items based on case situations. Answers and rationales are coded according to the stage of nursing process and the aspect of nursing care involved. Specific directions for scoring tests, diagnosing specific student learning needs, and planning for remedial work are included.
- The content and test format used are typical of other standardized and teacher-made validation examinations.
- Both the review content and test questions have been field tested with RN students in review sessions taught by the authors of this text at Indiana University School of Nursing.
- Audiotapes to facilitate auditory learning supplement and accompany the text. These tapes were made by faculty who taught the content in review sessions and who wrote the respective chapter(s) in the book.
- Bibliographies at the end of each unit serve to direct students needing a more in-depth review.
- A checklist for developing a study plan is provided to encourage active involvement of students in planning their own review.

The editors of the book wish to acknowledge Michael E. Scott, audiotape consultant and narrator, and the following individuals at the Indiana University School of Nursing who have contributed to the development of this project.

Dr. Charlotte Carlley, Assistant Dean for Continuing Education

RN students who attended the review sessions

Beverly Ross, Assistant Professor, chapter reviewer

LaVern Sutton, counselor, chapter reviewer

Helen Gullion, secretary
Carol Hash, secretary
Joy Hawkins, secretary
Sylvia Mason, secretary
Joyce Stout, secretary
Tracey H. Vibbert, secretary
Steffani R. White, secretary

Diane M. Billings, RN, EdD
Pamela R. Jeffries, RN, MSN
Carol H. Kammer, RN, EdD

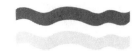

Contents

Unit I
Understanding and Preparing for RN Mobility 1

1 Introduction to RN Mobility 3
  What Is RN Mobility? 3
  What Is Validation? 3
  What Is Tested on Validation Examinations? 4
  How Are Examinations Administered and Scored? 4
  How Should I Prepare for Validation? 4

2 Study Skills and Test-Taking Strategies 6
  Studying Effectively 6
  Using Test-Taking Strategies 9
  Managing Test Anxiety 10
  Taking Validation Examinations 11

3 The Nursing Process 13
  Assessment 13
  Nursing Diagnosis 15
  Planning 15
  Implementation 18
  Evaluation 18

4 The Nurse as Communicator 21
  The Importance of Communication in Nurse/Client Relationships 22
  Models for Enhancing Communication 23
  Facilitation Skills 27
  Interviewing Skills 28
  Interpersonal Conflict Resolution Skills 30
  Interpersonal Skills to Promote Behavior Change 31

  Bibliography for Unit I 33

Unit II
Care of the Adult Client 35

5 Nursing Care of the Client Who Has a Deficiency in the Delivery of Oxygen to the Cells 37
  Cardiac Dysfunction 37
   Angina Pectoris 37
   Myocardial Infarction 40
   Congestive Heart Failure 43

Rheumatic Heart Disease   45
Mitral Stenosis   47
Heart Block   49

Vascular Dysfunction   51
Aneurysm   51
Thrombophlebitis   53
Pulmonary Embolism   55
Cerebrovascular Accident   56
Varicose Veins   58
Buerger's Disease (Thromboangiitis Obliterans)   59
Raynaud's Phenomenon   60
Arteriosclerosis   61
Hypertension   62

Pulmonary Dysfunction   64
Chronic Obstructive Pulmonary Disease   64
Neoplasia of Lung   66
Tuberculosis   68
Asthma   69
Acute Respiratory Infections   70
Adult Respiratory Distress Syndrome   71

6 **Nursing Care of the Client Who Has a Problem with Digestion, Metabolism, Elimination, and Providing Nutrients to the Cells**   74

Upper Gastrointestinal Dysfunction   74
Food Poisoning   74
Hiatal Hernia   75
Peptic Ulcer   76
Gallbladder Disease   78
Regional Enteritis (Crohn's Disease)   80

Large Bowel Dysfunction   81
Ulcerative Colitis   81
Cancer of the Colon   82
Hemorrhoids   83
Anal Abscess   85
Anal Fistula   86
Pilonidal Cyst   86
Appendicitis   86
Diverticulitis   87

Liver and Pancreas Dysfunction   88
Cirrhosis   88
Cancer of the Liver   91
Hepatitis   91
Pancreatitis   92

Metabolic Dysfunction   93
Diabetes Mellitus   93
Hyperthyroidism   96
Hypothyroidism   97
Addison's Disease   98

Blood Abnormalities and Related Conditions   99
Pernicious Anemia   99
Nutritional Anemia   100
Sickle Cell Anemia   101
Leukemia   102
Hodgkin's Disease   103
Ruptured Spleen   104

Integumentary Abnormalities   105
Herpes Zoster (Shingles)   105
Contact Dermatitis   105
Burns   106

7 **Nursing Care of the Client with Impairment in Sensorimotor Function**   108

Central Nervous System Impairment   108
Head Injury   108
Brain Tumors   109

Convulsive Disorders   111
Epilepsy and Seizures   111
Meningitis   112
Multiple Sclerosis   113
Myasthenia Gravis   114
Parkinson's Disease   116

Larynx Impairment   118
Laryngeal Tumors   118

Ear Impairment   119
Otosclerosis   119
Meniere's Syndrome   120

Eye Impairment   121
Glaucoma   121
Cataracts   122
Detached Retina   123

Nose Impairment 124
   Deviated Septum 124
Skeletal Dysfunction 125
   Fractures 125
   Spinal Cord Injuries 127
   Amputations 128
Joint Dysfunction 129
   Osteoarthritis 129
   Gout 130
   Rheumatoid Arthritis 131

8 Nursing Care of the Client with Dysfunction of the Genitourinary and Reproductive Systems 133

Female Reproductive Problems 133
   Uterine Fibroids or Uterine Leiomyomas 133
   Uterine Prolapse 134
   Pelvic Inflammatory Disease and Salpingitis 135
   Endometriosis 136
   Ovarian Cancer 138
   Breast Cancer 139
   Uterine and Cervical Cancer 140
Male Reproductive Problems 141
   Benign Prostatic Hypertrophy 141
   Cancer of the Prostate 143
   Cancer of the Testes 144
Sexually Transmitted Diseases 145
   Syphilis 145
   Gonorrhea 146
   Genital Herpes 147
   Chlamydia 148
   Acquired Immunodeficiency Syndrome (AIDS) 149
Renal Dysfunction 152
   Glomerulonephritis 152
   Renal Calculi 153
   Renal Tumor 154
   Acute Renal Failure 155
   Chronic Renal Failure 157
   Cystitis 159
   Bladder Tumors and Neoplasms 160

Bibliography for Unit II 161

Unit III
Care of the Client During Childbearing 163

9 Nursing Care During the Antepartal Period 165

The Client with a Normal Pregnancy 165
   Physiological Adaptations of the Conceptus 165
   Maternal Physiological Adaptations 165
   Health Promotion Needs 167
   Nutritional Care 167
   Fetal Assessment 167
   Developmental Tasks of the Expanding Family 168
   Preparation for Childbirth 168
The High Risk Prenatal Client 169
   Epidemiological and Other Risk Factors for Mother and Fetus 169
   Preexisting Medical Conditions as Risk Factors for Mother and Fetus 169
   Complications of Pregnancy 170

10 Nursing Care During the Intrapartal Period 173

The Client Undergoing Normal Labor and Delivery 173
   Assessment 173
   Support During Labor 175
   Delivery 176
   Immediate Care of the Newborn 176
   Maternal Physiological Assessments During Fourth Stage 177
The High Risk Labor Client 177
   Complications of Labor 177
   Dystocia 177
   Prolapsed Cord 177
   Induction of Labor with Oxytocin 177
   Episiotomy/Lacerations 178
   Indications for Forceps Delivery 178
   Premature Labor 178
   Precipitate or Emergency Delivery 178
   Uterine Rupture 178
   Inversion of Uterus 178

11   Nursing Care During the Postpartal Period   179

   The Normal Postpartum Client   179
      Physiological Adaptation: Assessment and Interventions   179
      Lactation and Breast-feeding   180
      Psychosocial Adaptation   181
      Educational Needs   181
   The High Risk Postpartum Client   182
      Assessing the High Risk Mother   182
      Complications of the Postpartal Period   182
      Hemorrhage   182
      Infection   183
      Thrombophlebitis   183
      Psychosocial Problems   183

12   Nursing Care of the Neonate and Family   184

   The Normal Newborn   184
      Physiological Changes   184
      Physical Assessment   184
      Nutritional Needs   185
   Complications That May Affect the Newborn   185
      Respiratory Problems   185
      Jaundice   186
      Feeding Problems   187
      Infection   187
      Congenital Anomalies   187
   Care of the High Risk Infant   187
   Effects of Maternal Problems on the Newborn   188

   Bibliography for Unit III   189

Unit IV
Care of the Child   191

13   Nursing Care of the Infant   193

   Growth and Development   193
   Health Promotion   193
   The Hospitalized Infant   196
   Health Problems of the Infant   196
      Myelomeningocele   196
      Hydrocephalus   196
      Cleft Lip and Cleft Palate   198
      Congenital Hip Dysplasia   199
      Strabismus   200
      Congenital Heart Disease   200
      Tracheoesophageal Fistula   201
      Acute Respiratory Infections   202
      Pyloric Stenosis   203
      Diarrhea and Dehydration   204
      Iron Deficiency Anemia   205
      Intussusception   206
      Hirschprung's Disease (Congenital Aganglionic Megacolon)   206
      Allergies   207
      Child Abuse   208
      Sudden Infant Death Syndrome   209
      Phenylketonuria   209
      Failure to Thrive   210

14   Nursing Care of the Toddler and Preschooler   212

   Growth and Development   212
   Health Promotion   212
   The Hospitalized Toddler and Preschooler   213
   Health Problems of the Toddler and Preschooler   213
      Tonsillitis and Tonsillectomy   213
      Otitis Media   214
      Cystic Fibrosis   215
      Ingestion of Poisonous Substances   216
      Celiac Disease   217
      Appendicitis   218
      Nephrosis   218
      Hemophilia   219
      Accidents   220

15   Nursing Care of the School-age Child   221

   Growth and Development   221
   Health Promotion   222
   The Hospitalized School-age Child   222

Health Problems of the School-age Child   223
   Accidents   223
   Helminthic Infections   223
   Mental Retardation   224
   Acute Lymphocytic Leukemia   224
   Brain Tumor   225
   Acute Glomerulonephritis   226
   Asthma   226
   Cystic Fibrosis   227
   Inguinal Hernia   228
   Appendicitis   228
   Acute Rheumatic Fever   229
   Sickle Cell Anemia   230
   Diabetes Mellitus   231
   Burns   231
   Fractures   232

16 Nursing Care of the Adolescent   234

Growth and Development   234
Health Promotion   234
The Hospitalized Adolescent   235
Health Problems of the Adolescent   235
   Accidents   235
   Obesity   235
   Bone Tumors   236
   Scoliosis   236
   Convulsive Disorder/Epilepsy   237
   Venereal Disease   237
   Drug Abuse   238
   Suicide   238
   Acne   239

Bibliography for Unit IV   239

Unit V
Care of the Client with a Mental Health Problem   241

17 General Psychiatric Nursing Treatment Modalities   243

Basic Assumptions of Nursing as a Practice Profession   243

Foundations of Psychiatric Nursing   243
Therapeutic Communication as Process   243
Psychotropic Medications   244
   Antipsychotic/Neuroleptic Agents   245
   Antidepressant Agents   246
   Antimania Agent: Lithium Carbonate   248
   Antianxiety Agents (Sedatives and Hypnotics)   250
   Antiparkinsonian and Antihistamine Agents   251
Electroconvulsive Therapy   253
Psychosocial Therapies   254
   Milieu Therapy   254
   Group Therapy   254
   Family Therapy   254
   Activity Therapy   254
   Behavior Therapy   254
   Crisis Intervention   254
   Suicide Intervention   255

18 Nursing Care of the Client with an Organic Mental Disorder   256

Delirium   256
Dementias Arising in the Senium and Presenium   257
Alcohol-induced Organic Mental Disorders   259
Barbiturate and Similar Sedative/Hypnotic Organic Mental Disorders   262
Opioid Organic Mental Disorders   263
Amphetamine and Similar Sympathomimetic Organic Mental Disorders   264
Cocaine Organic Mental Disorders   265
Mental Retardation   266

19 Nursing Care of the Client with a Mental Disorder from Psychological Causes 267

    Schizophrenia 267
    Bipolar Disorders 269
    Depressive Disorders 270
    Anxiety Disorder: Panic 271
    General Anxiety Disorder 271
    Obsessive Compulsive Disorder 272
    Somatoform Disorders 272
    Sexual Disorders 273
    Psychological Factors Affecting Physical Diseases 274
    Anorexia Nervosa 275
    Bulimia 275

20 Nursing Care of the Client with an Adjustment Disorder 277

    Assessment 277
    Nursing Plans and Interventions 278
    Drug Therapy 279
    Client/Family Teaching 279
    Evaluation 279

Bibliography for Unit V 279

Unit VI
Practice Tests 281

    How to Use the Practice Tests 283

Practice Test 1: Care of the Adult Client 286

    Answer Sheet—Test 1 315
    Answers and Rationales for Test 1 317
    Diagnostic Grid Test 1 327

Practice Test 2: Care of the Client During Childbearing 338

    Answer Sheet—Test 2 351
    Answers and Rationales for Test 2 352
    Diagnostic Grid Test 2 357

Practice Test 3: Care of the Child 363

    Answer Sheet—Test 3 377
    Answers and Rationales for Test 3 378
    Diagnostic Grid Test 3 384

Practice Test 4: Care of the Client with a Mental Health Problem 390

    Answer Sheet—Test 4 405
    Answers and Rationales for Test 4 406
    Diagnostic Grid Test 4 411

Practice Test Summary 417

Index 419

RN to BSN

Review and Challenge Tests

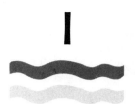

Understanding and Preparing for RN Mobility

1

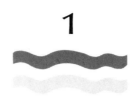

Introduction to RN Mobility

What Is RN Mobility?

RN mobility is the educational process that registered nurses use to attain advanced degrees in nursing. Many nursing schools offer RN mobility programs designed specifically to give credit for previously acquired nursing knowledge and experience. These programs commonly lead to a baccalaureate degree in nursing (BSN) and are called *RN completion* or *RN to BSN* programs. In addition, a few schools offer RN mobility programs leading toward a master's degree in nursing (MSN).

The number of RN students enrolled in RN mobility programs has steadily increased in the past 10 years. The most recent data show 41,112 RN students enrolled in baccalaureate nursing programs, representing 30% of the total baccalaureate nursing student enrollment. The number of RN students returning for BSN degrees has more than tripled in the 10-year period 1976–1986 (NLN, 1986).

RN mobility programs usually offer an opportunity for advanced placement in nursing courses, based on validation of previous nursing knowledge and experience. Many programs also have transition courses designed to bridge the knowledge and experience gap between RNs' previous and present nursing education.

What Is Validation?

Most RNs who are seeking an advanced degree hope to accomplish it as quickly as possible and to receive as much credit as possible for the knowledge, skills, and experience they have acquired in work settings and other nursing programs. Nursing programs want to recognize the competencies of RN students, but also need to maintain the integrity of their curricula in providing quality education. Therefore, schools of nursing must validate prior learning of RN students before awarding academic credit for advanced placement.

The specific validation process used by nursing schools varies, and may include such methods as course to course transfer credit, paper and pencil validation or challenge examinations, clinical performance examinations, and portfolio presentation of previous learning experiences. Some schools use examinations that are written by the faculty at that school, but a growing number of schools use standardized examinations to validate previously acquired nursing knowledge. The two standardized examinations most commonly used are the National League for Nursing (NLN) Mobility Profile II Examinations, and the American College Testing Program's Proficiency Examination Program (ACT/PEP).

What Is Tested on Validation Examinations?

Validation examinations written by faculty of individual schools vary greatly among schools. They may cover material taught in particular nursing courses, or cover more general knowledge. Usually, the faculty of a given school design the examination to test knowledge gained from courses taught at that school. Schools may provide study guides or course syllabi to help students prepare for these tests. The type of questions used on these tests also varies (*e.g.*, multiple choice or essay).

Standardized nursing validation examinations (NLN or ACT/PEP) typically include three or four individual tests covering the traditional content areas of adult, maternal/child, and psychiatric/mental health nursing. The tests are designed to assess knowledge of factors that reflect a client's health status, including those that suggest health problems and those that suggest normal growth and development. The examinations also measure understanding of how to use the nursing process in providing care to clients. NLN examinations also test knowledge of drug therapy, nutrition, and diet therapy.

The format of standardized examinations is multiple choice. The NLN tests utilize mostly case situations. The number of items per test varies from about 120 to 220 per test. Testing time is usually 2 to 4 hours per test, and 45 to 60 seconds are usually allowed per question. The individual tests may usually be taken at separate sessions if desired.

Study guides or informational booklets about the standardized tests are often available to students, from the school or the testing service. The booklets provide sample questions and a brief description of what is tested on the examination.

How Are Examinations Administered and Scored?

Policies regarding administration of validation examinations vary among schools. Students are usually charged a fee per test. The school or college testing department administers the test.

Scoring of validation examinations is done by either school faculty or a testing service. Scoring of standardized examinations is done by the testing service and reported to the student or school. The testing service furnishes schools with scoring data from students taking the tests in other schools, which is used to help establish minimum passing scores. Individual schools are responsible for determining the minimum passing score. The national average for the minimum passing score set by schools who use the NLN Mobility Profile II tests is a score of 90 to 92, which means that the student answered 58% to 67% of the items correctly (NLN, 1984). A recommended passing score on the ACT/PEP tests is 45, which means that the student answered 55% to 60% of the items correctly (ACT/PEP, 1985). Passing scores on examinations written by individual schools are determined by school faculty.

Individual schools determine how many times an examination may be taken and establish procedures for awarding advanced placement. Schools may allow students who have failed an examination to take it again, or to take an alternate form of the examination. Some schools require students who have failed an examination to enroll in courses.

How Should I Prepare for Validation?

You may have already taken the first step in preparation—talking with officials at the school of nursing where you plan to study. Information you will need to obtain includes:

- What program is available for RN students wishing to pursue a BSN or MSN? Ask for the current written materials describing the curriculum requirements and policies regarding admission, progression, and graduation.
- What is the school's current policy regarding validation? Specifically, what courses

must be taken? What method of validation is used and when are tests administered? What guidance does the school offer students regarding the process? What are the policies for repeating validation attempts if the first is unsuccessful?
- What happens if the school changes its policies regarding validation or any other requirements during your enrollment?
- If you plan a part-time course of study and do not enroll each semester, are there potential progression problems?
- What costs are involved for validation? Fees may be assessed for taking examinations and recording academic credit.
- When are academic credits awarded?
- How do validation credits transfer? What happens if you relocate and want to transfer to another school before graduating?

These questions are intended not to discourage you from pursuing your advanced degree, but to help you become an informed consumer of your education. Many RN students are nontraditional college students who work full-time or part-time and have family responsibilities that make planning and controlling an educational career very difficult. Some school programs, on the other hand, may be designed for full-time students who progress directly from high school and complete coursework in a predictable manner. Schools may not give you all the information you need to plan your progression. It is in your best interest to be informed about your school's policies, so don't hesitate to ask questions that will help you plan your course of study.

When you have obtained the necessary information from the school of nursing and enrolled in a course of study, it may be helpful to develop a validation progression plan. Chapter 2, on study skills and test-taking strategies, is designed to help you take the next step in preparing for validation—developing a study plan.

2

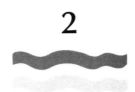

Study Skills and Test-Taking Strategies

Studying for and taking tests such as the validation examinations used in RN mobility programs require planning and preparation. Your time and energy can best be directed by making study time efficient, and learning effective test-taking strategies. In this chapter you will learn how to develop a study plan, use test-taking strategies, manage test anxiety, and take standardized or teacher-made validation examinations.

Studying Effectively

Studying for examinations is improved when resources such as time, energy, and study aids are focused and used wisely. A systematic approach includes assessing your study needs, creating a study plan, using study skills, and evaluating your progress.

Assessing Study Needs

The first step in developing a study plan is to appraise your knowledge of nursing practice in the content area or areas that will be tested. Knowing the strengths of your knowledge base will help you determine areas to study, and how to set study priorities. You can assess your knowledge by:

- *Reviewing clinical expertise.* The clinical area or areas of nursing in which you are currently employed or in which you have previous experience are likely to be areas in which you are knowledgeable. Studying these areas can be limited to review, so more concentrated study can be devoted to content areas in which you have less clinical experience.
- *Appraising success in nursing school.* Subjects in which you received high grades or that you found easy to learn will likely continue to be areas in which your knowledge is sound and thorough. Conversely, detailed review will likely be necessary in areas that you found difficult to learn.
- *Reviewing nursing knowledge content outlines.* The nursing knowledge base that is tested in most RN mobility or challenge examinations is presented in this book in an outline format to facilitate review. Skim the chapters to identify content that is familiar to you and content that will need concentrated study.
- *Taking practice examinations.* After reviewing the content outlines, take the practice examinations at the end of this book. These examinations can be used as a pretest for assessing your current knowledge in each clinical area. They will also help you assess your knowledge of pharmacology, nutrition, psychosocial aspects of nursing care,

CHECKLIST FOR DEVELOPING A STUDY ACTION PLAN

1. Assess study needs
   - ☐ Review individual clinical expertise—in which clinical areas do you have the greatest strength? _____
   - ☐ Reappraise nursing school success—in which subject areas did you perform best? _____
   - ☐ Review nursing knowledge content outlines. Skim the chapters of this book to identify familiar content and identify areas needing more concentrated study:

     Care of the Adult Client
     - ☐ Chapter 5   Nursing Care of the Client Who Has a Deficiency in the Delivery of Oxygen to the Cells
     - ☐ Chapter 6   Nursing Care of the Client Who Has a Problem in Digestion, Metabolism, Elimination, and Providing Nutrients to the Cells
     - ☐ Chapter 7   Nursing Care of the Client with Impairment in Sensorimotor Function
     - ☐ Chapter 8   Nursing Care of the Client with Dysfunction of the Genitourinary and Reproductive Systems

     Care of the Client During Childbearing
     - ☐ Chapter 9   Nursing Care During the Antepartal Period
     - ☐ Chapter 10 Nursing Care During the Intrapartal Period
     - ☐ Chapter 11 Nursing Care During the Postpartal Period
     - ☐ Chapter 12 Nursing Care of the Neonate and Family

     Care of the Child
     - ☐ Chapter 13 Nursing Care of the Infant
     - ☐ Chapter 14 Nursing Care of the Toddler and Preschooler
     - ☐ Chapter 15 Nursing Care of the School-age Child
     - ☐ Chapter 16 Nursing Care of the Adolescent

     Care of the Client with a Mental Health Problem
     - ☐ Chapter 17 General Psychiatric Nursing Treatment Modalities
     - ☐ Chapter 18 Nursing Care of the Client with an Organic Mental Disorder
     - ☐ Chapter 19 Nursing Care of the Client with a Mental Disorder from Psychological Causes
     - ☐ Chapter 20 Nursing Care of the Client with an Adjustment Disorder
   - ☐ Take practice exams—pretesting your current knowledge helps pinpoint areas for further study
2. Develop a specific study plan
   - ☐ Locate a quiet place to study
   - ☐ Draw up a study-time contract with yourself
   - ☐ Set priorities for study
   - ☐ Obtain needed study resources
3. Use study skills
   - ☐ Study to learn, not to memorize
   - ☐ Formulate questions and answers with rationales from the content
   - ☐ Study *common nursing measures*
   - ☐ Practice test-taking strategies
   - ☐ Simulate an examination through practice test-taking
4. Evaluate progress
   - ☐ Keep to a realistic schedule
   - ☐ Build confidence through positive self-feedback
   - ☐ Retake practice examinations
   - ☐ Identify the content areas you have mastered and focus on content problem areas

Figure 2-1.

and the nursing process. Each question is coded according to which of these content areas it tests, and which step of the nursing process it tests. Your subscores on these aspects of nursing care can be used to pinpoint areas for study.

Creating a Study Plan

Having identified areas for study, you can develop a specific study plan. Learners who develop a plan and study regularly have higher success rates than learners who wait until the last minute and "cram." Here are some suggestions for making a plan.

- *Identify a place for study.* The area should be quiet and have room for books and papers. Some learners designate an area in their home, others prefer a library.
- *Identify study times.* Establishing a time to study ensures a commitment to a study plan. Frequent and short study times of 1 to 2 hours are preferable to sporadic study times of 4 to 6 hours, because your concentration is more effective in short time periods. Make a contract with yourself; write the study time as a "date" in your calendar. Plan to finish studying a week before the examination. Last minute "cramming" can increase anxiety.
- *Set priorities.* Use the results of your assessment to develop a plan. Study those areas requiring the most preparation first.
- *Obtain needed resources.* Current textbooks, notes from previous classes, and study guides are helpful resources for studying. References and suggested readings are included at the end of each unit in this book; use them if you need suggestions for current resources.

Using Study Skills

Study skills enable you to acquire, organize, remember, and use the information you need to score successfully on the examinations you will be taking. Study skills include underlining, outlining, summarizing, listening, practicing test-taking, and studying with a friend or study group. Study skills can be learned and practiced.

You are probably familiar with study skills and know which ones work best for you. This review package has been designed to help you use several study skills, by presenting content in an outline format, and providing an audiotape and practice examinations. You can maximize the effectiveness of your study time by using these and other study skills. Other suggestions include:

- *Use study skills with which you are familiar and that have worked well for you in the past.* Some learners underline, others make notes. Some learn best by listening. Studying with a friend or study group may also be helpful.
- *Study to learn, not to memorize.* Most RN mobility or challenge examinations test application of knowledge. Study what you are learning in terms of how you would apply it in clinical practice.
- *Anticipate questions.* As you study, formulate questions that you think will likely be included on an examination. Practice giving rationales for your answers as well.
- *Study common nursing measures, not unique situations.* RN mobility or challenge examinations test a safe level of nursing practice. Do not overlook the common, accepted nursing practices to focus on less common nursing practices.
- *Practice the test-taking strategies and anxiety reduction strategies described in this chapter.* Make these strategies a part of your test-taking routine.
- *Simulate an examination.* Use the examinations in this book as post-tests to practice test-taking. These practice tests are similar to RN mobility and challenge examinations in terms of both length and the focus of the questions. Approximately 1 minute is allotted for answering each question, so you can time yourself to estimate your pace in taking an examination.

Evaluating Progress

As you implement your study plan, evaluate your progress and adjust your plan as needed. Points to consider include:

- *Keep on schedule.* Try not to let study time accumulate. This usually contributes to anxiety and can become a vicious cycle.
- *Give yourself positive self-feedback.* Build confidence.
- *Take the practice examinations again.* You should see your score(s) improving.
- *Make a review list.* Narrow the content area you have not mastered. Spend the rest of your time studying this content. Develop confidence in the content you have mastered and focus on content yet to be learned.

Using Test-taking Strategies

Researchers studying test-taking behavior have found that it is important not only to know the content, but also to know *how* to take an examination. The "how" of taking a test is called test-wiseness, and specific test-wise behaviors have been identified. These test-taking strategies can be learned and used to improve examination scores. Here is a list of strategies you may find helpful:

Understanding the Components of the Examination

Each examination is developed following a typical pattern. When you recognize these components, you can more easily discern the answer to each question.

- *Directions:* Each examination begins with directions that include information about the type of question (true/false, multiple choice, etc.), how the test is scored, and where to mark your answers. Your anxiety is likely to be highest at the beginning of the test; reading the directions carefully will prevent mistakes.

  Most examinations use computer answer sheets and computer scoring. When using computer answer sheets, it is important to use the appropriate pencil, and to align the test sheet and answer sheet so you are sure to mark the answer for each question in the right place on the answer sheet. Develop a habit of periodically checking alignment.
- *Situation:* The situation is a client-based scenario about which questions will be asked. The situation contains the information needed to answer the questions. Sometimes irrelevant data is included to test your ability to differentiate relevant from irrelevant data. Other times the situation may omit needed information and the question will ask you to determine what information is needed next. Several questions may relate to one situation, so you may need to refer back to that situation to answer a particular question.

  Read each situation carefully and base your answer on the data provided. Do not "read into" the situation information that is not there. Rather, select the answer that represents appropriate nursing care for the patient in that situation.
- *Stem:* The stem is the question. It may be a direct question such as "What should the nurse do first?" or an incomplete sentence such as "The nurse should . . ."
- *Options:* The options, or answers, are the possible responses to the stem. In typical multiple choice tests, there will be 1 correct option and 3 incorrect options, or distractors, for each question.

Using a Question Analysis Procedure

Skilled test-takers use a systematic approach to answer each question. Here is one format:

- Read the situation and stem to be sure you understand what the question is asking.
- Underline key words. Qualifiers such as "except," "but," and "not" can change the meaning of the question.

- Be sure you know the meaning of each word; decode unfamiliar words by breaking them into component parts.
- Check referents for pronouns (for instance, does "she" refer to the nurse, the client, or a family member?)
- Identify the step of the nursing process involved in answering the question: Do you need more data, are you setting priorities for planning, is this implementing or evaluating care?
- Answer the question before reading the options. If you understand the question clearly, a possible answer will probably come to mind.
- Read the options. Again, underline key words, including "except," "but," and "not."
- Find the option that matches your answer. If you do not know the answer, first reread the situation and question. Next, rule out incorrect options. If you are reasonably sure of an answer, and there is no penalty for guessing, make a guess. If you cannot make a reasonable guess, do not spend time deliberating. Put a question mark in the margin and come back to it later. There will be some questions in each examination that are difficult to answer. In these instances, give yourself positive self-talk and move on to the next question.
- Answers with words such as "never," "all," and "always" are usually incorrect responses.
- Answers that incorporate several other answers from the list of options are usually correct because they are most comprehensive.
- Answers should relate to the question. For example, if the question asks what to do first, the answer should reflect a priority nursing action; if the question asks what to have the *client* or family do, don't choose an option that indicates what the *nurse* should do.
- Answers should be based on nursing knowledge. The examination tests your knowledge of accepted nursing practice. Base item responses on nursing knowledge, not on what you *might* do, or on practices unique to your agency.
- Finally, mark the answer on the answer sheet. Be sure the answer number corresponds with the question number.
- Don't change an answer unless you are *certain* you have made a mistake. Test-taking research indicates a first response or guess is usually correct.

Monitoring Your Time

If you are a slow test-taker, be sure you are working steadily. Use the practice examinations in this book to identify your test-taking pace. Don't waste time on questions you find difficult; move on to those you find easier.

Managing Test Anxiety

Test anxiety refers to feelings of doubt and uncertainty about achieving satisfactory examination scores. Test anxiety can occur during study, immediately before the test, or even while taking the test. Test anxiety manifests itself in different ways with different people, but signs may include increased heart rate, labored breathing, sweating palms, dry mouth, and sleeplessness. While some anxiety is helpful to motivate study, excessive anxiety can decrease attention, alter perception, and inhibit your ability to respond correctly to test questions.

Being aware of test anxiety, identifying its source, and using strategies to manage it are helpful in improving study and test-taking skills. Just as different study strategies work well for different individuals, so do different test-anxiety management strategies work well for different test-takers. The key is to know which strategy or strategies work for you and use it or them when needed. Consider these strategies:

- *Mental rehearsal:* Mental rehearsal involves reviewing the events and environment related to the examination in your mind to consider how you will gain control of the situation and eliminate impulsive or negative behavior during the examination. During mental rehearsal you can anticipate how you will recognize and manage test anxiety, what the setting will be like, and what procedures you will use to take the test. Rehearsing these events during study and before the test will help you be organized and calm while taking the test.

- *Relaxation exercises:* Relaxation exercises involve tensing and relaxing various muscle groups to relieve the physical effects of anxiety. Systematic contraction and relaxation of muscle groups from the toes to the neck release energy for concentration. These simple exercises can be done during study and even while taking the examination.
- *Deep breathing:* Take deep breaths by inhaling slowly while counting to five, and exhaling slowly while counting to ten. This exercise decreases tenseness and increases the flow of oxygen to the lungs and brain, and can easily be done during study, as well as before and during examinations.
- *Visualize success:* Test-takers who expect success are more likely to attain it. Imagine a positive test-taking environment. Picture yourself taking the examination calmly. Expect high and passing examination results.
- *Positive self-talk:* Positive self-talk serves to correct negative thoughts ("I can't pass this test," "I'm too old [young, tired] to do this") about examinations, and reinforces a positive self-concept. If you find yourself giving yourself negative messages, convert those messages to positive ones. Tell yourself "I can do it," "I will pass," "I am a knowledgeable nurse, and a successful test-taker." This strategy is particularly useful if you become anxious or experience self-doubt during the examination.
- *Distraction:* Distraction involves thinking about something else and is a common and easy way to manage anxiety. Clear your mind. Think of something fun. Plan with a friend who is taking the test to talk about something besides the test.

Taking Validation Examinations

Now that you have studied, practiced test-taking skills, and learned anxiety management strategies, you are ready to take the validation examination. As the time to take the test approaches, there are several things you should consider doing before the test, during the test, and after the test. Thinking about them ahead of time is another way to prepare for the examination and manage inevitable test anxiety.

Before the Test

Before the test, be mentally and physically prepared. For example:

1. *Know the date, time, and place the test will be given.* If you have not been to the examination site before, find out where it is, how long it will take you to get there, and where you can park. Some nurses find it helpful to visit the examination site before the day of the test.
2. *Bring appropriate supplies.* If possible, know what supplies are required for the examination you will be taking. Most examinations require the use of a pencil or pen. Books are generally not needed, and are best left at home. Be certain to have enough money for meals or snacks. You may also need to pay examination registration fees. Some examinations require an admittance slip. Be sure to have it ready.
3. *Be physically prepared.* Get enough rest before the examination (don't stay up late cramming!) Fatigue can decrease your concentration, predispose you to illness, and diminish the effectiveness of anxiety management strategies. If you are working on a shift that is different from the time of the examination, try to adjust your work schedule to match the time of the test for

several days before the test, to synchronize your body rhythms. Don't use any drugs you usually do not use (including caffeine and nicotine). Avoid alcohol 2 days before the examination. Airline pilots follow this routine to improve concentration before a flight; it works for test-takers as well.

Dress comfortably. The temperature in the examination room will be variable; dress in layers that can be added or removed according to your comfort level.

Eat regular meals before the examination. If the test is in the morning, eat breakfast. High carbohydrate foods provide energy, but excessive sugar and caffeine can cause hyperactivity.

4. *Be mentally prepared.* Use mental rehearsal and visualize success. Arriving on time will help you feel relaxed and confident.

During the Test

The moment has come. Use the anxiety management strategies outlined in this chapter, and review test-taking protocol shortly before taking the test.

After entering the examination room, make yourself comfortable. If possible, sit in the part of the room where the lighting and temperature are best for you. Some test-takers prefer space around them, while others prefer to position themselves near the proctor or other test-takers. If other test-takers bother you, notify the proctor and ask to move.

Comparing answers with other test-takers during breaks usually increases anxiety. Don't think about questions you've already answered; instead, concentrate energy for the next test. Use distraction strategies.

After the Test

After the examination, you will be eager to know the results or scores. Find out how and when results will be reported. If possible, obtain the name of a contact person with whom you can discuss the test results. Many schools of nursing designate a counselor or faculty member for this purpose.

3

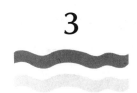

The Nursing Process

The nursing process is an organized, systematic approach to assessing a client's health status, identifying client needs or nursing problems, determining appropriate interventions to meet those needs, and evaluating the outcome of interventions. The major purpose of the nursing process is to provide an organizational framework for nurses to meet the individual needs of clients, families, and communities. The process allows nurses to determine desirable client outcomes, prescribe nursing action alternatives, and evaluate the results of nursing care. Since its origin in 1955, the nursing process has evolved into five sequential, interrelated steps—assessment, diagnosis, planning, implementation, and evaluation.

The purpose of this chapter is to promote an understanding of the nursing process. Although RN mobility and challenge examinations may or may not test understanding of the process, nurses should be familiar with each step and be able to choose nursing actions appropriate for each step. Table 3-1 summarizes actions and rationales related to each step.

Assessment

Assessment is the first step in the nursing process. It involves gathering, substantiating, and communicating data that together provide a comprehensive picture of a client's health status. Assessment begins with the nurse's initial contact with a client, and continues as long as the client needs nursing interventions.

The primary source of data is the client. The client provides data during the initial interview, the nursing history interview, and the physical examination. Other sources of data may include laboratory findings, medical records, and nursing notes.

The initial interview and nursing history interview involve gathering primarily *subjective* data; the physical examination involves gathering *objective* as well as subjective data. The client's experiences and perceptions (for instance, pain, nausea, emotions) are subjective because only the client can experience and describe them. No two persons experience pain in exactly the same way, for instance. Objective data refers to observations and measurements that any two persons would probably describe in exactly the same terms. Vital signs and laboratory results are examples of objective data.

The nurse should *report* all data as objectively as possible. For instance, the nurse can objectively report a client's subjective statement, "I feel awful today," by recording, "Mrs. S. said, 'I feel awful today.'" If the nurse instead wrote, "Mrs. S. is in a lot of pain today," she would be adding her own subjective per-

Table 3-1. **Components of the Nursing Process**

Steps	Nursing Actions	Rationales
Assessment Gathering data about an individual group, family, or community to identify actual and potential nursing diagnoses/problems	Gather, substantiate, and communicate data about the client Consider both subjective and objective data	Provides a comprehensive picture of the client's health status for identification of existing problems Other steps in the nursing process are based on findings made in assessment phase
Nursing Diagnosis Identifying an actual or potential health problem that nurses can legally treat independently, and initiating the nursing interventions necessary to prevent, resolve, or reduce the problem (Alfaro, 1986)	Analyze and interpret data collected during assessment to form basis of a plan of care	Identifies problems in order to develop a comprehensive plan of nursing care
Planning Developing a plan to direct client care	Establish priorities Determine client-centered goals (short term or long term) Define behavioral objectives List desired outcome criteria Plan appropriate nursing interventions	Provides a means to measure the client's progress Provides standards and a basis for evaluating client responses to nursing interventions
Intervention/Implementation Performing actions to maintain, promote, or restore the client's health and to prevent complications or illness	Perform client teaching Perform specific treatment actions Assist clients to perform activities and make decisions related to their health Consult other professionals as indicated	Provides a variety of nursing actions designed to promote comfort, prevent complications, and maintain and restore health
Evaluation Reassessing entire plan of nursing care	Assess to identify new problems and status of existing ones Establish outcome criteria for evaluation Evaluate goal achievement Modify or terminate nursing care as appropriate	Provides a basis for determining efficacy of nursing care plan, identifying necessary changes to improve client care, or demonstrating that problems have been resolved

ceptions to the report. (The client may have meant she feels awful about missing her daughter's birthday party because she is hospitalized.)

Data provides the foundation for identifying the client's potential problems, current health needs, and strengths. The other steps of the nursing process are based on findings made during the assessment phase.

Nursing Diagnosis

The second step in the nursing process is diagnosis. During this phase, the data that has been collected and compiled during the assessment phase is analyzed and interpreted. Diagnosis is a mechanism for arranging nursing knowledge so as to draw conclusions about the client's needs, problems, concerns, and responses to illness or injury.

A nursing diagnosis describes a client's healthy, unhealthy, or potentially unhealthy responses and the factors that sustain or contribute to each response identified. Medical diagnoses and nursing diagnoses differ in that medical diagnoses do not describe responses from the individual, family, or community but describe disease itself or the progress of disease, and guide treatment of the particular health problem. Both medical and nursing diagnoses are determined by using diagnostic analysis. Interview skills and a theoretical background are needed to derive either a medical or a nursing diagnosis. Each discipline is striving for the same goal—improving the client's level of health and promoting an optimal level of wellness—but the focuses of the two disciplines differ. Medicine's primary concern is health promotion through *cure*. Nursing's primary concern is *care*, although support of curative action is also an integral part of nursing's role in the care of clients.

A nursing diagnosis is written as a two-part statement. The first part consists of the diagnostic label or title. The second part names an etiological factor that has contributed to or sustained the identified problem. The two parts of the diagnosis are connected by the terms "related to" or "secondary to" to represent a complete nursing diagnosis. Table 3-2 provides several examples of diagnostic labels with corresponding etiological factors. Nursing diagnoses are evaluated regularly and altered periodically according to changes in the client's data base.

To standardize accepted nursing diagnoses, the North American Nursing Diagnosis Association (NANDA) has sorted and organized data into accepted specific nursing diagnoses (see Table 3-3). This standardization allows the nurse to describe a client's health status and communicate any deficits or potential deficits to other health care providers in an organized way. Furthermore, the comprehensive list of diagnoses enables nurses to explore all of a client's human needs and to recognize how one health-related problem may interrelate with another.

Planning

Planning is the third step of the nursing process. In order to develop an appropriate care plan for a particular client, the nurse must establish

Table 3-2. Examples of the Two Components of Nursing Diagnoses

Diagnostic Labels	*Etiological Factors*
Alteration in comfort	Lack of knowledge concerning pain management techniques
Anxiety	Feeling of powerlessness
Potential for infection	Interruption of the body's first line of defense
Impaired physical mobility	Loss of movement of the right leg

Table 3-3. Approved Nursing Diagnoses, North American Nursing Diagnosis Association, June 1988

Activity intolerance
Activity intolerance, potential
Airway clearance, ineffective
Anxiety
Aspiration, potential
Bowel elimination, alteration in: constipation
Bowel elimination, alteration in: diarrhea
Bowel elimination, alteration in: incontinence
Breathing pattern, ineffective
Cardiac output, alteration in: decreased
Chronic low self-esteem
Comfort, alteration in: pain
Colonic constipation
Communication, impaired: verbal
Coping, family: potential for growth
Coping, ineffective family: compromised
Coping, ineffective family: disabling
Coping, ineffective individual
Decisional conflict (specify)
Defensive coping
Diversional activity deficit
Dysreflexia
Family process, alteration in
Fatigue
Fear
Fluid volume alteration in: excess
Fluid volume deficit, actual
Fluid volume deficit, potential
Gas exchange, impaired
Grieving, anticipatory
Grieving, dysfunctional
Health maintenance, alteration in
Health seeking behaviors
Home maintenance management, impaired
Hypothermia
Ineffective breast-feeding
Ineffective denial
Injury, potential for
Knowledge deficit (specify)
Mobility, impaired physical
Noncompliance (specify)
Nutrition, alteration in: less than body requirements
Nutrition, alteration in: more than body requirements
Nutrition, alteration in: more than body requirements, potential
Oral mucous membrane, alteration in
Parental role conflict
Parenting, alteration in: actual
Parenting, alteration in: potential
Perceived constipation
Potential for disuse syndrome
Powerlessness
Rape trauma syndrome
Self-care deficit: feeding, bathing/hygiene, dressing/grooming, toileting
Self-concept, disturbance in: body image, self-esteem, role performance, personal identity
Self-esteem disturbance
Sensory-perceptual alteration: visual, auditory, kinesthetic, gustatory, tactile, olfactory
Sexual dysfunction
Situational low self-esteem
Skin integrity, impairment of: actual
Skin integrity, impairment of: potential
Sleep pattern disturbance
Social isolation
Spiritual distress (distress of the human spirit)
Thought processes, alteration in
Tissue perfusion, alteration in: cerebral, cardiopulmonary, renal, gastrointestinal, peripheral
Urinary elimination, alteration in patterns
Violence, potential for: self-directed or directed at others

priorities, goals, objectives, and outcome criteria based on the client's nursing diagnoses, and write nursing interventions (see Table 3-4). Planning begins as a mental process. In order to provide continuity of care, however, the plan must ultimately be documented.

The first step in planning is to establish priorities. *Setting priorities* helps the nurse make rational and accurate choices when confronted simultaneously with several problems or concerns while delivering care. Priority must be determined for nursing diagnoses, objectives, and interventions. Initially nursing diagnoses are ranked by means of a triaging or sorting process. Ranking determines which diagnoses must receive immediate, postponed, or no attention from health professionals delivering care to that client.

Priorities can constantly change. As the client's health status changes, so will the ranking of his or her diagnoses and needs. Priorities also change when a high-priority diagnosis or high-priority need is resolved—diagnoses that were lower on the list then shift upward.

Establishing *goals* related to each nursing diagnosis is another component of the planning phase. Goals direct nursing interventions, communicate the purpose of the plan to other caregivers, and establish the pace of activities for that client. Establishing goals allows the client to experience a sense of achievement when goals are met.

There are two types of goals, short term and long term. Short-term goals can be met quickly and usually have high priority. Long-term goals require a longer period of time to accomplish and frequently have lower priority. Long-term goals sometimes may be met by achieving a series of short-term goals.

A well-constructed goal is client-centered and includes a verb, a description of what is to be achieved, and the expected time when it will be achieved. Because goals are written in broad terms, they do not describe the exact process necessary to achieve what is desired. An appropriate goal might be worded, "JW's decubitus ulcer will have decreased in diameter to measure less than 1 cm by November 11."

Because goals are broad and general, *behavioral objectives* are needed to accurately measure the client's progress. A behavioral objective is a statement describing desirable, observable behaviors. Each nursing diagnosis generates at least one goal, which in turn generates several objectives that describe how the goal will be reached. Many variables help determine behavioral objectives, including the client's or family's input and the attitudes, knowledge, and educational background of health care professionals. A typical behavioral objective might be worded, "JW will describe three ways he can assist in decreasing the diameter of the decubitus ulcer."

Outcome criteria are standards used to determine the client's responses to nursing interventions. Sometimes, behavioral and other objectives themselves define these standards. Outcome criteria are important in the evaluation phase, but are developed in the planning phase. An outcome criterion might be worded, "The skin on JW's coccyx area will be pink, warm, and dry, with a decrease in diameter of the decubitus ulcer."

Table 3-4. Steps Involved in the Planning Phase of the Nursing Process (with Example)

Choose nursing diagnosis: Altered skin integrity related to impaired mobility.
Establish goal: Client will have improved skin integrity within 2 weeks.
Determine objective: Client will describe 3 ways to promote skin integrity by October 11.
Determine outcome criterion: Client's skin on coccyx area will be pink, warm, and dry without breakdown.
Perform nursing intervention: Teach client to turn to alternate sides every odd hour.

Nursing interventions also correspond to the client's nursing diagnoses. Interventions are nursing actions that help the client achieve goals and objectives. Nursing interventions focus on ways to maintain, promote, or restore the client's health. There are three types of nursing interventions: dependent, interdependent, and independent. Each type is characterized by the degree to which the nurse is independent in identifying and resolving problems.

Dependent nursing interventions are actions that carry out a physician's written medical orders. Diagnostic procedures, medication administration, hot and cold applications, and urinary catheterizations, for instance, are therapies usually controlled by physicians' orders and requiring dependent nursing interventions. Usually dependent nursing interventions cannot be initiated by the nurse without a written order from a physician. Although medical orders initiate dependent interventions, critical thinking and problem solving are still required by the nurse. For instance, a nurse who is instructed to give daily a.m. insulin to a client, but finds the client's fasting blood sugar is very low on a certain morning, should notify the physician of this finding before following the order.

Interdependent interventions involve those areas in which nurses collaborate with other health care professionals. For example, hypovolemia in a person with third-degree burns is both a medical and a nursing problem. The physician may focus on fluid replacement while the nurse focuses on assessing early response to treatment. These interventions are also legally a part of nursing care.

Independent nursing orders can legally be prescribed by and carried out by the nurse independently or without a physician's order. This dimension of nursing practice involves those clinical events or problems that are the direct responsibility of the nurse, who must implement the correct nursing action. Independent interventions address specific nursing diagnoses and provide the mechanism for achieving goals and objectives.

All nursing interventions should demonstrate certain characteristics. First, every intervention should be supported by scientific rationale from the nurse's knowledge base. Even though the relevant scientific principles are not included in the written nursing orders, the nurse must have a thorough understanding of those principles before prescribing an intervention. Second, nursing interventions must be individualized for every client. The client's strengths and weaknesses, the family's input, and the urgency of the situation must all be taken into account when writing nursing interventions. Finally, nursing interventions should take into account teaching strategies. The nurse must first determine the client's readiness to learn, however, by observing his or her condition and behavior, and considering variables that influence the person's ability to learn, such as education level, age, past experience, motivation, and state of health.

After formulating nursing interventions, the final phase of planning involves documenting priorities, goals, objectives, outcome criteria, and nursing interventions in an appropriate manner. A nursing care plan format (Figure 3-1) is usually used to document care.

Implementation

The implementation component of the nursing process is the actual delivery of nursing care as determined in the planning phase. It includes carrying out physicians' orders, following hospital protocol, and performing nursing interventions. Implementation of the nursing care plan allows for delivery of comprehensive care to the client, since the plan involves all aspects of care. Nurses can implement care plans in a variety of settings.

Evaluation

Evaluation is the last step of the nursing process. It is an ongoing, intentional activity that in-

Nursing Diagnosis: Altered skin integrity due to impaired mobility.
Goal: J. W.'s decubitus ulcer will be decreased in diameter to less than 1 cm, by November 11, 1989.
Outcome Criteria: J. W.'s skin on his coccyx area will be pink, warm, and dry with a decrease in diameter of the decubitus ulcer.
Evaluation: The goal for J. W. was achieved by November 11, 1989. Nursing interventions assisted in decreasing the diameter of the decubitus ulcer on the coccyx to .75 cm.

ASSESSMENT CRITERIA	PLANS/IMPLEMENTATION	EVALUATION
Objective Cues: . Decubitus ulcer on coccyx measures 1 cm in diameter.	1) Assess diameter of the decubitus ulcer every day.	1) Decubitus ulcer diameter assessed at the beginning of every shift; no increase in diameter noted.
. Client on strict bedrest per physician's orders.	2) Assess body position of client every 2 hours.	2) Client preferred to lay supine with very little position change.
. Skin intact around the decubitus ulcer—no further breakdown noted.	3) Turn and position client off of coccyx area every 2 hours.	3) Body position changed every two hours and recorded.
Subjective Cues: . Client complains of soreness in the area of the decubitus on the coccyx.	4) Massage around decubitus ulcer for 10-minute intervals every shift.	4) After massage, area around decubitus ulcer was pink and had increased warmth.
	5) Apply a flotation mattress on client's bed per order.	5) Client states flotation mattress is comfortable. No further skin breakdown is observed.
	6) Apply the heat lamp to decubitus ulcer for 20 minutes bid.	6) Heat lamp applied per order improving circulation to the area, therefore decreasing diameter of the decubitus ulcer.
	7) Arrange with dietician for nutritionally balanced diet high in protein and vitamin C.	7) After dietician consult, client's diet high in protein and vitamin C, promoting wound healing.
	8) Instruct client on importance of changing positions every 2 hours.	8) After client teaching, client staying off his coccyx area and rotating positions every two hours.

Figure 3-1. Nursing care plan.

volves the nurse, client, and other health team members in comparing the client's health status with the outcome criteria specified during the planning phase. Evaluation can be done in phases. Initially the nurse collects data about the client's health status by assessing several aspects of the client's condition: knowledge, emotional status, symptoms, appearance, and body functioning. After collecting this data, the nurse compares the results with the predetermined outcome criteria. Evaluation results in one of three possible judgments:

The client has achieved the outcomes.

The client has made progress toward achieving the outcomes.

The client has not achieved the outcomes and has made no progress toward achieving them.

Evaluation is an ongoing process. Aggressive efforts should be made to incorporate this important step of the nursing process in client care.

Conclusion

The nursing process is a problem-solving approach enabling the nurse to systematically examine a client's health status, identify client needs, determine approaches to meet those needs, and evaluate the outcomes of nursing interventions. The process consists of five steps—assessment, diagnosis, planning, implementation, and evaluation (Table 3-1). RN mobility or challenge examinations test the nurse's ability to utilize these steps, but questions about the steps themselves are not usually included. In the answers to the practice tests in this book, the step of the nursing process involved in each question is identified by a code for review. If you find you are having difficulty with one particular step, review this chapter for definitions and examples of each of these steps.

4

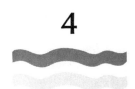

The Nurse as Communicator

The reality of the other person is not in what he reveals to you, but in what he cannot reveal to you.
Therefore, if you would understand him, listen not to what he says but rather to what he does not say.

Kahlil Gibran

Communication between the nurse and the client is the one element of nursing care that affects the outcome of all nursing activities. While technology has contributed to communicating information more readily, it has reduced the quality of nurse/client interaction. Mechanical devices such as the intercom have decreased the amount of time a nurse spends interacting personally with clients. Because the quantity of interactions has been reduced, quality becomes an even more critical component of nursing practice.

Individuals communicate something with every interpersonal interaction. Behavior as well as dialogue transmits information significant to the transaction. What is said, how it is said, and moreover, what is not said all affect interpersonal transactions. Communication with a client is an active process. Messages are constantly being transmitted and determine the course of the nursing process. Effective communication enhances the desired outcome of nursing care.

The increased complexity of health care delivery also requires a continuous exchange of information among all members of the health care team. However, the nurse is the primary connector among the members and is considered the significant communicator for the health care network of the client. Therefore, the quality of the nurse's communication with other professionals also affects the quality of care the client receives.

This chapter reviews concepts of interpersonal communication and explores the value of nurse/client interaction in delivering quality nursing care. The discussion includes variables that affect the quality of nurse/client relationships, models for understanding and improving nurse/client communication, and skills related to facilitating, interviewing, resolving conflicts, and promoting behavior change. The information may reinforce or clarify knowledge you already possess, or it may offer a new learning experience. It is intended to prepare you to respond accurately to examination questions related to interpersonal communication.

The Importance of Communication in Nurse/Client Relationships

Understanding the communication process is essential for developing an effective interpersonal relationship. First, consider the nature of *process*. A process is active, consists of a sequence of interdependent steps, and is directed toward an end. The concept of process is familiar to nurses since nursing practice is usually described in terms of the nursing process. Interpersonal communication is a dynamic, ongoing, and changing process involving two people interacting interdependently. It always occurs in the context of a relationship.

Interpersonal relationships always imply a reciprocal transaction. Each member acts and reacts according to the action and reaction of the other. Nurses should remember the importance of the cause and effect principle in communicating with clients. What the nurse says and does directly influences the client's response. Responsibility for the quality of a nurse/client interaction lies chiefly with the nurse.

Interpersonal transactions likewise imply a relationship. The quality of a relationship is determined by the way participants relate to each other. Of course, a number of other variables also affect the quality of an interpersonal relationship. Interactions between the persons communicating are affected by the emotional climate, physical disposition of both parties, and social circumstances prevalent at the time. The quality of a nurse/client relationship has a direct influence on the outcome of nursing care. Gerrard (1978) reviewed 27 studies in which the outcome of health care was assessed. Sixty-three percent of the studies demonstrated that beneficial physiological, psychological, or behavioral changes in clients resulted from health professionals' interpersonal skills.

According to Duldt, Giffin, and Patton (1984) there are three dimensions in an interpersonal relationship: the degree of involvement of both parties, the emotional tone or feelings, and the amount of interpersonal control maintained by each party. Degree of involvement between two people is determined by the value each places on the relationship, rather than by the amount of time spent together. A valued relationship includes self-disclosure and mutual consideration. Participants interact in an accepting manner.

Duldt, Giffin, and Patton state that the emotional tone of a relationship increases in importance as the degree of involvement increases. The emotional tone of a relationship is positive when participants feel closeness and mutual trust. It is negative when they experience rejection, hostility, uncertainty, or doubt. Both positive and negative emotions are experienced in all relationships; it is the degree and frequency with which each occurs that determine the overall quality of the relationship. Recalling the principle of cause and effect, the nurse should endeavor to promote the positive. Achieving a positive emotional tone requires attentive behavior, warmth, caring, and active listening.

The third component, interpersonal control, is most often overlooked in a health care relationship. Both parties need to maintain a sense of individual autonomy. Health professionals, however, habitually tell clients what they expect them to do. It might be said that this is an occupational habit, a behavior evolving from the frequent need to "do for" those under care. Furthermore, illness causes a change in a person's self-perception. It is not uncommon for a self-reliant, independent person to act submissive when ill. Submissive behavior in one person tends to create dominating behavior in the other. In other words, submissive people allow themselves to be controlled. However, this behavior often results in a breakdown in the nurse/client relationship. Interpersonal conflict develops when control issues are not recognized.

Models For Enhancing Communication

Knowledge of communication models enhances understanding of the communication process. Various communication models can help nurses improve the quality of their interpersonal interactions. This discussion will focus on selected communication models that emphasize the components of a health care interpersonal interaction.

Communication Model (Gerrard, Boniface, and Love)

Gerrard, Boniface, and Love's communication model (1980) describes five steps in a communication exchange. First, a message is formed in the sender's mind. Second, it is translated or *encoded* into a form that can be transmitted to the intended receiver. Third, the message is transmitted. Fourth, the receiver perceives the message, and finally (fifth), the receiver translates or *decodes* what is seen or heard to determine the meaning. When the message received is approximately the same as the message that was formed and sent, communication is considered successful. Conflict and misunderstanding result when the receiver perceives a different message from the one the sender intended. Stated another way, errors in encoding and decoding messages are often the cause of interpersonal stress.

The following example is a successful communication exchange:

- *Forming message:* Nurse wishes to know if the client needs pain medication.
- *Encoding message:* Nurse decides how to send the message (chooses words, tone of voice, facial expression, delivery in person or via intercom).
- *Transmitting message:* Nurse says, "It's been 3½ hours since I gave you a pain shot. Is your incision beginning to hurt you?"
- *Receiving message:* Client hears the nurse inquire about his pain.
- *Decoding message:* Client perceives the intention of the nurse to maintain his comfort. He then *encodes* and returns his message: "Yes, I think I'd better have another shot before it gets too bad."

An example of error in a communication exchange follows:

- *Forming message:* Nurse needs to ambulate a client.
- *Encoding message:* Nurse decides to go into the client's room with a very cheerful attitude and tell the client (in a happy sounding voice) that she needs to walk.
- *Transmitting message:* Nurse says, "It's time we got out of bed, Mrs. Peck."
- *Receiving message:* Client hears the nurse say she has to get up.
- *Decoding message:* Client translates what she has heard—"This nurse has no idea how painful it is for me to get out of this bed." She *encodes* a return message: "I don't want to get out of bed this morning."

In the above communication, an error occurred in encoding. The nurse failed to choose words, voice tone and manner that communicated caring to the client and wanting to help her walk because it would speed her recovery. The nurse also failed to acknowledge the client's pain. Consequently, the client misinterpreted the nurse's message. She perceived that she must get out of bed for the nurse's convenience, and that the nurse did not care about her pain. For this reason, the client is noncompliant and requires coercion to get out of bed.

In order for a message to be translated as the sender intended, the sender's tone of voice and body language must reinforce the verbal message. The nurse's behavior as well as words must depict care, concern, and genuine interest.

The message the speaker truly intended is often reflected more accurately in nonverbal behavior than in spoken words.

Rogerian Model

Carl Rogers (1951) maintains that a helping relationship should focus on clients: their needs, perceptions, feelings, and values. A successful outcome of therapeutic interaction between health professional and client depends on the health professional communicating with empathy, positive regard, and congruence. These three elements are integral components of a helping interpersonal transaction.

Empathy is being able to demonstrate with accuracy an understanding of the other person. Empathic behavior conveys verbally and nonverbally that one can put oneself in the position of clients and be sensitive to what they are experiencing. Gerrard, Boniface, and Love (1980) define empathy as active listening. *Positive regard* is demonstrating to clients that respect for them is genuine. *Congruence* is expressing oneself in such a way that behavior and statements complement each other accurately. When nurse/client interaction includes these components, the client feels understood and is better able to cope with health problems.

Forsythe (1977) has found that as the length of practice increases, nurses tend to lose empathic ability. Nurses can maintain this ability by assessing their interpersonal interactions, and by observing, listening, and assessing the interactions of others.

King's Interaction Model

Another model for describing effective communication is the interaction model developed by Imogene King. King (1971) describes interpersonal communication as follows:

> In the interactive process, as nurse and patient assess goals to be achieved, and mutually define health goals, a transaction occurs. This mutual agreement has an effect on the actions and judgments of the nurse and patient and influences each one's perception. A series of these kinds of acts takes place as the nurse and patient interact in a nursing situation (p. 92).

This model also supports the reciprocal nature of interpersonal interactions. Like the Rogerian model, it also implies that the transaction is client-centered.

Transactional Analysis Model

Transactional Analysis is a theory developed by Eric Berne, the psychiatrist who wrote the popular book, *Games People Play* (1964). According to Berne, there are three ego states in an individual's personality, each of which is actively reflected in interpersonal behavior throughout the life cycle. These ego states include the Parent, Adult, and Child egos. The *Parent* ego state incorporates all the behaviors and attitudes taught by parents, teachers, or other authority figures. These behaviors and attitudes are learned directly and indirectly as a person develops. The *Adult* ego state involves the ability to reason or behave rationally. It is logical. The *Child* ego state includes all the feelings a person experienced as a child, such as joy, fear, happiness, sadness, and anger. This state is also characterized by spontaneity and creativity. The Parent and Child ego states reflect past experiences and feelings associated with those events. Like a computer, the brain is a data bank that holds information about everything a person has experienced.

All three ego states alternate throughout a person's growth and development. Each relates to a way of behaving rather than a particular growth phase. Children and adults alike manifest all three ego states at different times. The logic and reasoning of a 3-year-old is an expression of the child's Adult ego state. Likewise, stubborn rebellion in a 40-year-old is a manifestation of the adult's Child ego state.

The Parent ego state also has two different aspects. When a person acts in an authoritative manner (for instance, being the "boss"), the *Critical Parent* ego state is functioning. When a person acts in a protective or nurturing way, the *Nurturing Parent* ego state prevails. Generally, when the *Parent* ego state prevails, a person demonstrates behaviors learned uncritically from others.

The Child ego state also includes three distinct aspects: *Natural Child, Rebellious Child,* and *Adapted Child.* Natural Child behaviors express the spontaneous feelings of happiness, joy, or pain of the natural, uninhibited child. The Rebellious Child reflects resistant, counterdependent behavior that usually was learned as a response to excessive parental demands. The Adapted Child ego state implies behavior adaptations or modifications learned in response to parental demands and social constraints. This ego state is characterized by compliance, withdrawal, crying, and suppressing spontaneous impulses.

The Child is the emotional part of the personality. Emotion reaches its greatest heights when the self is in danger or experiences satisfaction. Emotion reflects the personal meaning of an event being experienced at any given moment. The more personally meaningful an event is to a person, the more intense will be the associated feelings. When there is no personal meaning, there is no emotion. A person's mood at a given moment will also influence emotional response.

The Adult is not devoid of emotion or caring, but is reality-oriented and analyzes information before acting. The Adult ego state allows processing of information, through which judgments useful in solving problems, choosing alternatives, or considering options are made.

In interpersonal communication, people unconsciously recognize and respond to ego states reflected in each others' behavior. Certain types of transactions are common: for instance, people frequently respond to a Child ego state reflected in a person's behavior, by behaving in the Parent mode. The value in Transactional Analysis is learning to recognize an ego state in another person's behavior, and to respond in a way that reflects a complementary ego state. Successful communication involves what Berne calls a *complementary transaction,* in which the ego states of the two parties complement one another. A person in the Adult mode addresses the Adult in another person, for instance, while a person in the Parent mode addresses the Child in another. The following exchange, diagrammed in Figure 4-1, reflects a complementary transaction.

(1) Client: "What's in that IV I'm getting?"
(2) Nurse: "It's called Pitocin and it helps your uterine muscles to contract or tighten, and prevents you from bleeding excessively. You may also experience more cramping while you're getting it."
(3) Client: "I am having a lot of strong cramps, it's as bad as being in labor again."
(4) Nurse: "I'll give you some pain medication. You ought to feel more comfortable after the IV is completed. It has about an hour and a half to go."

This transaction reflects an Adult to Adult exchange. The client is asking for information in order to understand her treatment and cope with her pain, and the nurse responds by providing the information in a straightforward manner.

Communication difficulties can occur when the two parties' ego states do not complement one another. Berne calls exchanges such as the following (diagrammed in Figure 4-2) *crossed transactions.*

(1) Client (grimacing): "What's in that IV? I'm having worse pain now than I did in labor."
(2) Nurse: "Oh, it isn't that bad, now. Everyone gets this after delivery to prevent hemorrhage."
(3) Client: "I'll cry if I have to take much more of this. Can't you please give me something?"

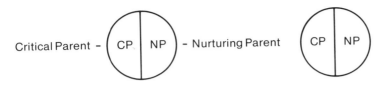

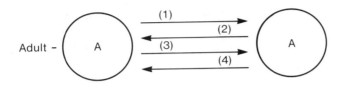

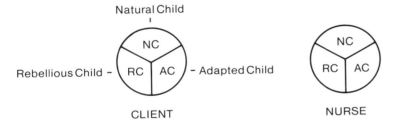

Figure 4-1. Complementary transaction. The numbered arrows refer to the numbered exchange between the nurse and the client in the accompanying dialogue. The client's Adult addresses the nurse's Adult (1). The nurse's Adult responds appropriately by addressing the client's Adult (2). The exchange continues between the nurse's and the client's Adult ego states (3 and 4).

(4) Nurse: "It's only been 3 hours since I gave you pain medication. You'll just have to bear with it for now. It's all part of being a mother."

In this transaction the client seeks comfort by asking for information and indicating a need. This is an Adult behavior. The nurse crosses the transaction by not responding with reason and understanding; that is, the nurse's Adult does not respond to the client's Adult. The nurse is in an authoritarian (Critical Parent) ego state, expecting an Adaptive Child response (compliance). The client's response reflects a Natural Child ego state (emotion associated with painful experiences). She attempts to gain relief by addressing the nurse's Nurturing Parent. But the nurse remains in a Critical Parent ego state, criticizing the client for complaining. Therefore, communication is blocked. The client did not receive the information and assistance she requested.

Interpersonal transactions can be greatly enhanced if the nurse recognizes the client's ego state as well as the nurse's own. Perceiving the client's ego state and responding with behaviors reflecting a complementary ego state allow the nurse to facilitate an effective dialogue.

Nurses must respect the value system of those with whom they work (colleagues as well as clients) in order to have open, reciprocal communication and promote trust. A person's value system is influenced by his or her cultural and ethnic heritage. Therefore, nurses must be cognizant of their own value systems and guard against transferring their own cultural expectations to the behavior of clients. A conflict in values generally results in crossed or ineffective communication. A breakdown in communication leads to decreased trust, limited disclosure,

The Nurse as Communicator 27

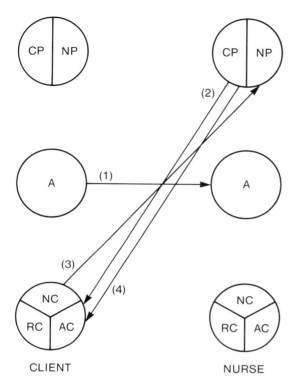

Figure 4-2. Crossed transaction. The numbered arrows refer to the numbered exchange between the nurse and the client in the accompanying dialogue. The client's Adult addresses the nurse's Adult (1); however, the nurse's Critical Parent responds (inappropriately) to the client's Adapted Child (2). The client's Natural Child then addresses the nurse's Nurturing Parent (3), but it is again the nurse's Critical Parent who responds (inappropriately) to the client's Adapted Child (4).

and a decrease in the quality of health care given.

Facilitation Skills

Interpersonal skills that promote trust and increase understanding are called *facilitation skills* (Gerrard, Boniface, and Love, 1984). To be understood and cared for is probably the key factor in a trusting relationship. Trust in the caretaker is essential if self-disclosure is to take place. Self-disclosure on the client's part helps the nurse understand and meet the client's needs.

Facilitation skills include listening, encouraging, and responding. They must be accompanied by accurate information and empathy. Empathy is demonstrated by expressing understanding of a client's feelings as well as the underlying cause of the feelings. Increasing one's ability to be empathic requires a conscious desire. Perception (of both clients' needs and one's own behavior) is a selective process, and perceptions depend on needs. Perceptions are interpretations of reality. For instance, some nurses may perceive themselves as sensitive caretakers while their clients perceive them as impersonal and methodical. If the nurse believes understanding a client is important, he or she will make an effort to do so. It is helpful to make an occasional mental assessment of one's ability to demonstrate sensitivity to clients.

Listening, encouraging, and responding skills can be developed with effort. Listening is more than remaining silent while another person is speaking. Feelings and thoughts are stimulated through listening; recall the communication model of Gerrard *et al* and note that translation occurs between both persons in the communication exchange. When one listens attentively, one hears with ears, eyes, and heart. Messages are translated as well as heard. Attentive listening can be learned with practice. A simple exercise is to look directly at the speaker, acknowledge interest by nonverbal gestures, and interpret for the speaker what was heard. Practicing this with someone with whom one has a close relationship is helpful.

Active listening is more than attentive listening. Active listening is hearing a message that was not explicit in the speaker's words and verbalizing that understanding back to the sender. Consider the following example.

Client: "You ought to quit smoking. When you are young there are other ways to receive pleasure. When you get to

Nurse: be my age, cigarettes are all you have."
Nurse: "You sound lonely today, Margaret. It must be hard to give up doing things you enjoy."
Client: "Oh, yes. There's nothing worse than losing your independence."

The preceding dialogue reflects active listening. The nurse sensed the feelings behind the client's verbal expression, as well as a possible cause for such feelings. When the nurse voiced understanding to the client, she was encouraged to disclose deeper concerns. Active listening requires conveying one's understanding of the client's feelings in one's own words. It promotes trust and self-disclosure and strengthens the nurse/client relationship.

The following dialogue is an example of *inattentive listening*.

Client (Bryan, 7 years old): "My mom and dad let me sleep with my light on."
Nurse: "Well that's nice. Would you like milk or juice before bed?" Moves around room, picking up things.
Client: "I don't want anything."
Nurse: "You don't? I thought all little boys liked to have a snack before bedtime." Puts light out. "I'll leave your door open a little. Call me if you change your mind."

Such conversations are not uncommon, especially when the nurse's workload is heavy. People often talk at each other rather than with each other, especially with children. Yet listening to and observing children's dialogue can offer some of the best learning experiences in interpersonal interactions. The nurse in the above example did not hear Bryan say he was afraid of the dark and was feeling lonely. Also, Bryan may have received the message that he was not valued because he was not like "all little boys." A more appropriate response is illustrated in the following dialogue.

Client (Bryan): "My mom and dad let me sleep with my light on."
Nurse: "Would you like me to leave your light on tonight? There are other children here who like their light on at night, too. It's hard to be away from mom and dad. I know you miss them, but they'll be back early in the morning. How about having some milk or juice now?"

The above response, when spoken with a gentle tone, physical closeness, such as holding the client's hand or gently stroking the forehead, and direct eye contact, reflects genuine caring. Children are astute interpreters of genuine feelings. They understand a message with remarkable clarity, especially the message the adult was not aware of sending. It is often said, "You can't fool a child." Perhaps it is so because children have not yet learned how not to be genuine.

Interviewing Skills

Learning and improving communication skills are essential to conducting successful client interviews. Evidence suggests that health professionals are ineffective in conducting interviews. Thompson (1986) indicates that only 10% of health care providers do an excellent job of history taking; 30% do an adequate job; and 60% do a poor job. These findings support the need for health professionals to learn effective interpersonal skills.

Typically, initial interviews are conducted when clients are admitted for service with health care agencies, and involve a structured questionnaire. Nurses must recognize that the initial interview is more than completing a nursing admission form. This first interaction makes a strong impression on the client. First impressions set the stage for further interactions. The client's perception of that first interaction is almost indelible, for it remains unless subsequent transactions alter it. Positive first impressions tend to leave a lasting positive impression. Less positive impressions require much effort and time to dispel.

The primary purpose of conducting an interview in the health care setting is to gather information for assessing the needs of the client. The needs assessment will become the basis for the nursing care plan. An interview requires that two people communicate in asking and answering questions. The nurse needs to be open to the client's questions so that any feelings of uneasiness on the client's part are allayed.

Stages of an Interview

Interviewing is a process with defined stages that if successfully completed, lead to a satisfying outcome. Stages include the introduction, the body, and the closing.

Stage One (Introduction)—Establishing Rapport. The introductory stage involves establishing rapport. It should include stating the purpose of the interview. It is also helpful to add a brief moment of "small talk." After greeting the client and making introductions, the nurse might remark on the weather or the client's attire. Casual conversation conveys warmth and demonstrates interest in the client as a person. Too often the interview begins abruptly with questions related to the health problem.

The nurse's introductory remarks should clarify the nurse's expectations as well as encourage clients to verbalize theirs. When expectations are not satisfied, both the nurse and the client experience frustration. Compliance and participation in health management increase when expectations are clearly understood.

Stage Two—Conducting the Body of the Interview. The body of an interview consists of the nurse's explicit questions and the client's responses. Questions may be *open-ended* or *closed*. Each type is necessary for an effective interview.

Open-ended questions allow the client to express feelings and concerns that otherwise might not be elicited. The question, "What kind of a night did you have?" allows the client to describe how he or she slept using his or her own words. Open-ended questions may lead to ambiguity; a *closed question* may be needed to redirect the discussion. A closed question such as "Did you sleep well?" limits the response.

Open-ended and closed questions can be effective when used in combination. For example:

Nurse: "Did you sleep well?" (closed question)
Client: "I slept pretty well but was awake since five."
Nurse: "What caused you to be awake since five o'clock?" (open-ended question)

Use of a *probe question* is another type of interviewing skill. Probing is simply asking for more explanation or clarification. It is not "delving into" unnecessarily. Probe questions are formulated in response to what the client is saying. Probing statements include "I'm wondering about . . . ," "Tell me more," and "Let's talk about that."

Transition is a technique that lets the client know the nurse needs to change the topic. Consider the following examples: "I believe I understand why you didn't seek medical attention sooner; let's go on to . . ." Transition statements allow for a smooth change in the discussion without causing clients to feel their disclosures are irrelevant.

Statements that may be perceived as evaluative can block disclosure. "When did you finally quit smoking?" may be perceived as an evaluative question. It can be rephrased more positively by asking "How long has it been since you quit smoking?" How the nurse asks a question may be more important than what is asked;

therefore, self-awareness on the nurse's part contributes to the strengths and limitations of interviews. When asking a question that the client may interpret as evaluative, it is important to use a tone of voice and facial expression that reflect the same genuine interest that other questions reflect. A nonverbal message, such as tone of voice or facial expression, may be perceived as approval or disapproval.

Stage Three—Closing the Interview. Closing the interview includes briefly summarizing the significant data obtained. After stating the essential findings, it is important to set the climate for the next interaction. This includes courteously acknowledging the client's cooperation, indicating what will be done to and for the client at this time, and explaining the time frame in which treatment will occur. A person experiencing a health problem is usually more sensitive to uncertainties. Explaining when tests and procedures will be performed gives the client a sense of timing.

Interpersonal Conflict Resolution Skills

One of the unique challenges a nurse must face is caring for a client who is angry. A number of studies have shown that health professionals have difficulty dealing with aggressive or angry clients. Anger is a strong emotion and ought to be given contextual consideration.

The nurse who recognizes when anger is displaced aggression will not take it as a personal attack. Using clarifying statements will help to validate the source of anger. There are times when it is therapeutic and valid for a client to express anger; however, when hostility creates an undesirable relationship, communication breaks down. Confrontation may serve to redirect the client's behavior. In terms of Transactional Analysis, hostility often reflects the client's *Child* or *Parent*, rather than *Adult*, ego state. For instance, a client might complain, "Don't tell me you can't leave my pills at my bedside. What do you think I am, a child?" The anger in this expression reflects the client's *Child* ego state. It represents hostile emotion.

An *active listening* response from the nurse's *Parent* ego state can help redirect the client's behavior. An effective response might be, "I know it upsets you to be told you can't do something that you are capable of doing, but I'm not allowed to leave my medications in the room." The nurse is offering legitimacy to the client's feelings and assuming responsibility for his or her action. There are situations, however, when a more direct confrontation is needed.

Confrontation skills help to promote a working relationship. Confrontation is best accomplished by being assertive. It involves not only expressing unwillingness to tolerate disrespectful behavior, but also stating that one expects consideration of one's feelings or rights, in a way that is not offensive to the other person. Consider the following confrontation.

Unit director:	"Tom, I need you to work again this weekend. Sarah's mother is sick and she can't come in." (Said in expectant tone of voice)
Nurse:	"I've worked two weekends in a row and notice I always get called when others have family problems that need them home. I'm not willing to always work but will help you out when I can." (Said in strong tone of voice)
Unit director:	"I thought I was doing you a favor since you need the extra money." (Said in defensive tone of voice)
Nurse:	"I appreciate that concern but it sounded to me like I didn't have an option." (Said in softer tone of voice)
Unit director:	"Then would you consider working this weekend?" (Said in appealing tone of voice)

Nurse: "I really need some time to get away. Thanks for your concern. You know you can rely on me most other times." (Said in soft, genuinely pleasant tone of voice)

Acting in an assertive manner also supports developing self-confidence and integrity. Confrontation through the use of assertiveness skills usually results in a winning situation for both the confronter and the person confronted.

Inappropriate forms of confrontation include using *blaming* statements. The following example illustrates *blaming*.

Nurse to coworker: "You said your child was OK when you went on break, but his IV ran out."
Coworker: "Are you kidding? I checked him before I left."
Nurse: "You knew his IV was a problem from morning report."
Coworker: "When you say 'you knew' I feel like I neglected my responsibility. When I left I told you he had 150 mL to go, and his rate was at 20 drops a minute. It upsets me to think I'm perceived as irresponsible."

In this exchange, the coworker's sense of being blamed provokes tension, which is defused by the coworker saying, "It upsets *me* to think *I'm* perceived as irresponsible." If the coworker had said, "*You* upset *me* when *you* say I'm negligent," tension and conflict would increase.

When nurses react to a tense situation, they, like most people, are apt to use words that do not reflect ownership of feelings. In order to resolve a conflict, it is best to express feelings or thoughts by using "I" statements. Saying "I feel . . ." or "I think . . . ," rather than "You make me . . ." or "You always . . ." demonstrates responsibility for the feelings expressed. When blaming statements are used, defensive responses will generate deeper conflict or outright hostility. "I" statements, accompanied by a moderate tone of voice and congruent body language, allow the other person to validate and clarify what was heard. Giving and receiving feedback is an effective way to resolve a conflict.

Interpersonal Skills to Promote Behavior Change

Occasionally, a change in behavior is the desired outcome of an interpersonal transaction. To effect change in a client's behavior—for instance, convincing a pregnant adolescent to improve her diet—identify variables that support the desired change and variables that impede the change. Communication models can be used to direct action. Consider the following example.

Nurse: "I noticed you're wearing a maternity top this month. It's very pretty. I remember last month's visit when you said you hoped you didn't have to wear these for a couple of months. What made you change your mind?" (open-ended question)
Client: "I've gained 4 pounds. I'm really porkin' out."
Nurse: "It's hard for a person as young and attractive as you to see yourself change so quickly. Tell me about your recent eating habits and let's see how we can control the weight gain."

In this dialogue, the variable that supports the desired change is a compliment. Adolescents are concerned about their body image; to recognize this concern with a sincere compliment is a way of saying "I like you." Criticism, on the other hand, can cause resistance to change. Criticism can be useful if expressed with a careful choice of words, and if the accompanying nonverbal behavior also reflects caring. Recall from the discussion on communication models that the person receiving the message will interpret it as he or she perceives it. Unless verbal and nonverbal messages are congruent, the intended message may be misrepresented.

Two skills helpful in facilitating change are information giving and support. Information giving satisfies the needs of some clients, but others also need support. To favor one particular method for effecting behavior change would be to deny the uniqueness of individual clients. For instance, a hypertensive client who needs to decrease sodium intake may need only to receive information on appropriate foods and their sodium content. The hypertensive condition acts as a support for a change in dietary behavior. However, the client who also needs to lose weight will need support and affirmation as well as information. In the latter situation, positive reinforcement is a significant adjunct to supporting behavior change. Attitudes rather than behavior may determine the way change will be initiated. Nursing literature is abundant with information related to change theory and provides evidence of the value of education in altering attitudes about health issues.

When a client feels valued by the nurse, he or she is inclined to accept desired change, that is, to comply with a prescribed health regimen. Listening to lay persons describe experiences related to health and illness management often provides cues to what they understand and value. People will usually accept suggestions for change from health professionals they like.

Key Terms

Active listening is a selective form of attentive communication. Empathy is most clearly demonstrated through active listening.

Closed questions are a type of interview question that limits an individual's response, for instance, "Do you like milk?"

Complementary transactions are communication exchanges in which the message is received by the ego state to which it was sent, and the receiver responds from that same ego state. Conversation lines are parallel and conversation flows comfortably.

Conflict is tension experienced by either or both persons in an interpersonal interaction. Conflict inhibits the development of an effective relationship.

Confrontation is the communication skill used to diffuse the tension resulting from interpersonal conflict. Interpersonal conflict needs to be confronted in order for individual integrity to be maintained.

Congruence in communication is achieved when a person's verbal statements and nonverbal behavior complement each other.

Crossed transactions are communication exchanges in which the person receiving the message responds from a different ego state from the one the speaker addressed. The ego states do not complement each other and communication difficulties may occur.

Emotional tone is the feeling dimension of an interpersonal relationship. Positive and negative emotions occur in all relationships.

Empathy is the ability to place oneself mentally in the other person's situation. It is a complex variable that helps the client to feel understood, accepted, and cared for. Empathy reduces misunderstanding and promotes accurate communication.

Facilitation skills are communication skills that encourage interpersonal trust. Communication is facilitated by listening attentively, showing warmth, demonstrating empathy through active listening, and being genuinely attentive. Facilitation skills are the hallmark of effective communication.

Interpersonal control is the dimension of an interpersonal relationship involving dominating and submissive behavior. Individuals need to achieve a balance that allows both parties to maintain a sense of autonomy.

Interviewing is the process of systematically questioning the client in order to collect data significant to planning nursing care. Inherent in the process of interviewing is the establishment of an interpersonal relationship. Interviewing skills include communicating concern for the client and recognizing the client's needs.

Involvement is the dimension of an interpersonal relationship determined by the value each person places on the relationship. Self-disclosure and mutual consideration occur when the relationship is highly valued.

Open-ended questions are interview questions that encourage the client to respond in any way desired, for instance, "What liquids do you like to drink?"

Probe questions are used in interview situations to encourage clients to give more information, for instance, "Tell me more about . . ."

Self-disclosure is the communicative process of revealing thoughts, feelings, and personal information. People are able to disclose information when they believe they are valued and protected. A safe environment facilitates self-disclosure.

Transactional Analysis is a theory about interpersonal behavior developed by Eric Berne. Communication occurs between the ego states of the sender and receiver. Ego states include the Parent, Adult, and Child.

Transition is a technique used in interviews to let the client know a change of topic is needed. It directs the client without implying that his or her comments are unimportant.

Trust is manifested in an interpersonal relationship when individuals feel comfortable relying on each other. In a nurse/client relationship, trust depends on the nurse avoiding evaluative communication. Statements that reflect acceptance of the client's viewpoint, values, and concerns support the development of trust.

Bibliography for Unit I
Understanding and Preparing for RN Mobility

Alfaro R: Application of Nursing Process: A Step-by-Step Guide. Philadelphia, JB Lippincott, 1986

Allen DW: Intentional Interviewing and Counseling. Monterey, CA, Brooks/Cole Publishing, 1988

American College Testing Program: ACT Proficiency Examination Program Technical Handbook, American College Testing Services, Iowa City, IA, 1988

Baer ED, Lowery BJ: Patient and situational factors that affect nursing students' like or dislike of caring for patients. Nurs Res 36(5): 298–299, 300–302, 1987

Berne E: Games People Play. New York, Grove Press, 1964

Carpenito LJ: Nursing Diagnosis: Application to Clinical Practice, 2nd ed. Philadelphia, JB Lippincott, 1987

Combs AW, Avila DL: Helping Relationships. Newton, MA, Allyn and Bacon, 1985

Duldt B, Giffin K, Patton, B: Interpersonal Communication in Nursing. Philadelphia, FA Davis, 1983

Elder J: Transactional Analysis in Health Care. Menlo Park, Addison-Wesley, 1978

Ellis DB: Becoming a Master Student. Rapid City, SD, College Survival, 1985

Gerrard BA, Boniface WJ, Love BH: Interpersonal Skills for Health Professionals. Reston, VA, Reston Publishing Co, 1980

Gordon M: Nursing Diagnosis: Process and Application. New York, McGraw-Hill, 1982

Griffith JW, Christensen PJ: Nursing Process: Application of Theories, Frameworks, and Models. St Louis, CV Mosby, 1982

Hunt R, Granzig W: Examinee strategies for increasing test scores. JOGN Nurs Sept/Oct 1975: 47–51

Iyer PW, Taptich BJ, Bernocchi-Losey D: Nursing Process and Nursing Diagnosis. Philadelphia, WB Saunders, 1986

King IM: Toward a Theory for Nursing: General Concepts of Human Behavior. New York, John Wiley & Sons, 1971

Kreps GL, Thornton BC: Health Communication. New York, Longman, 1984

Leininger MM: Care: The Essence of Nursing and Health. Thorofare, NJ, Charles B Slack, 1984

Long L, Prophit P: Understanding/Responding: A Communication Manual for Nurses. Belmont, CA, Wadsworth Publishing, 1981

Marriner A: The Nursing Process: A Scientific Approach to Nursing Care, 3rd ed. St Louis, CV Mosby, 1983

McCoy P: Further proof that touch speaks louder than words. RN November 1977: 43–46

Mitchell PH, Loustau A: Concepts Basic to Nursing, 3rd ed. New York, McGraw-Hill, 1981

National League for Nursing: Nursing Mobility Profile II Technical Manual, National League for Nursing, New York, 1984

Northouse PG, Northouse LL: Health Communication: A Handbook for Health Professionals. Englewood Cliffs, NJ, Prentice-Hall, 1985

Northouse PG: Interpersonal trust and empathy in nurse-nurse relationships. Nurs Res November–December 1979: 28:6: 365–368

Olson JK, Iwasiw CL: Effects of a training model on active listening skills of post-RN students. J Nurs Educ 26: 104–107, 1987

Phipps W, Long B, Woods N: Medical-Surgical Concepts and Clinical Practice, 3rd ed. St Louis, CV Mosby, 1987

Pinnell NN, de Meneses MD: The Nursing Process: Theory, Application and Related Processes. East Norwalk, CT, Appleton-Century-Crofts, 1986

Purtilo R: Health Professional/Patient Interaction. Philadelphia, WB Saunders, 1984

Riehl JS: Passing the State Board Examination. J Nurs Educ 23(8): 358–361, 1984

Rogers CR: Client-centered Therapy. Boston, Houghton Mifflin, 1951

Thompson TL: Communication for Health Professionals. New York, Harper & Row, 1986

Wlody GS: Communicating in the ICU: Do you read me loud and clear? Nurs Mgmt 15:9: 24–27, 1984

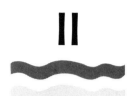

Care of the Adult Client

5

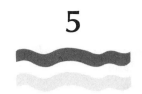

Nursing Care of the Client Who Has a Deficiency in the Delivery of Oxygen to the Cells

Cardiac Dysfunction

Angina Pectoris

Angina pectoris is chest pain of transient nature, associated with disruption of coronary artery blood flow to myocardial tissues. Transient chest pain is due to an imbalance of oxygen needed by and oxygen available to the myocardial cells. Decreased removal of the products of cell metabolism plays a role in myocardial cell health.

Assessment

Health Status

- Pain typically lasting 3–5 minutes; however, many clients have atypical symptoms (refer to comprehensive textbook for discussion of variant and unstable angina)
- Pain associated with physical exertion, exposure to cold, stress, or heavy meal
- Pain located midanterior chest, substernally or epigastrically, radiating to neck, back, arms, fingers, and jaw
- Pain diffuse, not pinpointed
- Pain described as tight, squeezing, heavy
- Pain similar from episode to episode
- Other findings: apprehension, dyspnea, diaphoresis, nausea, urge to void

Developmental Assessment

Atherosclerosis is the major cause of coronary artery disease (CAD), the predisposing disease of angina. It is characterized by the development of fatty plaques in the intima.

Risk factors include:

Elevated serum lipid levels
Elevated blood glucose levels
Hypertension
Cigarette smoking
Male sex, under age 65
Caucasian race
Family history of heart disease
Obesity
Sedentary lifestyle
Stressful lifestyle

Diagnostic Factors

History of chest pain in presence of risk factors
Electrocardiogram (ECG) shows evidence of ischemic tissue, *i.e.*, ST changes

Cardiac stress test shows diminished cardiac reserve and monitored ischemic changes

Coronary angiography demonstrates narrowing, obstruction, or vasospasm of coronary vessels as well as collateral vessels

Myocardial perfusion imaging with isotope may show ischemic areas as "cold spots"

Chest x-ray may show early evidence of congestive failure

Serum enzyme and isoenzyme (CPK, CPK-MB, SGOT, LDH) measurements rule out myocardial cell death (infarction)

Positive response to nitroglycerin (pain relief) test

Cardiac catheterization (see Table 5-1 for preoperative and postoperative care)

Psychosocial/Cultural Assessment

Most clients use denial in the early phase of angina.

Nursing Plans and Interventions

Goals

- Oxygen demands of myocardium will be reduced
- Acute pain and underlying disease process will be resolved
- Client will adapt to chronic disorder
- Client will be prepared for medical and/or surgical treatment (percutaneous transluminal coronary angioplasty [PTCA], coronary artery bypass graft [CABG])

Nursing Measures

- Administer prescribed medications
- Assess effect of drug therapy:
    Monitor vital signs
    Monitor ECG changes
    Watch for headache, facial flush, and tingling under tongue
- Assess for possible complications, myocardial infarction, unstable angina, dysrhythmia

Table 5-1. Cardiac Catheterization

A. Preoperative care
1. Make client npo
2. Prepare client for about a 2-hour procedure
3. Prepare client for possible uncomfortable sensations (palpitations, urgent need to cough, and a wave of heat sensation as contrast material is injected)
4. Encourage client to verbalize fears and anxieties, and provide reassurance and knowledge to reduce apprehension

B. Postoperative care
1. Monitor vital signs per protocol
2. Monitor and promote circulation in cannulated limb
   a. Immobilize extremity
   b. Assess quality of pulse, limb color, warmth, and sensation
   c. Maintain pressure dressing over insertion site
   d. Assess for hemorrhage or hematoma formation
3. Monitor for effect of heparinization
4. Monitor ECG for dysrhythmia
5. Assess I and O and maintain allowed hydration to promote renal clearance of contrast dyes
6. Assess for delayed hypersensitivity to contrast dye (rash, nausea)

- Reduce anxiety to reduce oxygen needs:
    Explain procedures
    Encourage client to verbalize concerns
    Administer sedatives
- Reduce activity to reduce oxygen needs:
    Provide physical care
    Provide oxygen
    Provide for safety from hypotension
- Support surgical treatment protocols if applicable and provide for client information needs

Medical/Surgical Treatment

Percutaneous transluminal coronary angioplasty (PTCA) is an invasive nonsurgical technique used in treating CAD. A balloon-tipped catheter is advanced to the lesion and inflated at the site, in order to reestablish blood flow to the ischemic myocardium.

Nursing measures include:

- Monitor vital signs and ECG
- Monitor and promote circulation in the cannulated limb
- Assess intake and output (I and O)
- Promote early activity
- Provide client teaching

Coronary artery bypass graft (CABG) is a graft consisting of the saphenous vein, internal mammary artery, or both, that revascularizes the distal portion of the stenotic coronary artery.

Nursing measures include:

- Maintain cardiac output, tissue perfusion, and stable vital signs
- Promote adequate ventilation and restoration of intrathoracic pressure
- Maintain renal perfusion and function
- Maintain adequate fluid and electrolyte balance
- Promote adequate nutrition
- Promote mobility
- Promote wound healing
- Provide client teaching

Drug Therapy

Nitroglycerin is mainstay of treatment to reduce oxygen use by heart and for pain relief (proper storage essential)

Oxygen is usually ordered to increase available oxygen in inspired air

β-adrenergic blocking agents may be added to reduce myocardial oxygen demand

Calcium channel blocking agents may be added to reduce oxygen demand

Antilipemics may be added to reduce blood lipids

Antiplatelet aggregates may be added to reduce thrombus formation

Nutrition Therapy

- Weight management to achieve ideal weight
- Low-cholesterol diet (avoid fried foods and animal fats–*e.g.*, eggs, red meat)
- Low-sodium diet (avoid processed foods)

Client/Family Teaching

Teach client to:

Recognize and prevent precipitating factors and events

Follow low-fat, low-sodium, appropriate-calorie diet

Follow individualized exercise program

Use medications (sublingual, transdermal nitroglycerin) correctly:

> Possible effects: sensations of fizzing and warmth under tongue, pounding headache, increased pulse, dizziness, and facial flushing
>
> May be used every 5 minutes for chest pain for a total of 3 tablets (if pain continues, seek physician assistance)
>
> Prophylactic use prior to exertional events that have been associated with chest pain in the past
>
> Importance of hypotension as a side-effect
>
> Store in a tightly capped dark glass (not in metal or plastic containers)

Evaluation

Client teaching is successful if client:

- Alters activity to reflect understanding of cardiac reserve
- Changes diet to indicate understanding of atherosclerosis
- Avoids physically and emotionally stressful situations
- Takes medications as prescribed, both prophylactically and if angina occurs
- Voices understanding of symptoms that require immediate medical attention
- Maintains appointments for reevaluation

Myocardial Infarction

Myocardial infarction occurs when ischemic changes of the myocardial cells become irreversible and the cells undergo necrosis.

Assessment

Health Status

- Persistent chest pain due to irreversible myocardial cell damage, caused by an imbalance of oxygen needed and oxygen available
- Typical pain of persistent episode longer than 20 minutes (atypical patterns occur, e.g., "silent" myocardial infarction, in which no episode of chest pain is reported)
- Pain not associated with precipitating events (e.g., work, stress)
- Pain located in substernal or retrosternal area, radiating into neck, arms, back, or jaw
- Pain described as heavy, crushing, viselike
- Pain diffuse, not pinpoint
- Pain not relieved by rest or nitroglycerin
- Nausea and vomiting due to stimulation of the vomiting center
- Cold, clammy, sweat and ashen color due to sympathetic stimulation and constriction of peripheral blood vessels
- Fever up to 102.2°F for first day to first week, due to inflammatory process of myocardial cells
- Extreme fatigue, weakness

Cardiovascular Signs

- Early increased blood pressure and pulse or late decreased blood pressure and pulse
- Decreased urine output
- Rales (crackles) noted in lung fields due to some degree of left sided congestive heart failure
- Hepatic engorgement and peripheral edema due to some degree of congestive heart failure (CHF)
- Distant heart sounds with split, indicating delay in ventricular response on the infarcted side; S_3, S_4, and murmurs may be heard

Cardiogenic Shock Syndrome (Pump Failure)

- Present in 10% to 15% of hospitalized acute myocardial infarction patients; associated with 45% damage to left ventricular muscle mass
- Occurs when the heart can no longer pump blood efficiently to all parts of the body
- May result from dysrhythmias and end stage congestive heart failure (CHF)
- See Table 5-2 for clinical manifestations

Developmental Assessment

Atherosclerosis is the major cause of CAD, the predisposing disease of angina. See angina pectoris discussion for associated risk factors.

Diagnostic Factors

- Serum enzyme and isoenzyme (CPK, CPK-MB, LDH and SGOT) evaluations indicate cellular death; CPK level rises within 6 hours of infarct and returns to near normal within 2–3 days; CPK isoenzyme MB is the most cardio-specific indicator of myocardial infarction damage; timing of samples is important (see Table 5-3)
- Twelve lead ECG over 6–96 hours is 80% accurate in diagnosing myocardial infarction and locating damage
- Chest x-ray is helpful in noting cardiac size and lung congestion (upper lobe venous distention indicates early left ventricular failure)
- White blood cell (WBC) levels elevate to 12,000–14,000 in response to myocardial inflammation
- Fasting blood sugar may increase up to 300 mg/dl or more in response to stress
- Nuclear imaging is a very sensitive indicator of myocardial damage
- Client history and presenting symptoms are also important considerations

Psychosocial/Cultural Assessment

Many clients deny that they might be experiencing a myocardial infarction (as many as 30%–40% of myocardial infarction clients die before reaching the hospital).

Table 5-2. **Manifestations of Cardiogenic Shock in Different Stages**

Manifestation	Early (compensatory)	Intermediate (progressive)	Late (irreversible)
Level of Consciousness	Restless, irritable, apprehensive; thoughts are oriented	Listless, agitated, confused; Response to pain is stimuli-oriented, but slowed	Unconscious; decreased reflexes, confused thoughts, incoherent speech
Skin Characteristics	Cool, pale	Cold, clammy, mottled, cyanotic	Cold, clammy, cyanotic
Heart Rate	Slightly increased (by 20 beats/min)	Tachycardia (rate 100–150 beats/min)	Slow
Heart Rhythm	Rhythm regular	Rhythm regular	Rhythm irregular
Blood Pressure			
Systolic	Normal or slightly increased	Below normal	Markedly below normal (may fall to zero)
Diastolic	Normal or slightly increased	Lower than normal Widening pulse pressure	May be absent
Respiratory Function			
Rate	Above client's usual rate	Rapid	Slow
Depth	Deeper than client's usual depth	Shallow	Shallow and irregular

Table 5-3. **Expected Time Pattern of Cardiac Enzyme Level Changes Following Acute Myocardial Infarction**

Enzyme	Onset	Peak	Return to Normal
CPK or CK	3–6 hours	12–24 hours	2–3 days
CPK-MB	2–4 hours	12–20 hours	48–72 hours
LDH	24 hours	48–72 hours	7–10 days
LDH_1 and LDH_2	4 hours	48 hours	10 days

Nursing Plans and Interventions

Goals

- Client will live and his or her condition will stabilize
- Pain will be controlled and area of infarction minimized
- Complications will be prevented (dysrhythmias, heart failure, cardiogenic shock, papillary muscle dysfunction, ventricular aneurysm, pericarditis, pulmonary embolism and Dressler's syndrome)

Nursing Measures

- Maintain oxygenation to vital tissues:
    Establish peripheral intravenous lines; central line may be established by physician
    Monitor arterial hemodynamics
    Monitor fluid and electrolyte status
    Assess heart and lung sounds
    Assess for other signs of heart failure
    Assess monitored ECG pattern
- Monitor for life-threatening dysrhythmias
- Lower oxygen needs:
    Decrease anxiety
    Decrease activity levels
    Promote normal elimination pattern
- Develop and support adaptive coping behaviors

Drug Therapy

Morphine sulfate intravenously (IV) for pain management

Nitroglycerin IV to decrease preload and afterload

Diazepam for sedation

Lidocaine to prevent dysrhythmias

β-blockers to reduce myocardial cell ischemic zone

Acetylsalicific acid (ASA) to reduce platelet aggregation and risk of recurrence

Oxygen to increase available oxygen in inspired air

Docusate sodium (Colace) for stool softening

Thrombolytic therapy is being used with selected clients to minimize myocardial damage by reducing the size of the infarction; streptokinase and tissue-type plasminogen activator (t-PA) are currently valuable agents.

Nutrition Therapy

- May be maintained on nothing by mouth (npo) status in early acute period
- Soft bland diet in late acute period
- Low-salt, low-fat diet to slow progression of arteriosclerotic process
- Reduced calorie diet to achieve ideal weight

Client/Family Teaching

Teach client to:

Follow low-fat, low-sodium, appropriate-calorie diet

Follow individualized exercise program

Use medication correctly

Understand physiologic changes associated with coronary artery disease

Comply with ongoing medical follow-up

Evaluation

Treatment and client teaching are successful if client:

- Maintains effectiveness of cardiovascular function
- Voices understanding of changed physiology and related treatments
- Alters activity to reflect understanding of how to improve cardiac reserve and collateral circulation, and of need for rest periods to prevent undue cardiac stress
- Maintains ideal weight through low-cholesterol, low-sodium diet
- Participates in rehabilitation program
- Can state drug schedule, including purpose, dosage, times, and parameters for measuring effectiveness and side-effects

Congestive Heart Failure

Congestive heart failure (CHF) is malfunction of the heart resulting in impaired pump performance.

Assessment

Health Status

Heart failure may occur in the right or left ventricular chambers.

Left ventricular failure results in the following clinical manifestations:

Pulmonary Congestion
- Auscultated rales
- X-ray changes
- Shortness of breath, paroxysmal nocturnal dyspnea
- Rapid breathing, 30–40/min (hyperpnea)
- Dry cough

Hypoxia
- Fatigue due to low cardiac output
- Decreased mentation due to hypoxia and hypotension
- Peripheral and central cyanosis
- Blood gases with low partial pressure of oxygen in arterial blood (PaO_2), high partial pressure of carbon dioxide in arterial blood ($PaCO_2$)

Cardiac Alterations
- Distant heart sounds
- Presence of third heart sound
- Decreased cardiac output
- Tachycardia

Right ventricular failure results in the following clinical manifestations:

Venous Congestion
- Neck vein engorgement with exaggerated pulsations
- Hepatomegaly and splenomegaly
- Dependent edema, especially in legs and sacrum
- Steady weight gain
- Congested gastrointestinal tract leading to flatulence, feeling of fullness, nausea, and anorexia

Hypoxia
- Peripheral cyanosis
- Prolonged circulation time

Developmental Assessment

Left-sided Failure Precursors

Coronary artery disease
Hypertension
Rheumatic heart disease
Valvular heart disease

Right-sided Failure Precursors

Left-sided failure
Pulmonary hypertension
Cor pulmonale caused by chronic obstructive pulmonary disease, pulmonary embolism

Precursors of Failure in the Unhealthy Heart

Dysrhythmias of the myocardium
Anemia
Thyrotoxicosis
Other increased work load demands
Dietary indiscretions such as increased sodium and water intake

Diagnostic Factors

Cardiovascular
- Chest x-ray shows cardiomegaly (enlarged heart)
- Auscultation reveals ventricular gallop
- Pulse of unequal volume and force
- ECG may show ventricular hypertrophy, prolonged PR interval
- Distant heart sounds on auscultation

Gastrointestinal
- Nausea and anorexia
- Distention and flatulence
- Weight gain history over short time frame

Psychosocial/Cultural Assessment

- Client may report immediate history of stressful events, excessive physical demands
- Client may report noncompliance with prescribed diet or medications

Nursing Plans and Interventions

Goals

- Underlying disease process will be controlled
- Acute exacerbation will be stabilized
- Client will adapt to possible chronic disorder

Nursing Measures

Promote physical and emotional rest:

- Encourage bedrest or chair rest
- Provide bedside commode
- Explain all procedures, reduce environmental stress
- Monitor vital signs frequently
- Provide stool softeners
- Provide small feedings to reduce work of heart for digestion

Promote normal fluid balance:

- Monitor body weight
- Administer prescribed diuretic therapy
- Monitor dependent edema by measuring ankle and girth
- Limit fluid intake if ordered
- Monitor intake and output (I and O)
- Provide low-sodium and low-fat diet
- Assess for electrolyte imbalance, especially hypokalemia due to diuretic therapy
- Assess integrity of edematous skin areas
- Reduce blood volume in circulation by using rotating tourniquets
  1. Mark peripheral pulses with X
  2. Place tourniquet cuff high on extremity
  3. Assess for arterial pulse with cuff inflated
  4. Set rotation schedule and monitor for correct function

Promote adequate cardiac output:

- Administer cardiac glycoside (digitalis) as prescribed
- Monitor apical heart rate; withhold drug if heart rate is below 60 beats/min, and notify physician
- Assess response to drug therapy
- Assess for toxic effects

Promote normal respiratory function:

- Position client in semi-Fowler's position
- Reduce skeletal muscle work by supporting arms with pillows
- Assess lung sounds every 4 hours
- Provide oxygen via nasal cannula

Provide support and encouragement for change in lifestyle:

- Teach about disease process and altered physiology
- Teach medication regimen and dietary modifications
- Encourage family involvement in planning care at home
- Teach specific manifestations of worsening condition that require prompt medical attention, such as shortness of breath at rest, increased edema, continuing weight gain of 2–4 pounds every 2 days, increased urinary frequency, resting heart rate increased by 20 beats/min

Drug Therapy

Digitalis to strengthen myocardial contractility and slow heart rate

Diuretic to reduce circulating blood volume

Vasodilators to reduce venous return of blood to the heart (preload) and reduce peripheral vascular resistance (afterload) to reduce work load of heart

Nutrition Therapy

- Low-fat, low-sodium diet
- Restrict fluid intake

Client/Family Teaching

Teach client to:

Understand physiologic changes related to CHF
Follow medication schedule
Follow low-sodium, low-fat diet
Follow activity schedule

Evaluation

Client teaching is successful if client:

- Modifies diet to reflect understanding of need to limit sodium and fluid intake
- Changes activity pattern to prevent recurrence of CHF
- Verbally identifies signs and symptoms indicating recurrence of CHF
- Voices understanding of dose, times, effect, and side-effects of prescribed medication
- Keeps appointments for monitoring drug therapy and medical reevaluation

Rheumatic Heart Disease

Rheumatic heart disease is heart damage resulting from rheumatic fever, an inflammatory disease involving all layers of the heart. Heart valve damage is characterized by scarring and deformity of the heart valves.

Assessment

Health Status

- Fever of 100.4°F or more
- Heart murmur over affected valve
- Cardiomegaly
- Signs of CHF (see congestive heart failure)
- Friction rub if pericardium is involved
- Tachycardia due to decreased cardiac output
- Migratory joint pain, swelling
- 5% show nonpurulent rash over trunk (erythema marginatum)
- Movable, firm, nontender subcutaneous nodules
- Mental changes, such as irritability and decreased concentration
- Anemia with fatigue

Developmental Assessment

Rheumatic heart disease is primarily a disorder of children and young adults, ages 11–22 years. Ninety five percent of cases follow group A β-hemolytic streptococcal infection.

Diagnostic Factors

-
- Increased antistreptolysin-O test (ASO) titer (greater than 250 IU/mL)
- Erythrocyte sedimentation rate greater than 15–20 mm/hr
- Positive C reactive protein
- Increased WBC count
- Echocardiogram demonstrates valvular damage
- Chest x-ray shows cardiomegaly
- ECG shows impaired AV conduction, low voltage QRS, ST segment and T-wave changes
- Increased cardiac enzymes

Psychosocial/Cultural Assessment

Depressed socioeconomic conditions contribute to:

- Poor nutrition
- Crowded living conditions
- Altered immune resistance

Cool damp weather may contribute to the disease.

Nursing Plans and Interventions

Goals

- Client will get physical and emotional rest, to reduce cardiac work load

- Reinfection will be prevented
- Heart damage will be prevented

Nursing Measures

- Administer antibiotic therapy, usually penicillin or erythromycin (prophylactic treatment should be continued for life if rheumatic carditis developed in childhood; prophylactic treatment with benzathine penicillin G usually continues for 5 years for those who develop rheumatic fever without carditis after age 18 years)
- Reduce fever and discomfort with salicylates
- Reduce inflammation with corticosteroids
- Maintain strict bedrest for 5–6 weeks, then slowly liberalize activity
- Provide diversional activity, especially school work, over bedrest period
- Provide supplemental nutritional support
- Monitor vital signs, auscultate heart sounds
- Maintain antiembolytic measures
- Prepare for surgical intervention (valve commissurotomy or valve replacement)

Medical/Surgical Treatment

Commissurotomy is an alternative to valve replacement. The leaflets are cut free from one another. Symptoms may recur, however, in which case valve replacement may be necessary.

Valve replacement involves removal of the original valve and the insertion of a prosthesis.

Preoperative Nursing Care

- Ensure client avoids ASA prior to surgery
- Discontinue digitalis 24–48 hours prior to surgery
- Support the client emotionally to reduce fear and anxiety, by teaching postoperative expectations (*e.g.*, IV lines, chest tubes in the case of valve replacement, urinary catheter, intubation and ventilator, need to use other means of communication, need for turning, coughing, deep breathing, and foot exercises)

Postoperative Nursing Care

- Monitor cardiac status, respiratory status, peripheral vascular status, renal function, fluid/electrolyte status
- Monitor and manage pain
- Assess for possible complications: decreased cardiac output, persistent bleeding, cardiac tamponade, cardiac failure, myocardial infarction, impaired gaseous exchange

Drug Therapy

Antibiotic therapy (penicillin or erythromycin) to reduce infective organisms

Salicylates to reduce inflammation

Long-term anticoagulation treatment

Nutrition Therapy

- High-protein, high-calorie diet
- Restrict fluid and sodium intake if signs of CHF are present

Client/Family Teaching

Teach client and family measures to prevent recurrence of infection, including:

Hygienic food preparation methods

Personal hygiene measures

Ensuring adequate rest

Complying with ongoing medical supervision and seeking immediate care if a sore throat develops

Prophylactic use of penicillin therapy

Evaluation

Client teaching is successful if client:

- Complies with prophylactic antibiotic treatment
- Plans activities of daily living to avoid fatigue and prevent reinfection
- Maintains oral hygiene practices to reduce risk of reinfection
- Keeps appointments for medical reevaluation as recommended

- Notifies other health care professionals, e.g., dentist, gynecologist, about need for prophylactic antibiotic treatment

Mitral Stenosis

Mitral stenosis is narrowing of the mitral valve caused by valvular abnormalities such as fibrosis and calcifications, which obstruct blood flow from the left atrium into the left ventricle, thereby producing increased left atrial pressure, increased pulmonary hypertension, right ventricular hypertension, and eventually, right-sided heart failure.

Assessment

Health Status

- Early rumbling diastolic heart murmur detected at apex
- Increased intensity of S_1 (as atrioventricular [AV] valve closes)
- Dyspnea on exertion, orthopnea, and paroxysmal nocturnal dyspnea
- Possible hemoptysis due to venous congestion
- Fatigue and weakness due to low cardiac output
- Atrial fibrillation with palpitations and possible systemic emboli
- Signs of right-sided CHF

Developmental Assessment

Predisposing factors include:

History of rheumatic heart disease (client may be asymptomatic 20–30 years)

Female sex (females more predisposed than males)

Presence of other congenital abnormalities

Predisposition to respiratory infections or history of frequent respiratory infections

Diagnostic Factors

Chest x-ray shows left atrial enlargement, enlarged pulmonary arteries, and mitral valve calcification

Echocardiogram shows thickened leaflets and narrowed lumen

ECG shows right axis deviation, left atrial hypertrophy, atrial fibrillation, and prolonged, notched P waves

Pulmonary capillary wedge pressure greater than 15 mm Hg

Nursing Plans and Interventions

Goals

- Recurrence of rheumatic heart disease will be prevented
- Symptoms of CHF will be reduced
- Atrial dysrhythmias will be eliminated
- Anemia will be resolved
- Infective disease will be prevented
- Valvular narrowing will be assessed on an ongoing basis, in preparation for surgery

Nursing Measures

- Promote adequate rest to reduce oxygen needs:
    Help client prioritize activities
    Help client conserve energy
    Plan rest periods in client's schedule
- Maintain cardiac function:
    Provide low-sodium diet to reduce body weight, if client is overweight
    Measure weight daily
    Monitor I and O
    Administer medications

Medical/Surgical Treatment

Mitral valve replacement or commissurotomy (see Rheumatic Heart Disease, Medical/Surgical Treatment, for pre- and postoperative nursing care)

Drug Therapy

Digitalis, diuretics, and electrolyte replacement to prevent CHF

Iron and folic acid to treat hemolytic anemia from valve damage on red blood cells (RBC)

Quinidine or procainamide hydrochloride (Pronestyl) for atrial fibrillation

Anticoagulant therapy to prevent embolism

Antibiotic therapy to treat infective processes

Nutrition Therapy

- Low-sodium diet

Client/Family Teaching

Teach client to:

Prioritize activities in order to conserve energy

Understand importance, purpose, and effects of prescribed medications

Comply with ongoing medical evaluation

Understand dangers of smoking

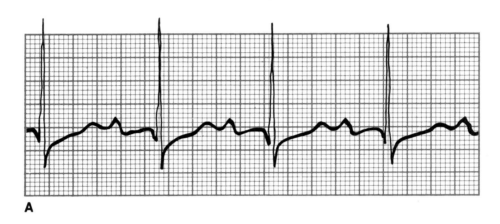

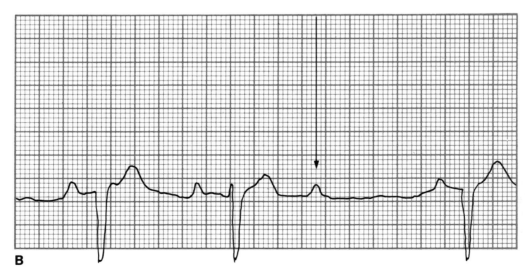

Figure 5-1. Assessment of heart block. (A) First degree AV heart block; (B) Second degree block—Mobitz I (Wenckebach). The arrow indicates the nonconducted P wave in this sequence. (C) Second degree block—Mobitz II. Arrows denote blocked P waves. (D) Third degree block (complete AV block). (Hudak CM, Gallo BM, Lohr T: Critical Care Nursing: A Holistic Approach, 4th ed. Philadelphia, JB Lippincott, 1986)

Evaluation

Client teaching is successful if client:

- Changes activity pattern to include periodic rest and prevent fatigue
- Maintains ideal weight to reduce cardiac work load
- Voices understanding of purpose, dose, time, desired effect, and side-effects of prescribed medication
- Keeps appointments for medical reevaluation

Heart Block (See Figure 5d)

Heart block refers to a delay or complete stopping of conduction of electrical impulses from the sinoatrial (SA) node to the ventricular tissues. First degree block results in the delay of impulses to ventricular conduction tissue without serious alteration in cardiac function. Second degree and third degree blocks usually require treatment to prevent serious cardiac dysfunction.

Assessment, Diagnostic Factors, and Medical/Surgical Treatment

First Degree Heart Block

First degree heart block is associated with rheumatic fever, chronic ischemic heart disease, acute myocardial infarction, hyperthyroidism,

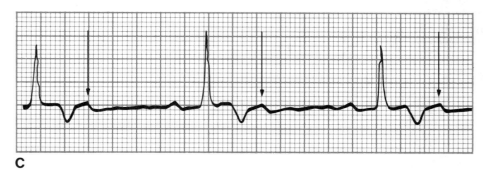

C

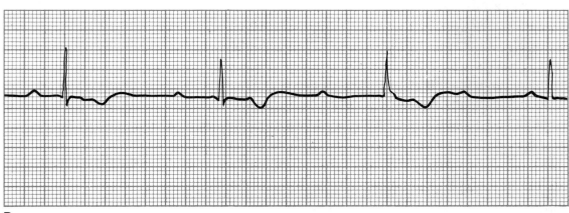

D

vagal stimulation and the use of certain drugs, *i.e.*, digitalis propranolol, IV verapamil.

- Normal rate
- Normal rhythm
- Normal P wave occurs before each QRS complex
- Consistently prolonged PR interval (greater than 0.20 seconds)
- Normal QRS contour, follows each P wave
- *Significance:* May lead to higher degree block
- *Treatment:* Monitor
- Client not aware of block

Second Degree Heart Block Type I

Second degree heart block type I (Mobitz I, Wenckebach) is characterized by the SA impulse having increasing difficulty conducting through the AV node until finally one impulse is stopped. The progression then repeats the pattern. Mobitz I is associated with diseases and drugs such as digitalis and propranolol that slow AV conduction by increasing parasympathetic tone.

- Normal atrial rate, but ventricular rate slower than atrial rate
- Ventricular rhythm usually irregular, with progressive lengthening of the PR interval
- Normal P wave
- PR interval contour lengthens progressively until QRS complex is dropped
- Normal QRS contour
- *Significance:* Transient in acute myocardial infarction; may lead to block of higher degree
- *Treatment:* None unless significant decrease in cardiac output (atropine or temporary pacer may be used if symptomatic)

Second Degree Heart Block Type II

Second degree heart block type II (Mobitz II) is serious because a certain number of SA node impulses are not transmitted to the ventricles. Normally, P waves are followed by QRS complexes in a 1:1 ratio. In the case of Mobitz II this ratio may be 2:1, 3:1, or 4:1. Mobitz II is associated with rheumatic or atherosclerotic heart disease, acute anterior myocardial infarction, and digitalis toxicity (as opposed to parasympathetic tone or drug effect).

- Normal atrial rate, but ventricular rate slower than atrial rate
- Regular atrial rhythm, but ventricular rhythm may be irregular
- Normal P wave contour
- PR interval may be normal, or prolonged on conducted beats and remaining fixed
- QRS complex may be normal or abnormally wide (greater than 0.12 seconds), because bundle-branch block is common
- *Significance:* Serious dysrhythmia leading to complete block may seriously decrease cardiac output and is usually associated with an organic lesion; this may have a poor prognosis
- *Treatment:* Temporary or permanent pacemaker; if client is very symptomatic an isoproterenol drip will increase the ventricular rate and increase cardiac output until a pacemaker can be placed

Third Degree Heart Block

Third degree heart block (complete heart block) is life threatening because no impulses from the atria are conducted to the ventricles, so the atria and ventricles beat independently. Third degree heart block is associated with acute myocardial infarction, rheumatic heart disease, Lev's disease as well as atherosclerosis.

- Sinus atrial rate usually 60–100 beats/min, but ventricular rate only 40–60 in the case of AV node block; in the case of Purkinje block, ventricular rate only 20–40 beats/min
- Both atrial and ventricular rhythms are regular but not synchronized
- Normal P wave contour
- PR interval cannot be measured because atria and ventricles are beating independently

- QRS complex normal if starting high as in the case of bundle-branch block; wide in the case of Purkinje block
- *Significance:* Markedly decreased cardiac output
- *Treatment:* Pacemaker (may try atropine, isoproterenol, or epinephrine) until pacemaker placed

Nursing Plans and Interventions

Goals

- Underlying condition will be resolved (using rapid recognition and treatment guidelines)

Nursing Measures

- Monitor clients at risk
- Assess unmonitored clients' vital signs frequently
- Ensure prompt treatment by keeping equipment ready
- Promote rest and comfort
- Assess blood, drug, and electrolyte levels for possible cause of block; monitor levels of digitalis and potassium especially
- Provide oxygen to reduce cellular hypoxia
- Assess tissue perfusion–problems indicated by:
  - Altered level of consciousness
  - Syncopal episode
  - Decreased urine output
  - Peripheral color changes
- Assess fluid balance by measuring:
  - I and O
  - Daily weight
  - Peripheral edema
- Assess and promote adequate pacemaker function by monitoring for:
  - Sensing and capturing failure
  - Signs of local and systemic infection
  - Cardiac function (by measuring vital signs)

Drug Therapy

First degree block: No drug treatment
Second degree block, type I: No treatment, or trial atropine
Second degree block, type II: Isoproterenol
Third degree block: Trial atropine, isoproterenol, or epinephrine

Nutrition Therapy

- Reduce elevated electrolyte levels (*e.g.*, by reducing potassium levels)
- Restrict caffeine intake

Client/Family Teaching

Teach client to:

Understand need for pacemaker
Recognize signs and symptoms of pacemaker malfunction
Comply with medical follow-up
Avoid high output generators
Monitor own pulse
Follow prescribed medication regimen
Recognize signs of local and systemic infection

Evaluation

Client teaching is successful if client:

- Modifies rest and activity patterns
- Voices understanding of purpose, dose, time, desired effect, and side-effects of prescribed medication
- Demonstrates skill in assessing own pulse rate
- Modifies diet to maintain adequate levels of calcium and potassium
- Seeks medical reevaluation as scheduled or if symptoms recur

Vascular Dysfunction

Aneurysm

Aneurysms are outpouchings or dilatations of the arterial wall. The aorta is commonly affected. Weakness of the muscle wall allows the intimal layer to bulge outward. Blood pressure within the vessel may also press the layer outward. The underlying process of disease is arteriosclerosis 95% of the time. Trauma, cystic medial necrosis, and syphilis may also be contributory.

Assessment

Health Status

- Palpable pulsating mass in periumbilical area
- Systolic bruit over aorta
- Reported tenderness on deep palpation
- Rarely causes decreased peripheral pulse or claudication unless emboli present
- Low back pain
- Hypertension may be contributory
- Pain may mimic renal calculi pain, lumbar disc pain
- Signs of shock in the case of peritoneal rupture
- Delayed signs of shock in the case of retroperitoneal rupture, because abdominal organs act as tamponade

Developmental Assessment

Most aneurysms occur between renal and iliac branches from the aorta.
Predisposing factors include:

Male sex (higher incidence than female sex)
Caucasian race
Age between 40–80 years

Diagnostic Factors

Aneurysms usually found accidently during routine physical examination or x-ray
Confirmed by ultrasound measuring size, shape, location
Abdominal anterior–posterior or lateral x-ray confirms 75% of all
Angioaortogram can locate and define condition of proximal and distal vessels

Nursing Plans and Interventions

Goals

- Client's condition will stabilize and he or she will be prepared for surgery (aneurysm repair)—prepare emergency equipment

Nursing Measures

Preoperative Care

- Monitor vital signs frequently
- Perform type and cross match test in preparation for blood administration
- Obtain blood for electrolyte, blood urea nitrogen (BUN) levels, creatinine levels, complete blood count (CBC)
- Evaluate ECG
- Monitor I and O and weight in preparation for surgery
- Be especially alert for acute renal failure
- Start antibiotic therapy

Postoperative Care

- Maintain fluid balance by IV and arterial lines
- Maintain respiratory status by monitoring changes recorded on the ventilator, arterial blood gas measurements (ABGs), skin color, breath sounds
- Monitor nasogastric (NG) tube function
- Assess bowel sounds and abdominal distention
- Assess urinary output
- Assess peripheral pulses distal to surgical site
- Assess blood loss by monitoring dressings
- Position for alignment and comfort
- Ambulate as soon as possible
- Provide pain relief by administering medications and performing nursing measures

Drug Therapy

Drugs used to support surgical intervention

Nutrition Therapy

- Usually npo postoperatively for a few days, then diet as tolerated
- Diet to slow progression of arteriosclerosis

Client/Family Teaching

Teach client to:

Avoid prolonged sitting or inactivity

Follow low-sodium, low-fat diet to slow progression of arteriosclerosis

Recognize symptoms that require immediate medical attention

Evaluation

Client teaching is successful if client:

- Maintains adequate circulation postoperatively
- Maintains appointments for reevaluation of circulation status, including laboratory monitoring

Thrombophlebitis

Thrombophlebitis is inflammation and thrombus formation that occurs in deep or superficial veins. Deep vein thrombosis is usually progressive and leads to pulmonary embolism. Alteration in the epithelial lining of vessels causes platelets to aggregate and is followed by fibrin entrapment of red blood cells (RBCs), white blood cells (WBCs), and other platelets.

Assessment

Health Status

Thrombi in Superficial Veins
- Visible and palpable veins
- Local heat and redness
- Local tenderness
- Local swelling and induration along length of vein

Thrombi in Deep Veins
- Severe pain
- Fever and chills
- Malaise
- Swelling and discoloration of affected extremity

Developmental Assessment

Causes of superficial thrombi include:

Local trauma
Local infective processes
IV drug abuse
Chemical irritation

   Causes of deep thrombi include:

Idiopathic factors
Endothelial damage
Accelerated blood clotting time
Decreased blood flow

   Other predisposing factors include:

Prolonged bedrest
Low abdominal surgery
Childbirth
Use of oral contraceptives
Estrogen replacement therapy

Diagnostic Factors

- Doppler study can amplify sounds of blood flow
- Plethysmography measures changes in calf volume resulting from obstruction of venous channels (helpful in deep vein measurement)
- Phlebography is an x-ray of injected vein with radiopaque dye
- Homans' sign is positive in 50% of cases with deep vein involvement
- Other diseases such as arterial occlusion, lymphangitis, cellulitis, and myositis must be ruled out

Psychosocial/Cultural Assessment

Habits such as crossing legs and wearing roller garters or constricting clothing may contribute to venous stasis.

Nursing Plans and Interventions

Goals

- Thrombus formation will be controlled

- Client's discomfort will be relieved
- Client will not experience complications and recurrence

Nursing Measures

- Promote venous return to the heart:
  - Provide bedrest to decrease tissue oxygen needs and reduce venous congestion
  - Elevate extremity to use gravity to improve venous return
  - Apply antiembolism stocking to apply uniform pressure over extremity
  - Provide warm moist soaks to increase thrombolysis
  - Maintain anticoagulation regimen to prevent enlargement of thrombus
  - Assess and monitor calf circumference and inflammatory signs
  - Provide adequate fluid balance to prevent hemoconcentration
- Promote comfort:
  - Administer analgesic to reduce discomfort; no ASA
  - Change position frequently
  - Encourage diversional activity
  - Teach leg exercises for nonaffected leg
- Monitor anticoagulant therapy:
  - Administer anticoagulant after considering results of laboratory tests: partial thromboplastin time for heparin therapy, prothrombin time for warfarin sodium crystalline (Coumadin) therapy
  - Have available specific antidote for anticoagulant used: protamine sulfate for heparin, vitamin K preparations for warfarin sodium crystalline
  - Monitor for signs of unusual bleeding in hematest stools, urine, vomitus, sputum, nasal mucus, oral cavity
- Provide a safe environment and use safe equipment
- Assess for pulmonary emboli, rales, dyspnea, hemoptysis, hypotension

Drug Therapy

Heparin, administered parenterally, either intermittently or continuously

Warfarin sodium crystalline, administered orally, usually daily, based on body weight and excretion rates

Monitor appropriate laboratory tests for each anticoagulant

Have available specific antidote for each

Monitor client for unusual bleeding

Assess diet and other medications for interaction with warfarin sodium crystalline:
- Effects of warfarin sodium crystalline are intensified by antibiotics, tolbutamide (orinase), salicylates, and dipyridamole (persantine)
- Effects of warfarin sodium crystalline are reduced by antacids, barbiturates, adrenal corticosteroids, oral contraceptives, and leafy green vegetables high in Vitamin K, such as cabbage and greens

Nutrition Therapy

- Ensure client avoids foods that interact with warfarin sodium crystalline (daily complete vitamin tablets, foods high in vitamin K)
- Maintain proper hydration

Client/Family Teaching

Teach client about:

Need for monitoring test as ordered

Purpose and side-effects of anticoagulant, and interactions with food and medications

Need to assess for unusual bleeding

Need to inform all caregivers of anticoagulant medications, wear med-alert jewelry, and carry information card

Ways to prevent accidental bleeding, *e.g.*, using electric shaver, foot coverings, gloves for work

Evaluation

Client teaching is successful if client:

- Expresses understanding of signs and symptoms of recurrence of thrombophlebitis, and of need for medical reevaluation
- Eliminates habits such as wearing constricting clothing, crossing legs
- Takes anticoagulant medications and voices understanding of appropriate anticoagulant precautions

Pulmonary Embolism

Pulmonary embolism is the obstruction of one or more pulmonary arteries by thrombi formed elsewhere in the venous system, including the right heart chambers. Thrombi from the venous system or right heart chambers lodge, usually during atrial fibrillation, in the more vascular lower lung lobe areas, thereby causing a ventilation/perfusion imbalance.

Assessment

Health Status

Clinical findings vary depending on the size of the area for diffusion of gases interfered with, and may include:

- Unexplained dyspnea
- Pleuritic chest pain and sense of impending doom
- Dry cough or hemoptysis
- Rales may be present
- Fever
- Distended neck veins
- Accentuated pulmonic heart sound (second heart sound)
- Decreased PAO_2, hypoxemia, cyanosis, and pallor
- Tachycardia
- Sudden respiratory and vascular collapse

Diagnostic Factors

Physical appearance: shock, pallor, and shortness of breath

ABG measurement shows decreased PAO_2

Radioisotope lung scan shows ventilation/perfusion defects

Pulmonary angiogram most revealing of blood filling defects

Nursing Plans and Interventions

Goals

- Adequate pulmonary function will be restored
- Recurrence of emboli will be prevented

Nursing Measures

Monitor vital signs by:

- Monitoring ECG for signs of right-sided failure
- Monitoring ABGs for signs of hypoxemia (low PaO_2)
- Assessing ventilatory effort
  1. Position in semi-Fowlers
  2. Ready mechanical ventilating equipment
  3. Administer oxygen
  4. Administer small doses of morphine to relieve anxiety and reduce oxygen needs

Give IV fluids to counteract shock and enhance right ventricular filling.

Administer parenteral anticoagulant to prevent extension of emboli or thrombus.

Monitor for unusual bleeding.

Prepare client for embolectomy, if this surgery is the selected treatment.

Medical/Surgical Treatment

Embolectomy is the removal of an occluding embolus from a vessel by means of a surgical incision into the artery, with the goal to restore blood flow.

Drug Therapy

Heparin therapy for 7–10 days

Warfarin sodium crystalline (Coumadin) therapy orally after 4–5 days of heparin therapy

Digitalis may be used to strengthen heart pumping

Vasopressor drugs may be used to improve blood pressure and treat vascular collapse

Thrombolytic drugs (streptokinase, urokinase, and tissue-type plasminogen activator [t-PA] may be used under investigational protocols

Nutrition Therapy

- Ensure adequate hydration
- Ensure client avoids foods known to interact with warfarin sodium crystalline (Coumadin)

Client/Family Teaching

Provide anticoagulant therapy information, including medication schedule and importance of:

Not skipping dose or "doubling up" if dose accidently skipped

Avoiding nonprescribed medications

Necessary laboratory monitoring tests

Monitoring self for unusual bleeding

Wearing medic-alert jewelry and notifying other health care professionals of condition

Avoiding prolonged inactivity, wearing constricting clothing, crossing legs

Evaluation

Treatment and client teaching are successful if client:

- Shows improved respiratory function
- Demonstrates knowledge of medication regimen
- Demonstrates knowledge of self-monitoring for unusual or prolonged bleeding

Cerebrovascular Accident

A *cerebrovascular accident* (CVA) is a neurologic deficit resulting from disruption of cerebral blood supply due to thrombus, embolism, stenosis, or hemorrhage. Blood circulation to brain structures is interrupted, producing areas of ischemia, infarct, edema, and congestion. These conditions lead to neurologic dysfunction.

Assessment

Health Status

- Depends on size and location of ischemic area
- Alteration and loss of sensory function
- Alteration and loss of motor function
- Impairment of mentation, memory, and speech
- Visual field deficits
- Bladder and bowel impairment
- Interference with protective reflexes, *i.e.*, cough, gag, blink, swallow

Developmental Assessment

Predisposing factors include:

Family history of CVA

History of transient ischemic attack (TIA)

Hypertension

Advanced age

Cigarette smoking

Estrogen therapy

Cardiac diseases

Diabetes

Diagnostic Factors

Computed tomography (CT) scan (x-ray with predetermined depth shows detailed cross-section)

Cerebral angiography (x-ray of blood vessels seen by radiopaque dye)

Echoencephology (ultrasound study of intracranial structures)

Carotid Doppler studies (measures velocity of blood flow through vessels)

Magnetic resonance imaging (MRI)

Nursing Plans and Interventions

Goals

- Brain edema will be reduced (to prevent extension of ischemia)

- Enlargement of causative factor will be prevented
- Cerebral circulation will be maintained or improved (to minimize damage)

Nursing Measures

Nursing measures involve promoting and monitoring vital functions, and include:

- Positioning to promote venous return from cerebral tissues
- Positioning to maintain patent airway
- Assessing neurologic function by monitoring:
    Level of consciousness and protective reflexes
    Pupillary signs and extraocular movements
    Spontaneous movements
    Respiratory pattern and rate (prepare for ventilator assistance)
    Body temperature
    Quality and rate of pulse
    Speech ability, especially if right-handed with left hemispheric lesion
- Maintaining hydration:
    Assess peripheral edema
    Monitor fluid losses as well as intake
    Monitor blood pressure
- Assessing comprehension and providing emotional support:
    Assess speech and comprehension
    Explain all procedures and equipment
    Explain what has happened
    Talk and listen to client to understand him or her
    Assess visual fields
    Promote functional control of bladder and bowel
- Promoting return of body function:
    Position for alignment and use of part
    Provide range of motion exercises
    Prevent flexion contractures
    Prevent dependent edema through position changes
    Teach muscle strengthening exercises
    Assess swallowing ability—semi-soft diet presented to nonaffected side best tolerated by client
    Assess residual deficits and plan compensating alterations
    Involve family members in care and support

Drug Therapy

Osmotic diuretics to reduce brain edema

Antihypertensives to reduce blood pressure

Maintain minimal hydration requirements to reduce edema

Corticosteroids to reduce inflammation

Anticoagulant therapy for nonhemorrhagic stroke, to reduce area of ischemia

Antiepileptics to stabilize neuron cell membrane

Nutrition Therapy

- May be initially npo
- NG tube feedings may be used to provide adequate calorie intake early
- When client is alert, with swallowing reflex, provide semi-soft diet to the nonaffected side of the mouth for safer management of eating and swallowing

Client/Family Teaching

Explain what has occurred

Mutually set realistic short-term goals emphasizing remaining abilities

Discuss with the family the client's fatigue and mental lability

Discuss adaptations at home to promote safety and ease of care

Encourage planning that allows adequate time for the client to do as much for himself or herself as possible

Discuss the need for ongoing medical evaluation

Discuss availability of community resources

Evaluation

Treatment and client teaching are successful if client:

- Participates in activities of daily living with assistance
- Participates in family and social relationships
- Communicates
- Participates in physical and speech therapy programs if appropriate
- Communicates understanding of dose, time, desired effects, and side-effects of prescribed medications

Varicose Veins

Varicose veins are irreversibly dilated, tortuous, and elongated superficial veins with incompetent venous valves.

Assessment

Health Status

- Reported feeling of leg heaviness
- Leg cramps, especially at night
- Dull, diffuse aching and discomfort in legs, especially with menstruation
- Easy fatigue
- Discoloration overlying vessel
- Dependent edema
- Incompetent venous valves

Developmental Assessment

Risk factors include:

Female sex, over age 40
Congenital weakness of the valves
Prolonged venostasis
Prolonged sitting or standing
Pregnancy
Obesity
Family history of varicose veins

Diagnostic Factors

Doppler ultrasound
Venogram
Venous outflow test and reflex plethysmography

Nursing Plans and Interventions

Goals

- Client will achieve ideal weight
- Legs will not be injured
- Client will not experience complications

Nursing Measures

- Monitor elastic bandage to maintain uniform pressure over entire limb from toes to groin
- Elevate entire length of affected limb about 30°
- Monitor sensation and circulation in affected limb
- Discourage sitting for long periods of time, dangling or crossing legs

Medical/Surgical Treatment

Vein ligation and stripping are carried out on enlarged, tortuous veins that cause great discomfort. The procedure reduces edema, pain, ulceration, and fatigue in the affected area.

Preoperative Nursing Care

- Instruct about need for early ambulation, frequent walking
- Explain that the evening before surgery, the surgeon will mark the veins with a felt-tipped pen, with client in standing position

Postoperative Nursing Care

- Assess pain in extremity on which surgery was performed
- Limited ambulation is usually encouraged on the first postoperative day
- Monitor for signs of infection
- Explain that some spotty leg numbness is common during the postoperative period
- Assess for bleeding every 2 hours

Nutrition Therapy

- Weight management to achieve ideal weight
- Maintain adequate hydration

Client/Family Teaching

Teach client about importance of:

Achieving ideal weight

Planning rest periods off feet throughout work period

Exercise program to enhance venous return

Avoiding prolonged sitting or standing and constricting clothing

Evaluation

Client teaching is successful if client:

- Modifies lifestyle to reduce associated and causative factors
- Modifies diet to achieve ideal weight

Buerger's Disease (Thromboangiitis Obliterans)

Buerger's disease is an inflammatory nonatheromatous occlusive condition of small and medium arteries. It causes decreased blood flow to the feet and legs. Diminished flow may lead to ulceration and eventually gangrene.

Assessment

Health Status

- Intermittent claudication of the instep aggravated by exercise and relieved by rest
- Exposure to cold causes feet to become cold, cyanotic, and numb; later reddened, hot, and tingly
- Diminished peripheral pulses
- Migratory superficial thrombophlebitis
- Late disease may show ulceration, muscle atrophy, gangrene

Developmental Assessment

Definite link with cigarette smoking

Hypersensitivity to nicotine may contribute

Men of Jewish ancestry, ages 20–40 years, who smoke heavily, most at risk

Diagnostic Factors

Physical examination and family history very helpful

Doppler ultrasound shows decreased blood flow

Plethysmography shows decreased blood flow

Arteriography useful to locate lesions and rule out atherosclerosis

Nursing Plans and Interventions

Goals

- Client will stop smoking
- Client's symptoms will be relieved and progress of disease prevented

Nursing Measures

- Support efforts to stop smoking
- Promote exercise program to use gravity to fill and drain veins
- Protect integrity of peripheral tissues:
    Provide foot cradle
    Wash affected area with mild soap, tepid water, rinse, and *pat* dry
    Wrap area with cotton batting
    Protect area from cold exposure
- Prepare for surgery if lesions do not heal

Medical/Surgical Treatment

Lumbar sympathectomy to improve circulation to skin

Amputation of gangrenous limb in the case of prolonged nonhealing lesions or intractable pain

Drug Therapy

No cigarette smoking

No nicotine ingestion

Nutrition Therapy

- Nourishing diet

Client/Family Teaching

Teach client about:

Need to stop smoking

Foot care practices
Need for ongoing medical supervision

Evaluation

Client teaching is successful if client:

- Stops cigarette smoking
- Expresses understanding of signs of infection
- Practices foot care activities to promote circulation and prevent injury
- Participates in individualized exercise program
- Keeps appointments for medical reevaluation

Raynaud's Phenomenon

Raynaud's phenomenon is primarily an arteriospastic disorder characterized by episodic vasospasm of small peripheral arterioles. Excessive sensitivity to cold temperature results in vasospastic occurrences.

Assessment

Health Status

- Arterioconstriction, usually in fingers, bilaterally
- Skin changes color from normal to blue, then white, and then red
- Pain in affected digits when red
- Numbness in affected digits when blue or white
- Ulceration of finger tips may result
- Application of external heat relieves episode
- Paronychia in long-standing cases

Developmental Assessment

Usually occurs in women ages 16–40 years
Stress may contribute

Diagnostic Factors

History of clinical color changes in affected digits
Vasospastic history longer than 2 years
Normal arterial pulses
Chronic arterial occlusive disease must be ruled out

Nursing Plans and Interventions

Goals

- Hand injury will be prevented
- Vasospasm episodes will be prevented
- Ulceration will not develop

Nursing Measures

- Prevent cold exposure
- Encourage client to wear protective mittens or gloves
- Discourage cigarette smoking, which causes vasoconstriction
- Administer vasodilator drugs

Drug Therapy

Varying success has been reported through the use of vasodilator drugs
Drug therapy usually reserved for severe cases

Nutrition Therapy

- Disorder has no known association with diet

Client/Family Teaching

Teach client about:

Importance of protecting hands from chemical, mechanical, or cold injury
Importance of stopping smoking
Importance of inspecting hands regularly for injury
Effect and side-effects of vasodilator drugs, if prescribed

Evaluation

Client teaching is successful if client:

- Stops cigarette smoking
- Modifies lifestyle to protect extremities from cold exposure

Arteriosclerosis

Arteriosclerosis is a pathologic process characterized by adhesion to the vessel wall of fatty material that hardens, narrowing the vessel lumen and causing lipid infiltration, thrombosis, and a change in vessel blood dynamics. Most symptoms are absent until the vessel lumen is 85%–95% narrowed.

Assessment

Health Status

- Exercise pain (intermittent claudication)–reproducible pain resulting from cell ischemia and products of anaerobic metabolism
- Rest pain occurs in the muscle at basal metabolic levels (may improve with leg in lowered position)
- Trophic changes:
    - Diminished peripheral pulse (pedal or posterior tibial)
    - Decreased amount and distribution of body extremity hair
    - Decreased skin thickness and taut, shiny skin in affected areas
    - Thickened nails
    - Ulcer lesions
    - Cold extremities
- Sexual dysfunction in approximately 30% of cases
- Numbness and tingling in extremity
- Dependent rubor, elevated pallor

Developmental Assessment

Risk factors include:

Advancing age
Male sex
Caucasian race
Elevated serum lipid levels
Elevated blood pressure
History of cigarette smoking
Elevated blood glucose level
Obesity
Sedentary lifestyle
Stressful lifestyle
Inherited predisposition
High-salt diet

Diagnostic Factors

Serum cholesterol greater than 250 mg/dL
Serum triglycerides greater than 150 mg/dL
Serum lipids elevated (especially low density lipids)
Hypertension
Doppler ultrasound measures velocity of blood flow through vessel
Oscillometry measures pulse waves
Ultrasound arteriography

Nursing Plans and Interventions

Goals

- Client will maintain activity level necessary to reduce progress of pathology
- Client will be as comfortable as possible
- Modifiable risk factors will be altered

Nursing Measures

- Encourage activities to promote arterial circulation:
    - Encourage walking to promote collateral vessel (slow progressive program)
    - Help client organize to include rest periods
    - Do *not* apply local heat (increases metabolism without increasing oxygen)
    - Prevent activities that produce vasospasm
- Help change modifiable risk factors:
    - Encourage dietary modifications
    - Reduce blood pressure by reducing emotional stress
    - Help client stop smoking
- Provide measures to protect the extremity:
    - Assess extremity frequently for color, warmth, pulse, sensation
    - Assess extremity for ulceration, injury

- Encourage client to wear properly fitting footwear and clothing
- Administer prescribed medications to modify serum lipid levels
- Prepare for surgical intervention if indicated

Drug Therapy

Modify serum lipids by administering:

Niacin to reduce production of lipoproteins and cholesterol

Clofibrate (Atromid-S) to reduce serum triglycerides

Cholestyramine (Questran) to reduce bile acid binding to reduce cholesterol

Cholestyramine (Questran) to enhance removal of lipoproteins

Colestipol hydrochloride (Colestid) to enhance removal of lipoproteins

Also administer:

Pentoxifylline (Trental) to reduce blood viscosity and increase RBC flexibility

Nutrition Therapy

- Weight reduction diet if appropriate
- Low-cholesterol, low-triglyceride diet
- Reduce sodium intake
- Diet to maintain normal glucose levels

Client/Family Teaching

Teach client about:

Dietary modifications

Risks of smoking

Exercise program to build collateral circulation

Proper care of extremity to maintain tissue integrity

Hazards of prolonged sitting, standing, crossing legs, or wearing constrictive clothing

Evaluation

Client teaching is successful if client:

- Modifies diet to reduce serum cholesterol levels
- Voices understanding of dose, time, desired effect and side-effects of prescribed medications
- Participates in exercise program to promote collateral circulation
- Practices hygienic activities to promote tissue integrity

Hypertension

Hypertension occurs when mechanisms that regulate arterial blood pressure are deranged due to unknown causes. A blood pressure of 140/90 represents borderline (mild) hypertension. Diagnosis is confirmed when blood pressure averages 140/90 or higher on two separate measurements.

Assessment

Health Status

- May be no symptoms in early stages
- Serial blood pressure readings reveal consistently elevated pressure, with diastolic pressure greater than 90 mm Hg
- Frequent morning headaches, nosebleeds
- Malaise and weakness, possible dizziness and syncope
- Muscle cramps
- Retinal hemorrhage, blurred vision
- Peripheral edema and peripheral pulse disparities
- Peripheral bruits
- Nocturia
- Palpitations and dyspnea

Developmental Factors

Predisposing factors include:

Family history of hypertension

Excessive sodium intake

Abnormal lipid levels

Cigarette smoking

Obesity

Black race (2:1 increased risk)

Male sex (males have higher incidence and earlier onset)

High-stress lifestyle

Excessive alcohol intake

Diagnostic Factors

Thorough history and physical examination

Chest x-ray to identify heart size

Funduscopic examination shows changes in vessels of retinas

Laboratory studies of both blood and urine, *i.e.*, BUN, creatinine, renin, and urine protein

Persistent elevated blood pressure, above 140 systolic or 90 diastolic on at least two separate measurements

Nursing Plans and Interventions

Goals

- Blood pressure will be reduced
- Client will comply with treatment on ongoing basis
- Complications will be prevented

Nursing Measures

- Administer prescribed medications
- Monitor blood pressure and vital signs
- Assess effectiveness of drugs related to vital signs
- Assess for side-effects of drug therapy, such as hypotension, dizziness, anorexia, nasal congestion, weakness
- Assess knowledge deficits and begin instruction about medications, diet, and activity (be sure to explain that no cure is available though symptoms may disappear)
- Provide a low-cholesterol, low-sodium diet and weight reduction diet if appropriate (teach client to avoid alcohol)

Drug Therapy

Treatment involves individualized stepped care, beginning with nonpharmacologic interventions, including:

Planned activity regimen

Reduced or no cigarette smoking

Step I pharmacologic intervention includes:

Thiazide, diuretic drug of choice for hypertensive clients over age 50: start at lowest effective dose and provide potassium replacements

β-adrenergic blocker such as propranolol hydrochloride (Inderal) may be initiated for those under age 50; sexual dysfunction may occur as side-effect

Step II involves adding adrenergic inhibiting agents, such as clonidine hydrochloride (Catapres), reserpine (Serpasil), and methyldopa (Aldomet), in small initial doses, if step I does not produce the desired response. Experimentation with one or several of these may be necessary to find the most effective drug.

Step III involves administering a peripheral vasodilator, such as prazosin hydrochloride (Minipress), hydralazine hydrochloride (Apresoline), captopril (Capoten), or minoxidil (Loniten). These drugs may increase heart rate and oxygen needs of the myocardium, and may produce side-effects of headache, palpitations, and tachycardia.

Step IV involves administering guanethidine (Ismelin). Guanethidine depletes stored norepinephrine, interacts with tricyclic antidepressants, and may cause serious hypotension, diarrhea, impotence, and retrograde ejaculation.

Nutrition Therapy

- Low-cholesterol, low-sodium diet
- Low-calorie diet if weight reduction is recommended

Client/Family Teaching

Teach client to:

Monitor own blood pressure

Understand pharmacologic treatment plan, including effects and side-effects

Follow low-cholesterol, low-sodium diet

Include foods high in potassium if client is taking diuretics

Follow regular activity program

Comply with medical reevaluation and treatment plans

Evaluation

Client teaching is successful if client:

- Maintains a low-cholesterol, low-sodium diet
- Maintains or achieves appropriate weight
- Avoids or reduces environmental stress
- Monitors own blood pressure
- Voices understanding of doses, times, desired effects, and side-effects of prescribed medications
- Voices understanding of signs and symptoms of change in health status that require medical reevaluation

Pulmonary Dysfunction

Chronic Obstructive Pulmonary Disease

Chronic obstructive pulmonary diseases (COPD) include several disease processes that result in irreversible obstruction of respiratory airways, including pulmonary emphysema and chronic bronchitis. Each client presents with varying combinations of excessive mucus production, infection, airway narrowing, and diminished gaseous exchange surfaces.

Assessment

Health Status

Emphysema
- Dyspnea
- Anorexia and weight loss
- Fatigue related to the work of breathing
- Cough more prominent with concurrent infection
- Hypoxemia and respiratory acidosis late in disease course
- Decreased airflow on exhalation
- Increased respiratory rate
- Barrel chest and flattened diaphragm
- Tripod position to enhance use of accessory muscles of respiration
- Decreased breath sounds with adventitious sounds present
- Decreased movement of chest on respiration

Chronic Bronchitis
- Infective/inflammatory process with persistent cough
- Early onset hypoxemia with possible right-sided failure of the heart
- Excessive sputum production
- Dyspnea and adventitious lung sounds
- Cyanosis and clubbing of digits late in disease course

Developmental Assessment

Higher incidence among males than among females; however, rate of incidence among females is increasing at a faster rate than rate of incidence among males

Usually develops slowly over 30–35 years

Cigarette smoking is the leading risk factor related to COPD

Incidence greater in urban than in rural areas

Incidence increases with aging

Air pollution and inhalation of pollutants contribute

Diagnostic Factors

ABG measurements

Physical examination

Excessive sputum with organisms

Pulmonary function tests

Nursing Plans and Interventions

Goals

- Client will reduce exposure to pollutants and inhaled irritants such as smoke, to promote ventilation and gas exchange
- Hydration will be maintained
- Respiratory secretions will be removed
- Client will maintain adequate nutrition
- Respiratory infections will be prevented

- Client will maintain adequate oxygenation
- Client will practice respiratory exercises to enhance effective ventilation
- Client will benefit from psychosocial support

Nursing Measures

- Maintain a pollutant-free environment for client (prohibit smoking by client or visitors)
- Provide adequate fluid to maintain liquified respiratory secretions (3,000–4,000 mL of fluid daily, within cardiac limits)
- Administer prescribed medications
- Reinforce effective coughing and diaphragmatic breathing exercises to lengthen the duration of expiration
- Monitor emesis and stool for occult blood
- Provide several small meals high in calories, protein, and fiber
- Provide low-flow oxygen via cannula for comfort and to decrease hypoxemia (obtain ABG measurements as needed to monitor respiratory acidosis and ventilation)
- Ensure supplies client needs are close at hand, to conserve energy (plan care within client's energy limits)
- Plan slowly progressive exercise and activity to improve physical conditioning and sense of well-being
- Promote a positive self-image and support constructive coping mechanisms

Drug Therapy

Sympathomimetic Bronchodilators

Epinephrine α, β, and β_2-receptor
Ephedrine α and β_2-receptor
Isoproterenol (Isuprel) β_1 and β_2
Metaproterenol (Alupent, β_2 Metaprel)
Albuterol (Proventil, Ventolin)
Isoetharine (Bronkosol)
Terbutaline (Brethine, Brethaire)

    Side-effects include:

Headache
Dizziness
Palpitations
Tremors
Restlessness
Arrhythmia
Tachycardia
Changes in blood pressure

Methylxanthine Derivative Bronchodilators

- Short-acting drugs:
  Slo-phyllin
  Aminophylline
  Oxtriphylline (choledyl)
- IV Drugs:
  Aminophylline
- Sustained release drugs:
  Theo-dur, Theo-dur sprinkles
  Cholydyl SA
  Duratab
- 24 hour drug:
  1 Theo 24

Cromones

Cromolyn sodium (Aarane, Intal): inhibits release of histamine and slow reacting substance of anaphylaxis (SRS-A) on mast cell to prevent antigen-antibodies response at mast cell

Mucolytics

Break down mucous protein viscosity
Acetylcysteine (Mucomyst)

Corticosteroids

Act as immunosuppression and antiinflammatory agents
Hydrocortisone (Solu-cortef)
Methylprednisolone (Medrol)
Prednisone
Beclomethasone (Vanceril, Beclovent)

Anticholinergics

Block action of acetylcholine to permit bronchodilation
Ipratropium (Atrovent)
Atropine

Expectorants

Help liquify respiratory secretions
Potassium iodide (SSKI)

Nutrition Therapy

- Small high protein, high calorie meals to provide energy for extra effort of breathing

Client/Family Teaching

Teach client about:

Efficient use of respiratory muscles through effective coughing techniques, diaphragmatic breathing, pursed-lip breathing to lengthen duration of exhalation

Use of hand-held aerosols or inhalers

Home use of low-flow oxygen

Signs and symptoms that should prompt immediate medical attention

Planning activities of daily living (ADL) to conserve energy (slowly increase activity)

Importance of exercise training

Evaluation

Client teaching has been successful if client:

- Expresses understanding of health teaching
- Demonstrates respiratory techniques such as effective coughing, pursed-lip breathing, and diaphragmatic breathing
- Voices understanding of signs and symptoms that indicate worsening COPD, such as increased sputum production, dyspnea, skin color changes, and mental confusion
- Demonstrates use of respiratory aids
- Voices understanding and demonstrates use of daily and prn medications
- Avoids exposure to sources of respiratory irritation and infection
- Participates in exercise program

Neoplasia of Lung

Bronchogenic cancer of the lung is a malignant tumor of the lung tissue arising from within the epithelial lining of the bronchus.

Assessment

Health Status

Four major cell types of cancer are recognized, including:

- Squamous cell
- Adenocarcinoma
- Small cell (oat cell)
- Large cell

Clinical findings include:

- Few symptoms in early stages
- Persistent cough or cough pattern change
- Hemoptysis
- Vague chest discomfort
- Frequent respiratory infections
- Weight loss, fatigue, anorexia
- Paraneoplastic syndromes

Developmental Assessment

Cigarette smokers at 25 times greater risk than nonsmokers

Steadily rising incidence worldwide

Exposure to industrial chemicals such as asbestos and chromium increases risk

Diagnostic Factors

Chest x-ray

Cystologic studies of sputum or pleural fluid

Bronchoscopy

Biopsy of regional lymph nodes

Pulmonary function studies

CT scan

Carcinoembryonic antigen studies

Nursing Plans and Interventions

Goals

- Depend on histologic report, progress of disease, and general physiologic condition of patient
- Client will benefit from support during diagnostic workup
- Client will benefit from supportive care for secondary effects of tumor and metastasis
- Treatment effects and discomfort from side-effects will be relieved
- Client will receive support during treatment regimen: immunologic, surgical, chemotherapeutic, or radiological

- Client will benefit from psychosocial support

Nursing Measures: Surgical Support for Lobectomy

Preoperative Care

- Promote alveolar ventilation and respiratory effectiveness
- Promote comfort, rest, and adequate nutrition
- Utilize efforts to reduce respiratory irritation and secretions
- Teach postoperative routines as tolerated

Postoperative Care

- Promote gas exchange and effective ventilation by monitoring:
    ABGs
    Breath sounds
    Placement of endotracheal tube
    Suction, until client can raise secretions
    For restlessness, an early sign of hypoxemia
- Monitor cardiovascular adequacy, including:
    Fluid replacement
    Vital signs
    ECG changes
    Characteristics of chest tube drainage
- Carefully monitor chest tube drainage system (glass bottles or three-chambered disposable system [Pleurovac] may be used):
    Check for air leak in system (continuous bubbling in underwater seal drainage means leak present)
    Check all connections and maintain taped seal
    Place two large hemostats for each chest tube at bedside
    Keep water seal bottles below client's chest level at all times
    Keep water seal bottles in upright position with glass tube underwater at all times
    Monitor fluctuation of water in the drainage tube on inspiration and expiration
    Maintain patency of chest tubes per physician order
    Prevent kinking of tubing
- Promote rest and comfort:
    Position to promote comfortable breathing and drainage (head of bed elevated 15–30°)
    Position to promote aeration of unaffected side to maximize base of breathing
    Splint incision for effective coughing techniques
- Promote bed activities to prevent complications
- Administer prescribed pain medications as appropriate

Nursing Measures: Nonsurgical Support

- Promote effective respirations:
    Position to improve ventilation
    Teach diaphragmatic breathing exercises and effective coughing technique
    Ensure hydration and provide medications to promote removal of sputum
- Promote adequate nutrition:
    Provide frequent small, high-calorie, high-protein meals
    Utilize multivitamin therapy
    Monitor I and O and body weight
    Monitor protein/calorie malnutrition and promote enteral or total parenteral nutrition if oral intake inadequate
- Monitor for complications, including:
    Infections: watch for change in vital signs and WBC
    Hemorrhage: low hemoglobin, low blood pressure, and tachycardia are indications
    Obstruction of major airway: Low PaO_2 and wheezing are indications
    Pleural effusion

Drug Therapy

Antineoplastic drugs (depending on histologic report)
Antiemetics

Analgesics
Replacement electrolytes and vitamins

Nutrition Therapy

- Frequent small meals
- High-calorie supplements
- Offer food at best times for client—late morning
- Total parenteral nutrition

Client/Family Teaching

Promote:

Coping strategies and use of personal resources

Involvement in daily activities, as much as possible

Comfort, through use and understanding of pain medication

Evaluation

Client teaching is successful if client:

- Modifies lifestyle to accommodate home care
- Demonstrates coping behaviors congruent with possible poor prognosis or death
- Voices understanding of available community resources
- Participates in medical reevaluation

Tuberculosis

Infection by *Mycobacterium tuberculosis*, usually of the pulmonary system but also of bone, the kidney, or the brain.

Assessment

Health Status

The disease has an insidious onset with few early symptoms. Clinical findings include:

- Cough
- Mucous purulent sputum
- Diffuse adventitious breath sounds
- Fatigue
- Weight loss
- Fever and night sweats
- Hemoptysis and dyspnea during late or extensive involvement

Developmental Assessment

Most predisposed are:

Children under age 2
Foreign-born persons in U.S. less than 1 year
Persons with diabetes
Persons with suppressed immune systems
Elderly, debilitated persons

Diagnostic Factors

Sputum culture positive for organism *Mycobacterium tuberculosis*

Gastric washing positive for organism

Chest x-ray may show cavitary lesions or Ghon complex lesions

Mantoux test reaction positive, or positive response to other screening tests

Nursing Plans and Interventions

Goals

- Disease process will be controlled
- Client will comply with treatment plan
- Transmission or relapse of disease will be prevented

Nursing Measures

- Administer prescribed antitubercular medications
- Assist in sputum collection techniques for culture
- Demonstrate proper techniques for disposal of secretions (bagging and handwashing)
- Provide measures that promote comfort, rest, and improved nutrition

Drug Therapy

First line antitubercular drugs include:

Isoniazid
Rifampin

Streptomycin
Ethambutol

Second line antitubercular drugs include:

Kanamycin
Ethionamide
Para-aminosalicylic acid

Preventative chemotherapy involves:

Isoniazid therapy for high-risk population, 300 mg daily for 9–12 months

Bacillus Calmette-Guérin (BCG) vaccine for immunity for population heavily exposed to tuberculosis

Nutrition Therapy

- Well-balanced diet
- Discourage alcohol use
- Appetite loss is side-effect of isoniazid therapy

Client/Family Teaching

Teach client and family about:

Necessity of long-term treatment regimen
Disease process and transmission
Side-effects of drug therapy
Respiratory hygiene techniques
Diet, rest, and activity to promote well-being
Need for follow-up; and plan follow-up
Need for family members to be evaluated and possibly treated

Evaluation

Client and family teaching is successful if:

- Client continues taking medications as prescribed
- Client and family voice understanding of doses, times, desired effects, and side-effects of medications
- Client modifies hygienic practices to control transmission of infection, by expectorating in tissues, bagging tissues, and using appropriate handwashing practices
- Client participates in exercise and diet programs to maintain body requirements
- Client keeps reevaluation appointments
- Family members participate in preventative drug treatment program if appropriate

Asthma

Asthma is characterized by widespread but *reversible* narrowing of airways due to hyperactive airways. This hyperactivity results from exposure to intrinsic and extrinsic stimuli. Allergic release of histamine and SRS-A cause bronchoconstriction, bronchospasm, increased capillary permeability, mucosal edema, and hypersecretion of mucus into the airways.

Assessment

Health Status

- Wheezing exhalation and bronchospasm
- Decreased breath sounds
- Flushing
- Prolonged exhalation (pursed-lip breathing)
- Tachycardia with paradoxical pulse
- Hypoxemia in late stage may lead to confusion and restlessness
- Excessive sputum
- Hyperventilation with carbon dioxide blown off until fatigue reduces ventilation, then carbon dioxide retained

Developmental Assessment

Prevalent in children with other allergic disorders

Adult causes less well understood

Diagnostic Factors

ABG measurements show low PaO_2, high $PaCO_2$ in late stage

Tachycardia

Right-sided heart changes

Pulmonary function studies show decreased

forced expiratory volume and increased residual volume

Chest x-ray shows hyperinflated lung

Nursing Plans and Interventions

Goals

- Secretions will be removed
- Client will maintain adequate hydration
- Client will conserve energy

Nursing Measures

- Assist positioning to enhance use of accessory muscles of respiration (best position is sitting up, leaning forward)
- Promote effective removal of thick copious mucus
- Administer bronchodilator medications
- Administer oxygen per cannula or by positive pressure
- Administer corticosteroid medications
- Be calm and reassuring, stay with client

Drug Therapy

Bronchodilators (adrenergics, noncatecholamines, methylxanthines)
Corticosteroids
Anticholinergic agents
Assess for ASA intolerance

Nutrition Therapy

- Well-balanced diet
- Food allergy may be causative factor

Client/Family Teaching

Teach client to:

Avoid known allergens

Follow medication regimen and understand side-effects of drugs

Understand relationship of fatigue and stress to asthmatic episodes

Adhere to healthy personal practices related to diet, rest, fluid intake, and activity

Avoid smoking and air pollution

Seek medical attention at first sign of respiratory or other infection

Evaluation

Client teaching is successful if:

- Voices understanding of physiologic changes
- Avoids identified precipitating substances and allergens such as smoke and air pollution
- Practices personal health habits that promote rest, adequate diet, and activity
- Voices recognition of signs and symptoms of respiratory irritation or infection that require medical attention
- Voices understanding of doses, times, desired effects, and side-effects of prescribed medications
- Demonstrates use of respiratory aids such as aerosol or inhaler

Acute Respiratory Infections

The most important acute respiratory infection is pneumonia, an infectious and inflammatory process of the lung parenchyma. In most cases, infectious agents are inhaled into the lower lung tissues due to lower respiratory defensive/protective mechanisms. Blood-borne infections are also possible.

Assessment

Health Status

Six cardinal indications are:

- Cough
- Sputum production
- Dyspnea
- Hemoptysis
- Pleuritic chest pain
- Wheezing

Other clinical findings include:

- Fever
- Chills

- Sweats
- Headache
- Fatigue
- Increased respiratory rate
- Change in breath sounds

Developmental Assessment

Most predisposed are:

Elderly, chronically ill, or debilitated persons
Young persons living in close quarters
Infants with immature immune systems

Diagnostic Factors

ABG measurements show decreased or increased $PaCO_2$
Chest x-ray shows extent and location
Fiberoptic bronchoscopy for specimen collection
Sputum culture reveals infective organism

Nursing Plans and Interventions

Goals

- Secretions will be removed
- Client will maintain systemic hydration
- Client will reduce energy needed for breathing and for ADL
- Vital signs will return to normal
- Client will receive adequate supplemental oxygen

Nursing Measures

- Position to increase ventilation
- Encourage breathing (five deep breaths every hour)
- Promote effective coughing
- Promote postural drainage
- Ensure adequate fluid intake
- Seek bedside humidification orders
- Monitor ABGs or color changes every 4 hours
- Administer prescribed medications
- Encourage client to comply with planned rest periods
- Provide frequent oral hygiene (every 2 hours)

Drug Therapy

Bronchodilators
Analgesics
Cough suppressants
Antibiotic therapy (specific to organism)
Expectorants

Nutrition Therapy

- Maintain adequate hydration
- Soft, regular, or high-calorie diet

Client/Family Teaching

Teach client about:

Pursed-lip breathing
Respiratory muscle strengthening (inspiratory)
Signs of infection via mucus changes
Medications and side-effects
Effective coughing techniques

Evaluation

Treatment and client teaching are successful if client:

- Has improved airway clearance
- Demonstrates less fatigue, increased energy
- Takes medications as prescribed
- Has adequate hydration
- Avoids known allergens and precipitating factors

Adult Respiratory Distress Syndrome

Adult respiratory distress syndrome (ARDS) is a descriptive term used to categorize a variety of acute and diffuse infiltrative lung injuries that cause refractory arterial hypoxemia and life-threatening respiratory distress of noncardiac origin. Adults without prior or preexisting lung disorder are most commonly affected.

Assessment

Health Status

- Onset of ARDS may be insidious
- Dyspnea, tachypnea, cough, and restlessness are early symptoms
- Fine, diffuse rales (crackles) may be auscultated
- Mild hypoxemia and respiratory alkalosis are usual early findings
- Progression of ARDS is characterized by
    Increased effort of breathing
    Noisy tachypneic and hyperpneic breathing
    Intercostal and suprasternal retractions
    Decreased lung volumes
    Tachycardia
    Diaphoresis
    Decreased mental functioning
    Pallor and cyanosis
    Progressive arterial hypoxemia in spite of aggressive oxygen therapy by endotracheal tube is diagnostic
    $PaCO_2$ may remain normal despite severe dyspnea and hypoxemia (high $PaCO_2$ indicates decompensation)
    Bronchial breath sounds occur in final stages, along with severe hypoxemia, hypercapnia, and metabolic acidosis

Developmental Assessment

No history of lung disease

Initial injury or trauma may predispose—e.g., chest trauma, prolonged hypotension, air or fat emboli, cardiopulmonary bypass, oxygen toxicity, acute pancreatitis, massive blood transfusion, aspiration pneumonia, viral pneumonia, inhaled irritants, drug overdose, near drowning, anaphylaxis, head injury

Diagnostic Factors

History of associated etiologic event
ABG abnormalities, especially refractory hypoxemia
Chest x-ray demonstrates consolidation and coalescing infiltrates, termed "white lung"
Pulmonary function tests reveal decreased lung volumes and diminished lung compliance
Pulmonary artery catheter wedge pressure within normal range, which indicates noncardiac cause

Nursing Plans and Interventions

Goals

- For high-risk clients, implement preoperative preventative measures (pulmonary function tests, ABG baseline measurements, efforts to optimize ventilation)
- Underlying causative or contributing factors will be treated
- Hypoventilation will be treated aggressively

Nursing Measures

- Assess respiratory function frequently and thoroughly, including:
    Rate
    Depth
    Breath sounds
    Secretions culture for sepsis
    Muscle involvement
- Monitor ABGs:
    Assess for low PaO_2 that is nonresponsive to oxygen therapy
    Assess $PaCO_2$ levels
    Assess pH
    Assess hemoglobin levels
    When PaO_2 level is 50–60 mm Hg, assess for oxygen saturation above 90%
- Assess cardiovascular function, including:
    Blood pressure (maintain at normal level for client)
    Pulse and rhythm pattern
    Hemodynamic status, especially if positive end-expiratory pressure (PEEP) is used
    Urinary output
- Provide and monitor mechanical ventilation efforts:

- Verify tidal volume setting (usually 10–15 ml/kg)
- Verify controlled rate settings to maintain normal pH
- Verify positive pressure and PEEP, and monitor cardiac output
- Verify fraction of inspired oxygen (FLO_2) setting to prevent oxygen toxicity
- Reposition endotracheal tube from side to side of mouth and maintain securely; auscultate for bilateral breath sounds; administer sedatives if ordered to reduce oxygen needs
- Suction endotracheal tube prn to maintain patent airway
- Administer inotropic drugs, *e.g.*, dopamine, to enhance cardiac output
- Provide judicious fluid administration:
  - Monitor hemodynamic status
  - Administer diuretics if ordered
  - Use microdrip administration sets to prevent overload
  - Monitor I and O hourly
  - Assess weight daily
  - Assess electrolyte reports for imbalance
- Provide appropriate hygienic and comfort measures

Medical Treatment

Mechanical ventilation

Continuous arteriovenous hemofiltration

Pharmacologic therapy

Supportive therapy

Administration of washed packed cells to improve oxygen carrying capacity of blood

Drug Therapy

Antibiotic if appropriate for cultured organism

Corticosteroid therapy to stabilize cell membranes

Sedation therapy to reduce oxygen needs of body

Diuretic therapy to reduce excessive fluids

Inotropic drugs to improve cardiac function

Nutrition Therapy

- Restrict fluid intake
- Enteral support

Client/Family Teaching

Explain treatments to client and family.

Evaluation

Treatment is successful if:

- Client shows improved lung compliance
- Client's PaO_2 level returns to normal range without mechanical ventilation
- Client can be weaned from mechanical ventilation
- Client avoids secondary complications

6

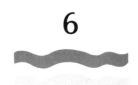

Nursing Care of the Client Who Has a Problem with Digestion, Metabolism, Elimination, and Providing Nutrients to the Cells

Upper Gastrointestinal Dysfunction

Food Poisoning

Food poisoning causes a severe gastroenteritis, usually self-limiting and usually not serious except in infants, and in elderly, debilitated, or chronically ill persons. The causative agent is commonly a virus, staphylococcus, or salmonella. Less common but potentially more serious is botulism, which can be fatal unless treated.

Assessment

Health Status

- Nausea, vomiting, and abdominal cramps (often violent), all usually occurring 2–4 hours after poisoning
- Botulism (symptoms appear 12–48 hours after eating contaminated food): muscle weakness and varying degrees of incapacity; ptosis and paralysis of extraocular muscles; in severe cases, paralysis spreads to respiratory muscles

Developmental Assessment

Assess when client ate in relation to onset of symptoms

Assess where client was and what he or she ate

Assess whether anyone else in family or group has same symptoms

Diagnostic Factors

Client history of nausea, vomiting and diarrhea

Physical examination may reveal fever, dehydration, and in case of botulism, muscle weakness and neurologic changes

Nursing Plans and Interventions

Goals

- Client will maintain adequate hydration
- Client will maintain adequate oxygenation in case of botulism

Nursing Measures

- Keep client npo until vomiting stops
- Assess for dehydration (skin turgor, mouth and mucous membranes, sunken eyes, scanty urine output)
- Administer intravenous (IV) fluids as ordered to maintain hydration
- Provide for bedrest
- Provide supportive treatment for clients with botulism (use respirator prn, and implement measures to prevent infection and complications of immobility)

Drug Therapy

In case of botulism, antitoxin on daily basis until symptoms subside

Antiemetics may be used when vomiting is severe and prolonged

Nutrition Therapy

- After vomiting stops, ice chips or sips of clear liquids (gatorade, broth, lemonade) to provide electrolytes and fluids
- Advance to regular diet as tolerated

Client/Family Teaching

Teach client and family to:

Refrigerate food promptly

Avoid mayonnaise-based foods at picnics during hot weather

Wash meats prior to storage and preparation, keep *cold*, use promptly

Avoid use of foods in bulging cans

Use pressure canner and have it checked professionally at regular intervals, if canning foods at home; follow canning instructions *exactly*

Evaluation

Treatment is successful if client:

- Has good fluid and electrolyte balance
- Is free of nausea, vomiting, diarrhea, and paralysis

Hiatal Hernia

Hiatal hernia is a weakness in the diaphragm (usually at the esophageal hiatus, the opening in the diaphragm through which the esophagus passes) that permits herniation of the stomach into the thoracic cavity. Hiatal hernia often causes incompetence of the cardiac sphincter, causing esophageal reflux. The esophagus has no protection against the effects of gastric juices, so inflammation results.

Assessment

Health Status

- Heartburn and epigastric pain after meals
- Bloating, belching, feeling full, nausea
- Symptoms become worse when lying down or bending over
- Symptoms subside as stomach empties (1–2 hours after eating)

Developmental Assessment

Often related to loss of muscle tone associated with aging

Can also occur due to trauma (assess for recent injury)

Diagnostic Factors

History and physical examination (H and P)
Barium swallow
Esophagoscopy
Esophageal motility studies

Nursing Plans and Interventions

Goal

- Client will be free of heartburn and indigestion

Nursing Measures

- Prepare client for diagnostic studies: client will receive local anesthetic for esophagoscopy, so assess for gag reflex when test is over before offering food or drink

- Condition is usually managed medically (surgery is last resort and not always successful)

Drug Therapy

Antacids may help

Metoclopramide (Reglan) to hasten gastric emptying

Nutrition Therapy

- Client may need to avoid highly seasoned or spicy foods
- Identify and eliminate foods that cause discomfort (on individual basis)

Client/Family Teaching

Teach client to:

Eat small, frequent meals

Sit or stand for at least 1 hour after meals

Avoid eating for at least 3 hours before going to bed

Put 6" blocks under head of bed (use reverse Trendelenberg position, in which gravity helps empty stomach)

Avoid bending over and lifting heavy objects

Avoid straining at stool

Evaluation

Client teaching is successful if client:

- Can describe ways to prevent reflux
- Understands actions and side-effects of medications and how to take them

Peptic Ulcer

Peptic ulcer is a sharply defined lesion caused by the action of acid secretions on the lining of stomach, duodenum, or esophagus. An ulcer often extends through the mucosa and submucosa into underlying muscle. It can infiltrate a blood vessel, causing bleeding; cause edema, which causes obstruction (especially of the pyloric sphincter); or perforate and release gastric secretions into the peritoneal cavity, causing peritonitis.

Assessment

Health Status

- Periodic and episodic pain, occurring on empty stomach, relieved by food or antacid, usually localized in midepigastric area but sometimes radiating to back

Symptoms associated with complications include:

- Bright red or coffee ground emesis and tarry stools (indicate bleeding)
- Early satiety, weight loss as client gradually decreases food intake, and emesis of foods eaten as much as 24 hours earlier (indicate obstruction)
- Sudden severe abdominal pain, shock, pallor, anxiety, and respiratory distress (indicate perforation)

Developmental Assessment

Often affects adults during most productive years

Can also affect children

Often associated with stressful lifestyle, fast pace, frequent deadlines, high-pressure jobs

Diagnostic Factors

H and P

Barium swallow

Endoscopy

Nursing Plans and Interventions

Goals

- Client will experience decrease in pain
- Ulcer will heal
- Client will experience no complications

Nursing Measures

- Assist in preparation and implementation of diagnostic tests

- Assist with management of bleeding (complication):
    Physician will insert nasogastric (NG) tube and iced saline lavage will be performed to control bleeding
    Physician will perform endoscopy to pinpoint source of bleeding
    Nurse will administer blood replacement as ordered
- Assist with management of perforation:
    Prepare for immediate surgery to repair leak
    Treat shock
    Offer supportive treatment as indicated
- Assist with management of obstruction:
    NG tube (low suction)
    Client may require preparation for surgery

Medical/Surgical Treatment

Surgical intervention is performed if conservative management fails or if complications become life threatening. Procedures include partial gastrectomy (approximately 60% of the stomach), often accompanied by selective vagotomy (dissecting the branch of the vagus that innervates the stomach).

Postoperative Nursing Care

- Manage NG tube: tube will drain blood—tinged drainage will progress to clear over 2–3 days; *do not* irrigate NG tube without specific physician's order; count any instilled fluid as *intake*; if NG tube not draining, instill air into blue pigtail or change client's position; if NG obstructed, call physician because buildup of secretions will put stress on suture line; assess for gastric distention
- Client on strict npo (offer no ice or water without physician's order)
- When NG removed, assess for nausea (N), vomiting (V), and distention
- Encourage client to "turn, cough, and deep breathe" (TCDB) to prevent atelectasis and pneumonia
- Ambulate client as ordered to:
    Promote lung expansion
    Promote peristalsis
    Promote circulation and decrease risk of clots
- Offer prn pain medication every 3–4 hours as ordered

Postoperative Teaching
Teach client about:

- Reduced stomach capacity—eat small, frequent meals
- Distressing symptoms related to dumping syndrome (weakness, diaphoresis, rapid pulse, decreased blood pressure)—will pass with time, in meantime, lie down after eating
- Possibility of developing tingling sensation in hands and feet—see physician because these symptoms may indicate pernicious anemia and need for vitamin B12 injections (symptoms will not develop until body uses up its stored supply of B12, which can take several months or even years)

Drug Therapy

Nonsystemic antacids: magnesium hydroxide (Gelusil, Mylanta), aluminum hydroxide (Amphojel):
   Most effective if taken after meals and on a regular schedule
   Can cause diarrhea if compound contains magnesium or constipation if compound contains aluminum; individual responses may vary so two different products may need to be alternated to minimize bowel side-effects
H_2-receptor antagonists (raise pH and decrease volume of gastric secretions: cimetidine (Tagamet), ranitidine (Zantac)
Carafate (Sucralfate) to coat and protect ulcers from effects of acid:

Give before meals
Follow instructions; it binds with some other medications (*e.g.*, cimetidine), so give 2 hours apart

Nutrition Therapy

- Begin with bland diet in small frequent feedings (keep food in stomach at all times to neutralize acidity)
- Progress to regular diet as tolerated
- Ensure client avoids beverages with caffeine (these stimulate acidity)

Client/Family Teaching

Teach client to:

Understand and comply with diet and medication regimen

If using chewable antacid tablet for convenience, drink glass of water to distribute medication over surface area of stomach

Avoid alcohol and aspirin (ASA) (gastric irritants)

Understand dangers of smoking and need to quit (predisposes to excess acidity); if unable or unwilling to quit, then smoke only after meals when stomach is full

If ever treated with steroid medications, report history of ulcer to prescribing physician

Identify life stressors and assess coping patterns (build on positive coping behaviors)

Build in rest periods during the day

Evaluation

Treatment and client teaching are successful if client:

- Is free of pain and complications
- Can verbalize understanding of important aspects of treatment regimen

Gallbladder Disease

Cholecystitis refers to inflammation and *cholelithiasis* to stone formation. Inflammation and stones can interfere with the ability of the gallbladder to concentrate, store, and secrete bile, which is necessary for fat digestion.

Assessment

Health Status

- Pain in right upper quadrant (RUQ) of abdomen and indigestion after meals
- May have chills and fever
- Flatulence and bloating, especially after high-fat intake

Developmental Assessment

Both sexes and all ages are susceptible, but those most prone to the disease are often "fair, fat, female, fertile, (and in their) forties." Incidence increases with age. Predisposing conditions include those associated with increased cholesterol (obesity, diabetes, and hypothyroidism).

Diagnostic Factors

H and P

Possible increased white blood cell (WBC) count; increased alkaline phosphatase

Abdominal ultrasound

Special x-rays:
Oral cholecystogram (see Table 6-1) assesses ability of gallbladder to fill, concentrate, and excrete dye
Cholangiograms used to visualize biliary tree (cystic, hepatic, and common bile duct)

Psychosocial/Cultural Assessment

- Incidence increasing in North America; high incidence in Sweden and among native Americans
- Low incidence in African and Oriental nations

Nursing Plans and Interventions

Goals

- Client will experience relief of pain and indigestion

Table 6-1. Preparation for Cholecystogram

Oral Method

The night before the test, the client is given a fat-free meal. Two to three hours later, 6 tablets containing radio-opaque dye are administered (tablets contain iodine so assess for allergy). Tablets should be taken 5 minutes apart with water. (If the client vomits after taking the tablets, the test will have to be rescheduled). The client is then to remain npo until the test. During the test, the client is given a high-fat drink. The gallbladder is assessed by x-ray for its ability to empty. If the gallbladder cannot be visualized, the test is repeated the following day, following administration of 12 dye tablets. If the gallbladder still cannot be visualized, cholecystitis or cholelithiasis are suspected.

IV Method

Client remains npo 6–8 hours before the test. Bowel preparation (may include castor oil and enemas) is done to permit clearer visualization of the biliary tree. During the test, a dye is injected intravenously. X-rays trace dye as it is excreted by the liver and passes through the hepatic, cystic, and common bile ducts.

T-Tube Method

Dye is injected via the T-tube during or after surgery to be sure there are no obstructions (i.e., stones, edema) in the common bile duct.

- Client will maintain fluid and electrolyte balance
- Client will understand purpose of tests and treatments
- Client will be free of postoperative complications

Nursing Measures

- Monitor NG tube (suctions to remove stomach secretions, which, if present, stimulate gallbladder (GB) to contract; also stops vomiting and relieves distention)
- Prepare client for diagnostic tests

Medical/Surgical Treatment

Cholecystectomy is the treatment of choice for an acute attack; it is also done as prophylaxis if "silent" gallstones present, especially for elderly and chronically ill persons, who are at high risk if an attack should occur. The gallbladder is removed, and if stones are present, the common bile duct is explored to be sure no stones remain lodged in the duct. A T-tube is placed in the common bile duct to keep edema (the result of surgical trauma) from obstructing the outlet for bile; the external arm of the T-tube is connected to a drainage bag in which bile is collected.

Nursing measures include:

- Assess the T-tube for patency; the amount of drainage should gradually decrease over 3–4 days as internal edema subsides and bile flows into duodenum
- Observe dressing around T-tube; if it becomes bile stained, T-tube may not be functioning (notify physician)

The T-tube is removed when client condition warrants, usually after assessment by T-tube cholangiogram. Clients may be discharged from the hospital with the T-tube still in place.

Special Nursing Considerations

- Cholecystectomy clients are at especially high risk for developing pneumonia postoperatively, so turning, coughing, and deep breathing are very important
- Clients are susceptible to gas pains on the second or third day after surgery when peristalsis returns; best action is to ambulate
- Clients need to know that the first bowel movement (BM) will be light color; stools will gradually become darker as bile resumes draining into duodenum
- After surgery, there may be temporary fat intolerance; in time, most clients can resume regular diet

Drug Therapy

Phenobarbital or nitroglycerin (NTG) to relax smooth muscle

Antibiotics if bacterial infection present

Nutrition Therapy

- For persons predisposed to GB attacks, low-fat diet and small, frequent meals
- Eliminate alcohol

Client/Family Teaching

Teach client about:

Foods to include and avoid in low-fat diet
Need for follow-up care
Pros and cons of cholecystectomy

Evaluation

Treatment and client teaching are successful if:

- Client understands any diet modifications.
- Surgical wound is free of redness, edema, and drainage
- Client understands how to care for T-tube at home

Regional Enteritis (Crohn's Disease)

Regional enteritis is a rare inflammatory disorder that can affect any portion of GI tract but most often affects the small intestine, especially at the terminal ileum. It is characterized by remissions and exacerbations, and decreases the absorptive capacity of the intestine, producing a general malnourished state. Onset may be sudden, but more often symptoms are mild and transitory at first.

Assessment

Health Status

- Abdominal pain
- Diarrhea
- Weight loss related to inability to absorb nutrients
- Abscess may develop, producing severe pain
- Fistulae form between one area of bowel and another or between bowel and bladder, bowel and vagina, bowel and rectum, or bowel and abdominal wall
- Extra-colonic symptoms:
  Arthritis
  Iritis
  Renal and biliary calculi

Developmental Assessment

May be genetic link, but this is unproven

Often occurs during early adulthood but can occur any time

Diagnostic Factors

H and P
X-ray shows lesions
Biopsy

Psychosocial/Cultural Assessment

- Occurs most often in urban, white-collar populations
- Higher incidence among Jews
- Was once thought to be psychosomatic in origin

Nursing Plans and Interventions

Goals

- Underlying inflammatory process will be controlled
- Client will be free of pain and other distressing symptoms
- Fluid and electrolyte balance will be maintained
- Nutritional status will be maintained
- Skin integrity will be maintained

Nursing Measures

- Provide rest to help decrease intestinal motility
- Record number of stools
- Keep accurate I and O records
- Provide general skin care to prevent excoriation from diarrhea (Sitz baths and protective skin coatings)

- Provide skin care and care of mucous membranes at fistula sites:
  - Use ostomy bag over fistula opening if location permits
  - Protect skin with zinc oxide, commercial skin protective substances or skin barriers (Stomahesive), aluminum paste, karaya gum, etc.

Medical/Surgical Treatment

Surgical intervention is required if abscesses develop, and is sometimes performed for fistulae, depending on their location. Affected areas of the intestine are removed. The client may or may not require ileostomy (this is avoided if possible because it is the nature of the disease to recur).

Drug Therapy

Anti-inflammatory agents (steroidal or nonsteroidal)

Antibiotics or antibacterials as indicated (*e.g.*, sulfasalazine)

Medication to provide bulk and decrease diarrhea (*e.g.*, psyllium hydrophilic mucilloid (Metamucil)

Nutrition Therapy

- Absorption is impaired; may require total parenteral nutrition (TPN) to assure availability of nutrients and to provide rest for intestine
- Elemental enteral feedings (*e.g.*, Vivonex) for easy digestion
- If on po intake, bland, low-fat, high-protein, high-calorie diet with supplemental vitamins

Client/Family Teaching

Teach client about:

Medication regimen, diet, symptoms that need reporting

TPN at home if indicated

Need for follow-up care

Evaluation

Treatment and client teaching are successful if client:

- Does not have diarrhea or abdominal pain
- Can verbalize understanding of specific foods to include in diet
- Can verbalize understanding of drug therapy
- Develops positive coping behaviors if ileostomy is necessary

Large Bowel Dysfunction

Ulcerative Colitis

Ulcerative colitis is a chronic inflammatory condition involving the large intestine. Lesions spread proximally from the rectum (in contrast to Crohn's disease, in which lesions skip). The disease is characterized by remissions and exacerbations like those of Crohn's disease, and by the same kinds of extracolonic disorders.

Assessment

Health Status

- Dehydrated, malnourished appearance
- Diarrhea accompanied by severe sense of urgency; often contains blood and pus
- Abdominal pain
- Pain and diarrhea worse after meals so client limits intake, contributing to weight loss and malnutrition

Developmental Assessment

More frequent in females than in males

Often begins in childhood; about 50% begin before age 30; another peak incidence around age 60

Diagnostic Factors

H and P

Anemia

Stool cultures done to rule out (RO) infectious agent

Barium enemas and sigmoidoscopy for definitive diagnosis, but must be used cautiously because of danger of perforation, especially during acute phase

Psychosocial/Cultural Assessment

- High familial occurrence
- Higher incidence among Jews

Nursing Plans and Interventions

Goals

- Inflammation will subside
- Pain associated with diarrhea and related skin excoriation will decrease
- Fluid and electrolyte balance will be maintained
- Adequate nutritional status will be restored and maintained

Nursing Measures

- Assess number, character, and frequency of stools
- Assess for abdominal distention, especially if accompanied by significant decrease in number of stools (may signal toxic megacolon)
- Provide for bedrest, with bedside commode or bedpan within reach
- Provide special skin care because client is debilitated
    Clean perianal area carefully and gently
    Use dibucaine hydrochloride (Nupercaine) ointment
- Assess temperature, WBC count, serum K levels
- Provide emotional support

Medical/Surgical Treatment

If attacks are frequent and severe, the rectum and the affected area of the colon may need to be removed, in which case the client will undergo a permanent colostomy. Surgery is curative, and is often done if the disease has been present 10 years or more, because the incidence of malignancy increases with the duration of the disease.

Drug Therapy

Antiinflammatory agents (steroids and nonsteroids)

Antibacterial agents for concurrent infection (sulfasalazine)

Sedatives or tranquilizers for anxiety

Antidiarrheal agents (used cautiously)

Ferrous gluconate for anemia

Nutrition Therapy

- May be npo or on elemental diet
- TPN during acute episodes
- High-protein, high-calorie, high-vitamin intake
- When diet resumed, include high-bulk, low-residue foods

Client/Family Teaching

Teach client about:

Importance of nutrition: examples of high-protein, iron-rich foods

Importance of sudden decrease in number of stools (may mean improvement in condition or can mean onset of toxic megacolon)

Need for frequent rest periods during day (will help decrease intestinal motility)

Need to see physician in case of mild attack (client can usually go about business if he or she takes medications and gets extra rest)

Evaluation

Client teaching is successful if client:

- Verbalizes understanding of diet and drug regimen
- Copes positively with alteration in elimination, if a colostomy has been performed

Cancer of the Colon

Cancer of the colon is the second most frequent cause of cancer death in the U.S. It usually occurs in the distal portion of the colon, from sigmoid to anus. The 5-year survival rate is 50%.

Assessment

Health Status

- Change in bowel habits persisting for 2 weeks should be evaluated
- Gradual decrease in diameter of stools
- Rectal bleeding
- Late symptoms include:
    Weight loss
    N and V
    Abdominal pain
    Palpable abdominal mass
    Bowel obstruction

Developmental Assessment

Men and women equally affected (colon more in women, rectum more in men)
Incidence increases with age
Diet may be major etiologic factor (diets high in fat and low in fiber may predispose)

Diagnostic Factors

One-third palpable on digital examination
Positive hematest of stool
Barium enema and sigmoidoscopy

Psychosocial/Cultural Assessment

- High incidence in many developed countries
- Low incidence in Japan, India, Africa
- Possibly related to diet

Nursing Plans and Interventions

Goals

- Tumor will be removed prior to metastasis
- If colostomy necessary, client will cope effectively with changes in elimination and changes in body image
- Client will cope effectively with anxiety

Nursing Measures

- Provide emotional support: client will have high anxiety level; will need opportunity to ask questions and express concerns
- Explain tests and procedures and what to expect
- Provide pre- and postoperative care (see Tables 6-2 and 6-3)

Evaluation

Treatment is successful if client:

- Is able to look at stoma and participate in its care
- Is able to discuss concerns with professional staff and with significant others

Hemorrhoids

Hemorrhoids are varicose veins in the rectum and anus. Internal hemorrhoids are above the internal sphincter. External hemorrhoids are outside the anal sphincter. The problem is secondary to congestion in the hemorrhoidal veins. Factors contributing to congestion are hereditary predisposition, constipation and straining, long periods of standing or sitting, and pregnancy.

Assessment

Health Status

- Bright bleeding
- Pain if hemorrhoids are irritated or thrombosed

Diagnostic Factors

External hemorrhoids are visible
Internal hemorrhoids are palpable by rectal examination

Nursing Plans and Interventions

Goals

- Client will experience pain relief
- Client will experience no further blood loss

Nursing Measures

Initial conservative management includes:

- Sitz baths for comfort
- Local application of analgesic ointments

Table 6-2. Preoperative and Postoperative Care of the Client Having Colon Surgery

Preoperative	Postoperative

1. Provide thorough explanation of what an ostomy is
2. Give client a chance to ask questions and express concerns
3. Have consent signed
4. Bowel preparation
   a. Low residue or liquid diet 24–48 hours preoperatively (npo after midnight on day of surgery)
   b. Antibiotics that have local effects on bowel
     (1) Neomycin
     (2) Certain sulfonamides
   c. Cleansing enemas: if cramping occurs, temporarily stop flow, then lower bag
   d. NG tubes for decompression
5. Skin preparation prior to surgery
   a. Thorough cleansing with antibacterial preparation (i.e., hexachlorophene or chlorhexidine gluconate [Hibiclens])
   b. Several scrubs at specified intervals
   c. Hair removal
     (1) Dipilatory if client not sensitive
     (2) Shaving (if needed) should be done in OR immediately before incision made (risk of infection less than if client shaved several hours before)
	1. NG tube will be in place and attached to low suction until bowel sounds return; client will remain npo until flatus is expelled
	2. Client will have abdominal incision; may also have perineal wounds, drains, and dressings
	3. An ostomy bag will be in place over the stoma: at first, only mucus and air will be expelled (be sure to open bag periodically to release air build-up); when fecal drainage begins, be sure it does not come in contact with incision; empty bag when it is 1/3 full; if leakage occurs around bag, replace with a new bag (taping around old bag usually will not seal the leak)
	4. When applying a new bag leave 1/8–1/16 inch around stoma for expansion during peristalsis; no nerve endings are present so client will not know if it is too tight, so could cause necrosis; protect skin around stoma—apply protective barrier (e.g., stomahesive)
	5. Assess stoma: should be bright red; may even have areas of pinpoint bleeding; dark color indicates impaired blood supply—report *stat*

Medical/Surgical Treatment

Injections to sclerose veins

Ligation with rubber bands (causes necrosis and sloughing of affected veins)

Surgical excision

Postoperative Nursing Care

- Assess for hemorrhage (bleeding may be internal in rectum and not readily obvious)
- Assess for voiding:
  Client may have difficulty because of edema
  Provide Sitz bath to stimulate voiding
- Implement measures for pain control:
  Provide Sitz baths to promote comfort
  Client will anticipate and fear pain with first BM (may experience dizziness and faint at the thought); to avoid possible injury stay with client until he or she is seated
  Give analgesic as soon as client feels urge to defecate

Drug Therapy

Stool softeners

Narcotics in early postoperative phase

Bulk laxatives or mineral oil

Nutrition Therapy

- Aimed at preventing constipation

Table 6-3. Client Teaching for Ostomy Care

- No special diet; you will learn to avoid foods that are poorly tolerated; may want to avoid gas-forming foods
- Drink plenty of fluids (especially important for ileostomy clients); drink extra in hot weather; call physician if N and V occurs because you are at special risk of dehydration
- No laxatives except as ordered by physician
- Stoma will gradually shrink to about ¼ its postoperative size, over several months—postpone fitting for permanent appliance until this occurs
- Irrigation procedure (if applicable; irrigations are performed for sigmoid colostomies for regulation purposes, ostomies higher in tract cannot be regulated—stool too liquid)
- Two crushed aspirin tablets in the ostomy bag may help control odor; commercial odor control preparation also available

---

- Fruits and vegetables (raw and cooked), whole grain cereals, nuts, high-fiber foods
- 8 glasses of water every day

Client/Family Teaching

For Clients Who Do Not Have Surgery

Teach client to:

Avoid constipation and straining
    Eat high-fiber diet
    Drink 8 glasses of water daily
    Use stool softeners
    Take time for daily BM (regular time best)
    Get regular exercise
After defecation, wash area gently and pat dry (avoid vigorous rubbing)
Have regular examinations, because bright bleeding is also a symptom of cancer of rectum (do not assume hemorrhoids are cause)

Postoperative Teaching

Teach client to:

Continue Sitz baths
Eat high-fiber diet
Follow habits listed above to avoid constipation

Evaluation

Client teaching is successful if client:

- Is able to describe diet and personal habits that prevent constipation
- Understands need for follow-up care if bleeding recurs

Anal Abscess

Anal infection and abscess formation are usually caused by a crack in the mucosal lining of the anal canal. The crack is usually caused by passing hard stools, or by anal trauma.

Assessment

Health Status

- Throbbing local pain and redness, inflammation at site
- Difficulty sitting or standing, because of discomfort

Medical/Surgical Treatment

Goal

- Infection will be eradicated

Nursing Measures

- Care for incision and drainage of abscess:
    Observe for urinary retention
    Provide dressing (can be held in place by T-binder)
- Provide Sitz bath after each BM

Drug Therapy

Analgesics
Antibiotics
Stool softeners

Nutrition Therapy

- High-fiber diet to prevent constipation
- 8 glasses of water every day

Anal Fistula

Anal fistulas are often due to a ruptured anal abscess. The term refers to an abnormal passageway between the anal canal and the rectal mucous membrane or between the anal canal and the external perineal area.

Assessment

Health Status

- Periodic drainage that stains underclothing

Nursing Plans and Interventions

Nursing Measures

The client will have a fistulectomy or a fistulotomy. Nursing measures include:

- Provide Sitz baths after each BM
- Provide care similar to that previously discussed in anal abscess section

Drug Therapy

Stool softeners or mild laxatives

Nutrition Therapy

- Diet to prevent constipation

Evaluation

Treatment and client teaching are successful if:

- Client can verbalize ways to prevent constipation
- Fistula heals without complications

Pilonidal Cyst

A pilonidal cyst is a hair-containing cyst and sometimes a sinus tract occurring at the base of the sacrum; the skin folds in but hair continues to grow. The client may be asymptomatic unless infection occurs, which is likely because of the proximity of the cyst to the rectum.

Assessment

Health Status

- Pain
- Swelling
- Discharge

Developmental Assessment

Occurs most often in young adult men with a lot of hair

Diagnostic Factors

History
Physical examination

Nursing Plans and Interventions

Goal

- Surgical wound will heal without infection

Nursing measures after the surgical excision of a cyst include:

- Provide wound care to avoid contamination
- Administer oil retention enema or lubricating laxative before first BM to decrease strain on suture line
- No special drug or diet therapy except to prevent constipation

Client/Family Teaching

Teach client about:

Wound care (healing is slow)

Measures to prevent constipation

Evaluation

Treatment and client teaching are successful if client:

- Can verbalize ways to keep area clean
- Experiences no wound infection

Appendicitis

Appendicitis is inflammation of the appendix, often secondary to kinking, obstruction, bowel wall edema, or adhesions.

Client/Family Teaching

Teach client ways to prevent constipation as outlined in hemorrhoids section

Assessment

Health Status

- Acute, abdominal, wavelike pain; begins around umbilicus and moves to right lower quadrant (RLQ) of abdomen; in small children and in the elderly, pain may not be "characteristic"; clients draw legs up and "guard" abdomen
- Vomiting and nausea
- May feel flatus is "trapped" and feel need to have BM; may take laxative or enema—these are *contraindicated* because can cause rupture and peritonitis

Diagnostic Factors

H and P
Increased WBC
Rebound tenderness when abdomen palpated

Nursing Plans and Interventions

Goal

- Appendix will not rupture

Nursing Measures

- Keep client npo; observe and report symptoms
- If hospitalized, client may have IV
- Apply ice bag to abdomen for pain relief

Medical/Surgical Treatment

Surgery may be necessary on an emergency basis. Recovery is usually fast and uncomplicated unless the appendix has ruptured. In the case of rupture, there will be a drain in the incision; wet-to-dry dressing will likely be ordered.

Drug Therapy

Narcotics for pain relief after diagnosis and in the early postoperative period
IV antibiotics if appendix has ruptured

Nutrition Therapy

- npo prior to surgery and postoperatively until nausea subsides and peristalsis resumes
- Clear liquids progressing to regular diet as tolerated

Client/Family Teaching

Teach clients in the community the characteristics of appendicitis pain and the importance of not using laxatives, enemas, or heat.

Evaluation

Treatment is successful if client is free of postoperative complications.

Diverticulitis

Diverticula are small outpouchings of the intestine caused by weakness in the musculature of the colon. These are blind pouches in which small pieces of undigested food or fecal particles can become trapped and start an inflammatory process. Diverticulosis is the presence of diverticula without inflammation.

Assessment

Health Status

- History of constipation or constipation alternating with diarrhea
- Severe diarrhea; may have blood and pus in stool
- Abdominal cramps, usually in lower left quadrant (LLQ) of the abdomen, aggravated by eating
- Fever

Developmental Assessment

Seldom seen until midadulthood; after that incidence increases with age

Diagnostic Factors

H and P
Elevated WBC
Barium enema

Psychosocial/Cultural Assessment

- Higher incidence in highly developed countries; probably associated with low fiber intake

- Lower incidence in Japan and nonindustrialized countries

Nursing Plans and Interventions

Goal
- Pain will subside
- Fluid and electrolyte balance will be maintained
- Nutritional status will be maintained

Nursing Measures
- Provide bedrest and clear liquids to rest the bowel
- Administer IV fluids as ordered
- Provide blood replacement as ordered

Medical/Surgical Treatment

Surgical intervention is required if conservative treatment fails or if diverticula perforate. The affected area of colon is resected, and the remaining bowel segments may be anastomosed, or a temporary or permanent colostomy may be created. For pre- and postoperative care related to colon surgery, see Tables 6-2 and 6-3.

Drug Therapy

Antispasmodic agents, such as dicyclomine hydrochloride (Bentyl), or propantheline bromide (Probanthine)

Analgesics for pain (avoid morphine)

Antibiotics until attack subsides

Neomycin preoperatively to sterilize bowel

Nutrition Therapy
- Clear liquids; then bland, low-residue diet until attack subsides
- When acute attack subsides include vegetable and cereal fiber; unprocessed wheat bran or psyllium hydrophilic mucilloid (Metamucil) optional

Client/Family Teaching

Teach client to avoid repeat attacks by:

Complying with diet

Avoiding activities that increase intraabdominal pressure (bending, lifting)

Drinking 8 glasses of water a day

Controlling weight (reducing if obese)

Following prescribed regimen to avoid repeat attack

Evaluation

Treatment and client teaching are successful if:

- Client is able to describe diet modifications
- Unpleasant symptoms subside
- Client is able to explain signs and symptoms that require medical attention

Liver and Pancreas Dysfunction

Cirrhosis

Cirrhosis is inflammation and fibrosis of liver cells, usually associated with chronic alcoholism but also with hepatitis, bile duct obstruction, and interruption of blood supply. Cirrhosis is a major problem because the liver is a vital organ that performs functions affecting virtually every system. A relatively small percent of chronic alcohol abusers develop cirrhosis, possibly because of individual variations in metabolism. Alcohol is known to cause edema in the biliary–pancreatic ductal system and to cause fatty changes in the liver. The adverse effects on liver cells are reversible if alcohol intake or other causative agent is stopped in time, because liver cells are capable of regeneration.

Assessment

Health Status
- Jaundice (usually proportional to amount of liver damage)
- Bruising tendency
- General malnourished state (muscle atrophy, weakness, anemia)
- Vague gastrointestinal (GI) complaints initially; later anorexia, weight loss, flatulence
- Concurrent infections
- Gynecomastia, vascular skin lesions, hair loss, palmar erythema (secondary to disrupted estrogen metabolism)

- Ascites
- Dependent edema
- GI bleeding due to esophageal varices and other weakened collateral vessels (result of portal hypertension)
- Prominent veins on abdomen
- Neurologic symptoms that signal impending hepatic coma
- Peripheral neuropathy

Diagnostic Factors

H and P

Enlarged liver

Abnormal liver function test results

Liver biopsy—performed only if prothrombin time (PT) and partial thromboplastin time (PTT) adequate

Nursing Plans and Interventions

Goals

- Liver function will be maximized and no additional damage will occur
- Nutritional status and fluid and electrolyte balance will be maintained
- Client will experience no complications

Nursing Measures

- Provide supportive treatment
- Provide bedrest to promote diuresis and decrease ascites
- Assess fluid balance (including ascites):
    - Monitor I and O
    - Monitor daily weight
    - Measure abdominal girth
- Provide skin care (edematous skin prone to break down, jaundice causes itching):
    - Avoid harsh soaps; use soap only in crucial areas, otherwise clear water
    - Keep nails short
    - Administer medications to control itching—cholestyramine, diphenhydramine hydrochloride (Benadryl), cimetidine
- Monitor emesis and stool for blood
- Provide for client safety in light of peripheral neuropathy

Nursing Care in Relation to Special Procedures

Nursing care for *liver biopsy* includes:

- Instruct client to hold breath for 5–10 seconds while needle is inserted
- Lie on right side for 2 hours after biopsy, to decrease risk of bleeding
- Monitor vital signs closely
- Provide bedrest for 24 hours
- Check site for bleeding or hematoma
- Check sheets under client for blood

Nursing care for *paracentesis* (performed if ascites so severe that it interferes with respirations) includes:

- Administer povidone-iodine (Betadine) skin preparation prior to procedure
- Have client void immediately before procedure
- Position client sitting on chair with feet flat on floor

Medical Treatment for Complications

Hepatic Coma

Hepatic coma occurs because of the diseased liver's inability to break down ammonia, which is toxic to the central nervous system (CNS). Ammonia is produced as intestinal bacteria act on protein.

Goals

- Serum ammonia levels will return to normal
- GI bleeding will be controlled (blood is protein)

Nursing Measures

- Administer lactulose as ordered (prevents ammonia formation)
- Administer mineral oil or laxatives as ordered to remove protein from intestine
- Administer enemas as ordered
- Assist with hemodialysis as necessary to reduce serum ammonia levels

GI Bleeding

GI bleeding is a frequent complication of cirrhosis and is an emergency—50% of clients die because they are bleeding and cannot manufacture clotting factors.

Goal

- GI bleeding will be controlled

Nursing Measures

- Assist with placement of Blakemore-Sengstaken tube (special NG tube with balloons that are inflated after insertion to put pressure on bleeding varices; iced saline lavage is administered through lumen of NG tube; bleeding may resume when balloons deflated and tubes removed—dislodges clots)
- Assist with blood replacement as ordered
- Administer Vitamin K as ordered if liver can utilize

Long-term management of varices is accomplished by:

Injection sclerotherapy: sclerosing agent instilled into varices to seal them and prevent blood flow through them, thus controlling bleeding; only moderately successful

Shunt procedures to reroute blood around liver, bypassing high pressure area; about 1/3 of clients develop hepatic coma postoperatively

Drug Therapy

Dosage of all drugs will be decreased: administer narcotics and sedatives in small doses, and monitor serum levels of digoxin and antibiotics

Supplemental vitamins (may be poorly utilized, even in large doses)

Vitamin K subcutaneously (will be effective only if liver cells functioning well enough to use)

Salt-poor albumin: replaces albumin (diseased liver cannot synthesize albumin) and helps restore fluid balance; client at risk for circulatory overload as albumin pulls fluid back into vascular space

Diuretics, such as spironolactone and furosemide (Lasix): assess potassium levels and hydration status

Lactulose or neomycin to control serum ammonia levels; will cause diarrhea (must continue medications anyway)

Nutrition Therapy

- Restrict sodium and water
- Provide bile salts supplement as required
- High-calorie, low-fat diet
- Protein intake depends on serum ammonia levels: if normal, provide large amounts of protein; if high, restrict protein to as little as 40 g/day (just a little over 1 ounce)

Client/Family Teaching

Teach client to:

Report weight gain or increasing abdominal girth

Avoid alcohol

Avoid over-the-counter (OTC) medications, especially acetaminophen (Tylenol), which can be toxic to liver

Operationalize amount of protein permitted in diet (*e.g.*, 40 g is one egg or 1 1/3 oz. hamburger)

Prevent or control bruising and bleeding:
    Avoid aspirin
    Avoid forceful nose blowing
    Do not wear tight, restrictive clothing
    Use electric razor
    Avoid invasive procedures (intramuscular injections, catheterization, enemas, suppositories)

Control exposure to infection if possible; pay prompt attention to cuts and scratches

Recognize signs and symptoms that should be reported to physician, including:
    Increasing abdominal girth
    Nervousness, lack of coordination, drowsiness, abnormal muscle tremors in hands, impaired attention span, delayed response, changes in speech

patterns (all these neurological symptoms indicate impending hepatic coma)

Bleeding via emesis or stool

Evaluation

Treatment and client teaching are successful if client:

- Can verbalize understanding of diet and drug regimen
- Understands that taking medications is important even if side-effects unpleasant
- Does not experience complications

Cancer of the Liver

Cancer of the liver can be a primary tumor, but the vast majority of liver cancers are metastatic lesions. Their effect is similar to cirrhosis in that liver functions are disrupted, depending on the extent of the tumor.

Assessment

Health Status

- Client with history of cancer elsewhere becomes anorexic; experiences weight loss and pain in RUQ
- Increasing abdominal girth
- Jaundice
- Bruising and bleeding
- Symptoms associated with cirrhosis; degree may vary

Diagnostic Factors

Enlarged liver

Increased alkaline phosphatase

Factors associated with cirrhosis

Nursing Plans and Interventions

Goals

- Tumor will be removed prior to metastasis (possible only if it is primary tumor localized to one lobe—very rare; lobectomy possible since liver can regenerate)
- Client will be as comfortable as possible

Nursing Measures

There is no known cure for cancer of the liver, and the prognosis is poor. Chemotherapy may produce temporary regression of the tumor.

- Employ supportive measures similar to those used with clients with cirrhosis
- Provide for client comfort

Evaluation

Treatment and client teaching are successful if client:

- Is as comfortable as possible
- Understands therapy and procedures

Hepatitis

Hepatitis is inflammation of the liver caused by a virus, bacteria, or toxic substance. Type A, type B, type non-A non-B cause similar symptoms but are caused by different organisms and differ in severity and mode of transmission.

Assessment

Health Status

- Number and severity of symptoms vary (depend on amount of liver damage)
- Early symptoms include anorexia, lethargy, and fever, and are flulike in nature
- Jaundice occurs later (first evident in sclera); urine becomes dark
- Over time, stools become light and clay colored

Developmental Assessment

Type A transmitted by fecal-oral route (associated with poor personal hygiene), by direct contact, or by eating shellfish from contaminated water; can also be transmitted by food handlers

Type B and Type non-A non-B associated with history of drug abuse or recent blood transfusion (virus transmitted by blood or body secretions)

Toxic hepatitis can occur after exposure to hepatotoxic drugs or chemicals; not communicable

Diagnostic Factors

Enlarged liver

Elevated serum bilirubin levels, prolonged PT time

Elevated alkaline phosphatase level

H and P

Psychosocial/Cultural Assessment

Risk factors include:

- Poor hygiene practice
- Drug use
- Crowded living conditions

Nursing Plans and Interventions

Goals

- Liver cells will regenerate
- Client will not suffer relapse, progress to chronic state, or develop cirrhosis
- Client will not transmit disease to others

Nursing Measures

- Ensure bedrest to slow metabolism to promote cellular regeneration
- Provide skin care to relieve itching (see notes in cirrhosis section)
- Follow Centers for Disease Control (CDC) for Blood and Body Fluid Precautions to prevent transmission of organisms (see Table 8-1)

Drug Therapy

Immunoglobulin to other exposed persons (warn them to expect tenderness at injection site)

Same antihistamines for itching as for cirrhosis

Antiemetics

Vitamin K subcutaneously

Nutrition Therapy

- Client will have experienced a change in eating habits due to anorexia
- 3000 mL fluid intake daily
- High-protein, high-carbohydrate (CHO), low-to-moderate fat intake

Client Teaching

Teach client to:

Get extra rest and restrict activity (even when feeling better) until liver function test (LFT) results normal

Avoid alcohol

Avoid oral and sexual contact until LFT results are normal (virus transmitted in saliva, semen, and vaginal secretions)

Practice adequate personal hygiene: keep hands away from face and mouth and wash hands after using toilet

Never donate blood again

Get Hepatitis B vaccine if in high-risk group (*e.g.*, health care workers, dialysis patients)

Get periodic LFTs

Evaluation

Client teaching is successful if client:

- Can explain isolation precautions and how these will be carried out in hospital or at home
- Can explain diet and activity regimens
- Makes plans for follow-up care

Pancreatitis

Pancreatitis is acute or chronic inflammation of the pancreas. It occurs when pancreatic secretions are activated within the pancreas instead of in the duodenum. Pancreatitis can be acute or chronic; either condition can damage islet cells, resulting in diabetes mellitus. Permanent insufficiency of pancreatic digestive enzymes can also result.

Assessment

Health Status

- Severe pain in epigastric area radiating to back and flank
- Symptoms of shock
- Fever
- Abdominal distention (possible rigid abdomen)

Diagnostic Factors

H and P

Elevated serum amylase and serum lipase levels

Developmental Assessment

Associated with alcoholism

Occurs more often in men than in women

Associated with gallstones

Can occur as a result of trauma

Sometimes no known cause

Nursing Plans and Interventions

Goals

- Inflammatory process will subside
- Nutritional status and fluid and electrolyte balance will be maintained

Nursing Measures

- Maintain on npo status (no ice chips or water)
- Use NG tube to suction
- Administer IV fluids; often TPN
- Provide comfort measures

Drug Therapy

Meperidine hydrochloride (Demerol) for pain (do not use morphine—may cause spasm of sphincter of Oddi)

IV Cimetidine to decrease volume of gastric secretions, which are stimuli for pancreatic secretions

May require insulin

Nutrition Therapy

- Maintain on npo status until serum amylase level falls
- Begin with clear liquids and progress to bland, low-fat diet; resume regular diet gradually as tolerated
- May require pancreatic enzyme supplements temporarily or permanently

Client/Family Teaching

Teach client about:

Importance of npo status to provide rest for pancreas

Need to avoid alcohol

Evaluation

Treatment and client teaching are successful if:

- Client remains free of pain
- Serum amylase levels return to normal
- Cause of pancreatitis is identified and removed

Metabolic Dysfunction

Diabetes Mellitus

Diabetes mellitus results from inadequate insulin production, causing disruption in CHO, fat, and protein metabolism. Type I or insulin-dependent diabetes mellitus (IDDM) occurs when pancreatic islet cells produce little or no insulin. Type II or non–insulin-dependent diabetes mellitus (NIDDM) occurs when islet cells produce small, inadequate amounts of insulin. Type II can be controlled by diet and exercise alone or in combination with oral hypoglycemic agents. Diabetes is associated with vascular changes that ultimately affect vision, kidney

Table 6-4. Metabolic Acidosis and its Occurrence with Diabetes*

Diabetic Acidosis (Ketoacidosis)	Hypoglycemia
Pathophysiology	
Without insulin, blood glucose level rises because glucose cannot enter cells; glucose exerts osmotic pull, causing loss of cellular fluids and electrolytes, and leads to dehydration	Blood sugar levels drop below normal (often occurs at or near peak action time of insulin)
Also, cells are starving for glucose, so body starts mobilizing fat reserves, an inefficient process which increases glucose levels but also produces large amounts of acidic waste products (ketones)	Often caused by insufficient dietary intake accompanied by usual insulin dosage; may be related to excessive physical activity
Body buffering systems strive to maintain pH in normal range; bicarbonate is depleted (reflected by CO_2 levels: do not confuse with pCO_2)	Brain cells need glucose to function; autonomic nervous system is activated and epinephrine is released in effort to mobilize stored carbohydrate
When bicarbonate reserves are gone, client will die without immediate medical intervention	Client will die unless he or she receives glucose
Symptoms	
Polyuria, polydipsia, polyphagia Deep, rapid respirations (Kussmaul's) Fruity odor to respirations Dry, flushed skin Weight loss Stupor progressing to coma	Hunger Weakness, tremulousness Diaphoresis (often profuse) Tachycardia Elevated BP Headache, drowsiness Mental confusion or irritability Coma
Treatment	
IV fluids Regular insulin IV Careful monitoring of glucose and potassium levels (insulin drives potassium back into cells) ECG monitoring because of initial hyperkalemia and eventual possible hypokalemia	Orange juice Cola drink (regular, *not* diet) Candy Honey Jelly — *If client is awake enough to swallow* 50% glucose solution IV Glucagon S.C. if IV not possible immediately Note: With treatment, recovery is rapid and dramatic

* *Hyperglycemic, Hyperosmolar, Nonketotic Coma (HHNK) is a potential complication of type II Diabetes. Blood sugar levels become very high, but because some insulin is being produced, ketoacidosis does not develop. Dehydration does occur and can be life threatening without treatment.*

function, and peripheral circulation, causing a peripheral neuropathy. Metabolic acidosis and dehydration are potential complications.

Assessment

Health Status
- Polyuria
- Polydipsia
- Polyphagia
- Weight loss
- Increased susceptibility to infection
- Poor wound healing
- Peripheral neuropathy: client loses sensation in feet (not aware of blisters and foot injuries)
- Diabetic ketoacidosis (See Table 6-4)

Developmental Assessment

Both types can occur at any age. Type I usually occurs before age 15. Type II usually occurs after age 40. There may be a hereditary component. The disease has a low incidence in underdeveloped countries (possibly because these populations consume a high-fiber diet and do not have access to refined, processed foods).

Diagnostic Factors

High blood glucose levels when fasting and under other controlled conditions
Glycosuria
H and P

Nursing Plans and Interventions

Goals
- Blood glucose levels will remain within normal limits
- Client will not experience complications
- Client will control weight (if obese, return to normal weight can decrease or eliminate need for exogenous insulin)

Nursing Measures
- Assess for symptoms that distinguish acidosis from hypoglycemia (see Table 6-4)
- Remember that an insulin injection can kill; sugar intake on a one-time basis cannot
- Provide care during acidosis (See Table 6-4)

Drug Therapy

Insulin carries glucose into the cells. It is derived from beef or pork pancreas or manufactured using recombinant DNA technology (*e.g.,* Humulin insulin) Manufactured insulin is not interchangeable with insulin of beef or pork extraction.

Regular: the only form of insulin that can be administered IV; used during emergency treatment of acidosis; also may be administered subcutaneously as part of total insulin regimen

Intermediate (NPH or Lente): administered subcutaneously; peak action 8–12 hours later (when hypoglycemia is most likely)

Longer-acting insulins are available but not commonly used (*e.g.,* Ultralente)

Oral hypoglycemic agents, such as chlorpropamide (Diabinese), tolbutamide (Orinase), and glyburide stimulate the pancreas to produce insulin, and are used in Type II diabetes.

Nutrition Therapy
- Modifying diet very important to control diabetes
- Food can be weighed in exact portions; older diabetic clients may be more accustomed to this method
- *American Diabetic Association (ADA) Exchange Diet* most widely used—classifies foods into various groups, within which foods can be exchanged or substituted for one another (example: group that includes bread also includes cereal and starchy vegetables—client can choose slice of bread or specified amount of potatoes or cereal as bread exchange for a certain meal)
- Diet must supply adequate nutrients and also keep blood glucose levels constant; in-

cludes regular meals and scheduled snacks; includes most carbohydrate calories from complex starches, not refined sugars

Client/Family Teaching

Teach client:

How to draw up and administer insulin, and not to change brand of insulin without medical supervision

To follow diabetic exchange diet

How to check blood sugar levels (use of glucometers)

Importance of maintaining constant blood glucose levels (which may delay or minimize circulatory and neurologic complications)

To wear medic-alert tag

Importance of foot care: how to care for calluses (best done by professionals), and to inspect feet daily, using mirror if necessary

Relationship of diet and exercise to insulin requirements: calorie requirement increases, insulin requirement decreases with exercise

Signs, symptoms, and treatment of hyperglycemia and hypoglycemia

Importance of regular eye tests

Evaluation

Treatment and client teaching are successful if:

- Client's blood sugar levels remain within normal range
- Client inspects feet daily and promptly seeks medical attention for cuts or blisters
- Client maintains quality of life
- Client avoids complications

Hyperthyroidism

Hyperthyroidism is caused by overactivity of the thyroid gland, resulting in an excess of the thyroid hormone. The condition results in an increase in body metabolism.

Assessment

Health Status

- Agitation, irritability
- Rapid pulse
- Tremulousness, even at rest
- Ravenous appetite but weight loss anyway
- Diaphoresis; intolerance to heat; in extreme cases, thyroid storm develops—can be fatal

Diagnostic Factors

H and P

Elevated serum thyroid levels

Elevated radioiodine uptake

May have a goiter and exophthalmos (toxic goiter is Graves disease)

Nursing Plans and Interventions

Goals

- Thyroxin levels will stabilize
- Complications (*e.g.*, corneal injury if exophthalmos exists) will not occur
- Hypermetabolic state and dehydration will be avoided

Nursing Measures

- Provide quiet, restful environment
- Keep room cool
- Assess vital signs, activity level
- For exophthalmos, tape eyelids at night to prevent corneal ulceration
- Monitor daily weight

Medical/Surgical Treatment

The client may be treated with radioactive iodine, concentrated in the thyroid gland to destroy thyroid cells. Surgical removal of the thyroid may be necessary. Radioactive iodine is the isotope of choice because it is automatically attracted to and concentrated in the thyroid

Preoperative Nursing Care

- Administer antithyroid medications *e.g.*, propylthiouracil or methimazole (Tapazole)

to suppress hormone secretion and keep metabolic rate at safe level
- Administer potassium iodide (SSKI) or Lugol's Solution to decrease vascularity of gland
- Administer β-blockers to control tachycardia and palpitations

Postoperative Nursing Care (In Addition to Routine Care After Any Major Surgery)

- Check respirations (local edema can obstruct respiratory passages)
- Watch for bleeding (check behind neck)
- Monitor calcium levels (may drop if parathyroids accidentally removed during surgery); note twitching movements, especially when tapping face in front of ear, and note complaints of tingling in extremities; keep ampule of calcium gluconate at bedside for emergency use
- Support client's head upon movement

Drug Therapy

Client will suffer hypothyroidism and require hormone replacement, *e.g.*, sodium levothyroxine (Synthroid) postoperatively if entire gland is removed.

Nutrition Therapy

In hyperthyroid state, client needs high-calorie, high-protein, high-CHO diet and supplemental vitamins.

Client/Family Teaching

In the case of exophthalmus, teach client to:

Wear dark glasses to help keep dust and dirt out of eyes

Tape lids at night if necessary

Elevate head of bed (HOB) at night to decrease edema behind eyes

Teach client that while in hyperthyroid state, he or she must report infections promptly, because they can precipitate thyroid storm.

Evaluation

Treatment and client teaching are successful if:

- Client avoids postoperative complications
- Client can verbalize ways to prevent corneal injury
- Client's vital signs remain in normal range

Hypothyroidism

Hypothyroidism is caused by underactivity of the thyroid gland and insufficient amounts of thyroid hormone, which lead to a decrease in metabolism and a slowing of body processes. *Cretinism* refers to severe thyroid deficiency in infants (low hormone levels beginning *in utero*), causing defective development and mental retardation. *Myxedema* refers to thyroid deficiency in adults.

Assessment

Health Status

- Decreased pulse
- Lethargy, malaise, apathy
- Dry skin and hair
- Weight gain
- Sensitivity to cold
- Slowed physical and mental reactions

Developmental Assessment

Causes include:

Genetic defects

Low dietary iodine intake

Pituitary dysfunction

Subtotal or total thyroidectomy (always occurs after latter unless client takes hormone replacement)

Clients may become so apathetic and listless they cease to bathe and work, and do not seek help for themselves.

Diagnostic Factors

H and P

May have goiter (gland enlarges in effort to compensate for decreased secretion)

Low serum thyroxin levels

High serum cholesterol level

Nursing Plans and Interventions

Goals

- Thyroid hormone will be replaced

Nursing Measures

- Client may need subtotal thyroidectomy if goiter present and pressing on trachea—provide supportive care until hormone takes effect

Drug Therapy

Daily thyroid replacement, *e.g.*, sodium levothyroxine (Synthroid)

Nutrition Therapy

- Low-calorie diet until hormone levels rise and weight stabilizes at lower level
- Necessary caloric intake to maintain weight in appropriate range

Client/Family Teaching

Teach client:

Importance of taking thyroid replacement every day

To wear medic-alert bracelet or carry information about condition on person

Evaluation

Treatment and client teaching are successful if client:

- Increases physical and mental activity
- Maintains weight at normal level
- Shows improved skin turgor

Addison's Disease

Addison's disease involves primary adrenocortical insufficiency, resulting in inadequate amounts of glucocorticoids, cortisol, aldosterone, and androgens. The result is fluid and electrolyte imbalance, which can progress to dehydration and vascular collapse. CHO metabolism is altered, resulting in insufficient energy for body processes.

Assessment

Health Status

- Weakness, exhaustion
- Anorexia, N and V, weight loss
- Emotional disturbance
- Low blood pressure (BP), rapid pulse, shock state

Developmental Assessment

Addison's disease may be caused by a tumor or autoimmune disorder. It is more common, however, in clients receiving long-term steroid therapy if treatment stops abruptly, dose is decreased too rapidly, or if the client is under severe stress. These clients develop sudden weakness and shock and will die unless they receive steroid replacement quickly.

Diagnostic Factors

H and P

Series of 24-hour urine tests for 17 ketosteroids and 17 hydroxycorticosteroids

Nursing Plans and Interventions

Goal

- Hormone will be replaced

Nursing Measures

- Watch vital signs carefully for signs of circulatory collapse
- Assess client's condition preoperatively to see if he or she has been receiving steroid

therapy: if so, dose should be increased prior to surgery and decreased to original dose after surgery

Drug Therapy

Cortisone po (or IV in emergency)

Antacid to counteract ulcer-causing effects of steroids

Client/Family Teaching

Teach client to:

Take cortisone with meals to decrease GI irritation

Take medications as prescribed

Control exposure (avoid infection)

Wear medic-alert tag

Evaluation

Client teaching has been successful if client can verbalize understanding of need to take steroid medications as prescribed.

Blood Abnormalities and Related Conditions

Pernicious Anemia

Pernicious anemia is caused by deficiency of intrinsic factor, which causes inability to absorb vitamin B12. The condition often follows gastrectomy, in which many intrinsic-factor–secreting cells are removed, and also occurs in gastric atrophy. Without treatment, permanent neurologic impairment will occur.

Assessment

Health Status

- Sore mouth, beefy red tongue
- Weakness and pallor
- Fatigue
- Palpitations
- Weight loss
- Neurologic symptoms (tingling and numbness in hands and feet)
- Irritability and depression
- Jaundice (red cells are large and abnormal and are broken down more quickly, releasing heme, which becomes part of bilirubin)

Diagnostic Factors

Anemia

Morphological changes in RBCs

Elevated indirect bilirubin level

Elevated lactate dehydrogenase (LDH)

Schilling test

Therapeutic response to injections of vitamin B12

Nursing Plans and Interventions

Goals

- Client's tolerance to physical activity will increase
- Neurologic damage will be prevented
- Client will experience relief of symptoms

Nursing Measures

- Provide rest
- Provide blankets for warmth

Drug Therapy

Vitamin B12 injections every month for life (note that if administered orally, vitamin will not be absorbed without intrinsic factor, and even then absorbed erratically; injections ensure consistent dose)

May need iron supplements (because B12 stimulates RBC production, iron stores may be depleted)

Nutrition Therapy

- Well-balanced diet
- Supplemental vitamins

Client/Family Teaching

Teach client about:

Need to continue treatment even if feeling better

Course of disease—peripheral nerve functioning usually improves, but any spinal cord or brain damage will be permanent

Evaluation

Treatment and client teaching are successful if:

- Client experiences increased stamina and vitality
- Neurologic symptoms disappear

Nutritional Anemia

Nutritional anemia involves an anemia with nutritional factors. RBCs need iron, B complex vitamins and trace minerals to develop. Absence of any of these, whether due to decreased intake, or decreased utilization will cause anemia. When RBCs wear out and are broken down, the iron they contain is reused. Blood loss can be the cause of iron deficiency anemia.

Assessment

Health Status

- Fatigue
- Weakness
- Pale conjunctiva and mucous membranes
- Palpitations
- Dizziness
- Stomatitis
- Sensitivity to cold

Developmental Assessment

Most predisposed are:

Children in formative years (growth causes an increase in need for iron and vitamins)

Women of reproductive age (at risk for iron deficiency due to blood loss during menses and childbirth)

Elderly persons, if intake or utilization of iron and vitamins impaired

Diagnostic Factors

RBC count and hemoglobin level less than normal

Morphologic changes in RBCs provide clues about particular nutrient deficiency

History of blood loss or poor dietary habits

Psychosocial/Cultural Assessment

- Older people living alone may not be able or motivated to buy nutritious foods
- Vegetarians are at risk unless they plan diets with special care

Goals

- Nutritional deficiency will be identified and its cause eliminated

Nursing Measures

- Plan client's activities to conserve energy and allow for rest
- Provide extra warmth (blankets to conserve body heat; avoid heating pads)

Drug Therapy

Vitamin supplements and iron as needed (oral or parenteral)

Supplemental iron and vitamins as preventive measure when need is high (*i.e.*, in pregnant or menstruating women, children and adolescents)

Nutrition Therapy

- Basic four food groups
- Green, leafy vegetables
- Organ and muscle meats
- Yeast breads
- Citrus fruits

Client/Family Teaching

Teach client about importance of proper diet, including taking supplemental iron and vitamins.

Evaluation

Treatment and client teaching are successful if:

- Client demonstrates increased strength and vitality
- RBC count and hemoglobin level remain in normal range

Sickle Cell Anemia

In sickle cell anemia, a genetic defect in hemoglobin molecules causes RBCs to assume bizarre, distorted shapes during the deoxygenated stage. The alteration in shape interferes with the ability of the RBCs to move through tiny capillaries, and results in infarctions, pain, and tissue damage. Organs that are frequently damaged include the kidneys and brain.

Assessment

Health Status

- Episodes of severe pain due to hypoxia (called sickle cell crisis)
- Growth alteration during childhood
- Impaired renal function that often progresses to uremia
- Predisposition to cerobrovascular accidents (CVAs)

Developmental Assessment

Sickle cell anemia is a disease of childhood that limits a person's lifespan. Most clients do not survive beyond early adulthood.

Diagnostic Factors

Electrophoresis or special blood smears identifies hemoglobin S
Low hemoglobin level
Elevated reticulocyte level
Elevated bilirubin level
Hepatosplenomegaly

Psychosocial/Cultural Assessment

Sickle cell anemia primarily affects blacks, but also affects populations whose ancestors lived in areas where the incidence of malaria is high (*e.g.*, the Middle East).

Nursing Plans and Interventions

Goals

- Clients and parents will be able to identify and control factors that precipitate crises (imbalance between oxygen supply and demand)

Nursing Measures

- Provide supportive care during crisis
- Maintain high fluid intake to decrease blood viscosity; supplement oral intake with IV fluids if necessary
- Implement measures to control pain
- Provide oxygen therapy

Drug Therapy

Narcotics for pain relief during crisis
Sodium bicarbonate to correct the acidosis that develops during crisis
Daily folic acid supplements

Nutrition Therapy

- Balanced diet
- Supplemental vitamins

Client/Family Teaching

Teach client or family that client should:

Notify physician if fever, nausea and vomiting occur (can precipitate crisis)
Maintain fluid intake of 3000 mL/day
Keep immunizations current
Avoid extreme cold and high altitudes
Avoid pregnancy (poses very high risk)

Teach parents that:

Affected children are likely to be bedwetters because their kidneys may lose ability to concentrate urine
Genetic counseling is available; sickle cell trait can be identified, and if both parents carry

the trait, each child has 25% chance of having the disease

Evaluation

Treatment and client teaching are successful if client:

- Participates in many activities that are normally associated with his or her age group
- Remains free of pain and crisis

Leukemia

Leukemia is abnormal proliferation of immature, nonfunctioning WBCs. There are acute and chronic forms of the disease. Long-term remissions have been achieved in afflicted children. Remissions tend to be shorter in adults, and without a successful bone marrow transplant, the disease is fatal.

Assessment

Health Status

- Very high susceptibility to infection (often the cause of death)
- Severe anemia
- Petechiae, bruising, and bleeding due to low platelet count
- Pain resulting from infiltration of leukemic cells into organs and bones
- Hepatosplenomegaly

Developmental Assessment

The cause is unknown; the disease may involve a hereditary factor, and is sometimes associated with exposure to radiation and certain chemicals.

Diagnostic Factors

Very high WBC count
Low RBC count, hemoglobin level, and platelet count
Bone marrow biopsy confirms diagnosis

Nursing Plans and Interventions

Goals

- Client will achieve remission of disease process
- Client will be free of infection and hemorrhage

Nursing Measures

Chemotherapy is the treatment of choice to induce remission. Dose is limited by toxicity to bone marrow.

- Chemotherapy affects normal as well as abnormal cells—acts by interfering with cells' mitosis or reproduction; encourage use of half strength hydrogen peroxide mouth wash to reduce bacterial population and risk of infection
- Ensure high fluid intake because chemotherapy often causes nephrotoxicity

Nursing Care for the Client Receiving Chemotherapy

- Maintain constant infusion rate
- Watch IV site carefully; if infiltration occurs, remove needle and follow agency policy about application of ice to site; call physician so infusion can be restarted

Avoid contact between skin and chemotherapeutic agents by:

- Wearing gloves when handling infusion bags and equipment and following Centers for Disease Control (CDC) guidelines (see Table 8-1) when handling client's excretions (urine, stool, emesis); in case of contact, wash skin as soon as possible with soap and water

Control infection by:

- Restricting contact with visitors and staff who have active infections
- Arranging for private room
- Remembering handwashing before client contact

- Wearing gloves, mask, gown when caring for client (protective isolation) in some cases
- Permitting no live plants, flowers, or unpeeled fruits or vegetables in client's room

Control bleeding by:

- Avoiding invasive procedures (IMs, catheters, rectal temperatures, enemas, suppositories)
- Perform hematest on urine, stool, emesis
- Having client use soft toothbrushes or toothettes, electric razor
- Avoiding uncooked or unpeeled fruits and vegetables
- Instructing client to avoid forceful nose blowing
- Applying direct pressure to needle puncture sites for a minimum of 5 minutes, longer if oozing persists
- Assessing for increased intracranial pressure (may indicate intracranial hemorrhage)
- Assisting with platelet transfusions as ordered

Provide comfort by administering:

- Narcotics as ordered
- Anesthetic preparations, *e.g.*, viscous lidocaine (Xylocaine) for mouth lesions
- Antiemetics to control nausea

Provide opportunity for rest (client may be extremely fatigued due to low RBC count and hemoglobin level).
Encourage fluid intake.
Provide emotional support.

Drug Therapy

Chemotherapy: specific agents used depend on cell type and on research protocols
Antibiotics and antifungals as needed
Antiemetics
Narcotics
Allopurinol (controls serum uric acid levels, which rise as result of massive cellular destruction due to chemotherapy)

Nutrition Therapy

- High-calorie diet and high-fluid intake (both hard to maintain because of nausea caused by chemotherapy)
- May require TPN

Client/Family Teaching

Teach client about:

Terminology he or she will hear used
Purpose of treatment and what can realistically be expected
Ways to control infection and bleeding

Evaluation

Treatment and client teaching are successful if:

- Client achieves remission
- Client is able to discuss feelings with health care professionals or with significant others
- Bone marrow rebounds after chemotherapy

Hodgkin's Disease

Hodgkin's disease is a malignant condition in which abnormal cells replace the normal cells in the lymph nodes.

Assessment

Health Status

- Weakness and fatigue
- Generalized pruritus
- Painless, enlarged lymph nodes
- Unexplained fevers, night sweats, weight loss

Developmental Assessment

Most common in men between ages 20–40

Diagnostic Factors

H and P
Mediastinal mass may show on chest x-ray
Positive lymph node biopsy

Nursing Plans and Interventions

Goal

- Client will achieve permanent remission (possible if disease is diagnosed early)

Nursing Measures

- Provide care for client receiving chemotherapy as discussed in leukemia section
- Implement measures to control itching

Drug Therapy

Nitrogen mustard is commonly used chemotherapeutic agent—causes nausea, vomiting, diarrhea, and sore mouth; rarely causes alopecia

Nutrition Therapy

- Balanced diet
- Supplemental vitamins

Client/Family Teaching

Teach client:

That permanent sterility can result from chemotherapy—men may want to consider sperm banking prior to treatment
Ways to minimize side-effects of chemotherapy

Evaluation

Treatment and client teaching are successful if client:

- Maintains fluid and electrolyte balance while on chemotherapy
- Verbalizes understanding of how to prevent infection while bone marrow is suppressed
- Verbalizes concerns to health care professionals or significant others
- Remains free of Hodgkin's Disease after treatment

Ruptured Spleen

Ruptured spleen usually results from trauma (*e.g.*, auto accident, gunshot wound, severe blow) or from diseases that may weaken spleen (infectious mononucleosis and malaria). The problem is complicated by hemorrhage.

Assessment

Health Status

- Abdominal pain
- Symptoms of shock: elevated pulse and respirations, decreased BP
- Apprehension
- Restlessness
- Pale, clammy skin

Diagnostic Factors

H and P
Computed tomography (CT) scans

Nursing Plans and Interventions

Goals

- Hemorrhage will be controlled (usually by removing spleen)

Nursing Measures After Splenectomy

- Keep client npo until peristalsis resumes; can rinse mouth but cannot chew on ice chips or drink water
- Assess vital signs (VS) frequently because of danger of hemorrhage
- Measure urine output hourly (client will have had large blood loss—be sure kidney is adequately perfused)
- Assess level of consciousness (LOC) and orientation—will indicate improvement if good; restlessness can mean anoxia
- Assess for pulmonary complications of anesthesia
- Assess for infection

Drug Therapy

Analgesia for pain

Client/Family Teaching

Teach client that:

Other organs can assume functions of spleen
He or she will be more susceptible to pneu-

moccocal infections; physician may recommend vaccine

Evaluation

Treatment and client teaching are successful if client:

- Remains free of postoperative complications
- Verbalizes understanding of postoperative activity restrictions and need for follow-up care

Integumentary Abnormalities

Herpes Zoster (Shingles)

Herpes zoster (shingles) is a painful but self-limiting infection caused by a herpes virus. Vesicles and later crusts form on the skin, following the path of nerve routes. Lesions ultimately disappear, usually within 2 weeks. The virus lies dormant and causes recurrent attacks during times of stress or immunosuppression.

Assessment

Health Status

- Painful vesicular lesions

Diagnostic Factors

H and P
Physical examination

Nursing Plans and Interventions

Goals

- Lesions will heal without development of secondary infection
- Virus will not be transmitted to others.

Nursing Measures

- Implement comfort measures: cool soaks to lesions, antipruritic lotions
- Wear protective gloves when touching lesions

Drug Therapy

Antipruritics
Acyclovir to treat lesions (used prophylactically if client is immunosuppressed)
Analgesics for pain

Nutrition Therapy

- Balanced diet
- No dietary restrictions

Client/Family Teaching

Teach client about:

Importance of handwashing
Communicability of disease

Evaluation

Treatment and client teaching are successful if:

- Lesions heal and client experiences no pain or complications
- Client can verbalize ways to avoid infecting others

Contact Dermatitis

Contact dermatitis is caused by an irritant or allergen that comes into direct contact with skin or mucous membrane. Common causes are soaps, solvents, plants, hair dye. An example of contact dermatitis is poison ivy.

Assessment

Health Status

- Fine red rash, papules, and vesicles
- Weeping skin lesions
- Severe itching

Diagnostic Factors

H and P
Find specific causative irritant by trial and error

Nursing Plans and Interventions

Goals

- Lesions will heal without secondary infections

- Causative agent will be identified and reoccurrence prevented

Nursing Measures

- Provide wet soaks for 20 minutes 4 times a day to weeping lesions (Burow's solution often used)
- Provide colloidal baths to help control itching

Drug Therapy

Topical corticosteroids to dry lesions

Systemic steroids in severe cases

Antibiotics if secondary infection develops

Antipruritics, sedatives, and tranquilizers for itching

Client/Family Teaching

Teach client:

That condition can result from direct contact with irritant, including touching an animal or clothing that has contacted the irritant; can also occur as a result of inhaling smoke that contains the irritant

To avoid known irritants

To wash affected areas with alkaline soap and rinse well, if contact occurs

Evaluation

Client teaching is successful if client:

- Can describe ways to prevent infection in lesions
- Can describe steps to take in case of repeat contact with causative substance

Burns

Burns can be caused by heat, chemicals, radiation, or electric current. Burns interfere with functions normally carried out by the skin, which include providing a barrier to infection; conserving body heat and fluids; certain excretory and sensory functions; and providing a sense of personal identity (face). Burns may be accompanied by smoke inhalation, which can lead to edema of respiratory passages and suffocation.

Assessment

Health Status

- *First degree:* painful erythema (*e.g.*, sunburn)
- *Second degree:* pain, large blister formation; healing takes 2–4 weeks
- *Third degree:* entire dermis destroyed, including nerves and underlying muscle; no pain; requires grafting to heal; pain occurs as healing progresses; assess respirations to determine if smoke was inhaled

Nursing Plans and Interventions

Goals

- Extent of burn will be minimized (stop burning process)
- Fluids will be replaced
- Infection will be prevented

Nursing Measures

First Aid

- Stop burning—if person on fire, should "stop, drop, and roll"
- Flush with cool water, *not* ice
- Remove metal jewelry
- Do not remove adherent clothing
- *Do not* apply vaseline or ointment
- Assess and maintain airway
- Wrap in cleanest covering available (*e.g.*, clean sheet)

Minor Burns (Treated at Home)

- Clean burned area
- Apply topical ointment per physician's order
- Apply sterile dressings

Moderate and Severe Burns (Treated in Hospital)

- Insert airway if smoke has been inhaled
- Clean burned area (may debride also), and treat as above

- Replace fluid and electrolytes (client is losing massive amounts)
- Insert central line to take central venous pressure (CVP) reading to estimate circulating blood volume—helps calculate need for fluid replacement—take reading with client in same position each time, with zero point on manometer at level of right (R) atrium (4th intercostal space [ICS] and midaxillary line)
- Assist with wound coverings (often skin grafts from another species (*e.g.*, porcine) to provide temporary protection against infection, loss of body fluids and heat; eventually replaced with grafts of client's own skin)
- Provide support during extensive, painful physical therapy (PT) rehabilitation
- Apply pressure garment (Jobst stocking) over healing areas to control scar formation
- Provide emotional support; anger is a normal response that client needs to express

Drug Therapy

IV narcotics for pain control—area adjacent to burns very painful, especially during debridement, and later as nerves regenerate; pain is associated with the required extensive range of motion (ROM) exercises

Antibiotics

Tetanus prophylaxis

Human plasma protein fraction (Plasmanate) as part of IV intake (helps expand fluid volume; helps replace loss of proteins and thereby helps control additional fluid shifts)

Nutrition Therapy

- *High* caloric intake required (7000–8000 calories daily)
- Supplemental TPN may be required
- Oral intake started when peristalsis returns
- High-protein, high-CHO, high-iron diet (include spinach, organ meats, milkshakes)
- Vitamin supplements

Client/Family Teaching

Teach client about:

Need for painful procedures

Diet

Prevention:
    Install smoke detectors
    Use precautions while cooking
    Test water temperature before bathing, especially for small children
    Supervise children at all times
    Turn off Christmas tree lights at night and when away from home

Evaluation

Treatment and client teaching are successful if:

- Client's vital signs are in normal range
- Client's pain is controlled
- Fluid, electrolyte, and nutritional status are restored and maintained
- Client develops positive coping behaviors during recovery process
- Skin heals with minimum scarring and permits full range of motion

7

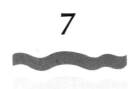

Nursing Care of the Client with Impairment in Sensorimotor Function

Central Nervous System Impairment

Head Injury

The category of head injury includes any injury to the head or brain. *Concussion* is transient paralysis of nerve function without any damage to cerebral tissues. *Contusion* is bruising of brain tissue characterized by coup/contracoup signs. *Coup* refers to bruising of brain at the site of injury. *Contracoup* refers to bruising or laceration of the brain opposite the site of injury.

Assessment

Health Status

- Change in level of consciousness
- Change in mental status
- Pupillary changes
- Changes in vital signs:
    Widening pulse pressure
    Elevated systolic pressure
    Decreased pulse rate
    Increased respirations
    Seizures
    Abnormal posturing
    Aphasia, hemiparesis, hemiplegia
    Projectile vomiting

Developmental Assessment

Males more at risk than females
15–40 years is age range at greatest risk

Diagnostic Factors

Computed tomography (CT) scan
Skull x-rays
Usually no lumbar puncture
Magnetic resonance imagery (MRI)

Nursing Plans and Interventions

Goals

- Intracranial pressure will decrease
- Complications from increased intracranial pressure will be prevented
- Client will achieve as much independence as possible

Nursing Measures

- Maintain patent airway with good respiratory exchange
- Position client supine with head above bed, elevated 30–45° or as ordered

- Maintain neutral head position
- Monitor for signs and symptoms of increasing intracranial pressure (use Glasgow coma scale):
    - Change in level of consciousness
    - Widening pulse pressure
    - Change in motor functions
    - Change in pupillary size, equality and accommodation
- Ensure client does not perform Valsalva maneuver
- Maintain seizure precautions (see convulsive disorders section)
- If clear oozing from nose or ear, test for presence of glucose
- Monitor intake and output (I and O) and laboratory values
- Maintain normothermia
- Maintain as quiet and unstimulating an environment as possible; ensure complete bedrest
- Administer prescribed medications

Medical/Surgical Treatment

Common sequelae to head injuries include:

Epidural hematoma—life threatening

Subdural hematoma (may be acute, subacute, chronic)—surgical intervention necessary

Subarachnoid hemorrhage—may need surgical intervention

Drug Therapy

Corticosteroids, such as dexamethasone (Decadron), to decrease cerebral edema; side-effects include impaired wound healing, headache, mood changes

Osmotic diuretics, such as mannitol, to decrease cerebral edema; side-effects include headache, dizziness, convulsion; administer IV through a filter; monitor for congestive heart failure (CHF)

Anticonvulsants for seizure control; side-effects include confusion, slurred speech, nystagmus

Ventilatory therapy: hyperventilating to decrease CO_2 in arterial blood to decrease cerebral vasodilation; PCO_2 is a potent vasodilator, as is lactic acid

Client/Family Teaching

Teach client about:

Potential for seizures as sequelae to trauma

Medications (dosage, purpose, side-effects)

Aids to independence if deficits result

Evaluation

Treatment and client teaching are successful if:

- No complications result
- Client is independent in activities of daily living (ADL)
- Intracranial pressure remains within normal limits

Brain Tumors

A brain tumor is a tumor or neoplasm that arises from any tissue within or outside the cranium or spinal cord. Brain tumors can be gliomas, meningiomas, pituitary adenomas, acoustic neuromas, hemangiomas, or dermoid cysts.

Assessment

Health Status

- Occur in great variety, so signs and symptoms depend on location, size, and invasive qualities of tumor
- Headache
- Visual disturbances, including papilledema
- Olfactory disturbances
- Abnormalities in other cranial nerves
- Difficulty with coordination or movement
- Seizures (without history of trauma)
- Changes in behavior, personality
- Decrease in mental functioning
- Dizziness and vertigo
- Projectile vomiting or other signs and symptoms of increased intracranial pressure (see head trauma section)

Developmental Assessment

May occur at any age, but generally highest incidence is between 40–70 years of age

Not usually hereditary except for tumors of neurofibromatosis

Diagnostic Factors

CT scans

Positive emission tomography (PET) scans

Skull x-rays

Electroencephalogram (EEG)

MRI

Arteriography

Brain scan

Lumbar puncture (except where contraindicated)

Echoencephalography

Psychosocial/Cultural Assessment

- High incidence of lung cancer metastasizing to the brain
- Cigarette smoking direct link with brain tumors

Nursing Plans and Interventions

Goals

- Intracranial pressure will remain within normal values
- Functioning will be maintained or restored
- Complications will be prevented
- Client will achieve as much independence as possible

Nursing Measures

- Monitor vital and neurologic signs
- Monitor I and O
- Monitor for changes in sensorimotor functioning, personality, behavior, mood
- Maintain seizure precautions (see convulsive disorders section)
- Provide emotional support
- Explain radiation/chemical therapy (dosage, effects, side-effects)
- Monitor laboratory values (complete blood counts if having chemotherapy)
- If client receiving chemotherapy, monitor for neurotoxicity, nephrotoxicity, cardiopulmonary toxicity, alopecia, bleeding
- If client receiving radiation therapy, perform skin assessments and provide skin care

Postoperative Care

- Position according to surgery (neutral head position): infratentorial—bed flat; supratentorial—head of bed at 30° angle
- Monitor for syndrome of inappropriate antidiuretic hormone (SIADH) and diabetes insipidus (DI)
- Monitor for seizures
- Assess for signs and symptoms of increased intracranial pressure and infection
- Prevent client from performing the Valsalva maneuver

Drug Therapy

Osmotic diuretics, such as mannitol, to decrease cerebral edema; side-effects include headache, dizziness, convulsion; administer IV through a filter

Corticosteroids, such as dexamethasone (Decadron), to decrease cerebral edema; side-effects include impaired wound healing, headache, mood changes

Antacids

Anticonvulsants such as phenytoin (Dilantin), used prophylactically for up to 1 year; side-effects include gingival hyperplasia

Nutrition Therapy

- May be anorexic—offer small, frequent meals, favorite foods
- May be fluid restricted

Client Teaching

Teach client about:

Radiation/chemotherapy effects, side-effects, dosage

Safety measures during and after seizure activity
ADL aids
Community supports
Signs and symptoms of increased intracranial pressure

Evaluation

Treatment and client teaching are successful if:

- Intracranial pressure remains within normal values
- No complications occur
- Client performs ADL independently
- No seizure activity occurs

Convulsive Disorders

Epilepsy and Seizures

Epilepsy and seizures result from excessive discharges of electrical impulses in the cerebral cortex.

Assessment

Classification of Convulsive Disorders
Focal or partial seizures
Generalized
Unilateral
Unclassified
Paroxysmal

Health Status
- Automatisms (automatic behavior or actions performed without conscious intent or knowledge)
- Change in level of consciousness
- Sensory or motor dysfunctions
- Asymmetry in body movements, reflexes
- Absence spells (brief temporary loss of consciousness)
- Incontinence

Developmental Assessment
Early adult years (18–35): convulsive disorders most commonly caused by trauma, neoplasms, epilepsy, alcohol, drug addiction
Middle adult years (35–60): convulsive disorders most commonly caused by neoplasms, alcohol, drug addiction, vascular disease
Older adult years (over 60): convulsive disorders most commonly caused by degeneration, tumors, vascular disease

Diagnostic Factors
EEG
Skull x-rays, CT scans
Serologic and spinal fluid examinations

Nursing Plans and Interventions

Goals
- Seizure activity will be controlled
- Injuries will be prevented

Nursing Measures

Assess and document seizure activity in early state by noting:

- Prodromal warning sign (aura)
- Epileptic cry

Assess and document activity in the ictal state by noting:

- Date, time, duration of seizure activity
- Site of onset and sequence of progression of seizure activity
- Pupillary size and reaction
- Loss of consciousness (how long)
- Deviation of head, eyes
- Tonic-clonic movements
- Clenching of teeth or jaw
- Biting of tongue or cheek
- Drooling or frothing at mouth
- Incontinence of urine or feces
- Diaphoresis
- Loss of consciousness

Assess and document activity in the postictal state by noting:

- Patency of airway, vital signs
- Memory impairment, headache, sleepiness, change in level of consciousness
- Injuries, *e.g.*, bruises, lacerations
- Paresis or paralysis of extremities

Protect from injury by:

- Padding side rails
- Raising side rails
- Maintaining bed in low position
- Inserting bite block or padded tongue blade immediately prior to onset of seizure
- Maintaining a clutter-free room

After a seizure:

- Reorient client and provide emotional support
- Assess for precipitating factors for seizure activity
- Monitor and administer anticonvulsant medications
- Explain lifestyle restrictions

Drug Therapy

Most Common Anticonvulsant Medications (Used to Control Seizure Activity)

Phenytoin (Dilantin) to control generalized seizures; side-effects include gingival hyperplasia, photosensitivity; continue medication even if client seizure-free

Carbamazepine (Tegretol) to control focal seizures and decrease neuronal excitability; side-effects include effects on neurologic, cardiovascular, renal, and digestive systems

Minor Tranquilizers

Diazepam (Valium) to depress the subcortical level of inhibition of electrical impulses; side-effects include drowsiness, dizziness, fatigue

Client/Family Teaching

Teach client about:

Lifestyle restrictions: driving, swimming, water activities

Medication: Dose, purpose, side-effects

Self-care

Evaluation

Treatment and client teaching are successful if client:

- Suffers decreased or no seizure activity
- Suffers no injuries
- Can name medications and state dose, effects, side-effects
- Can state lifestyle restrictions
- Is knowledgeable about condition and treatment

Meningitis

Meningitis is inflammation of the meninges of the brain and spinal cord due to invasion by bacteria, virus, or fungal organisms.

Assessment

Health Status

Types of Meningitis

- Aseptic: due to viral infection or irritation
- Septic: due to bacterial infections
- Tuberculous: due to tubercle bacillus

Signs of Meningeal Irritation

- Nuchal rigidity
- Severe headache
- Opisthotonic positioning
- Photophobia

Other signs include:

- Change in mental status
- Hyperirritability
- Seizures
- Skin rash
- Nausea, vomiting

Developmental Assessment

More frequent in children

In adults, caused by trauma or neoplasm

Diagnostic Factors

Skull x-rays of head and sinuses

Chest x-rays

Examination of cerebrospinal fluid
Lumbar puncture

Nursing Plans and Interventions

Goals

- Client will be as comfortable as possible
- Client will not suffer long-term deficits
- Nutritional and electrolyte statuses will be maintained

Nursing Measures

- Assess vital signs, level of consciousness and neurologic signs and symptoms
- Ensure appropriate infection control (respiratory isolation)
- Give tepid sponge baths, administer antipyretics, hypothermia blankets
- Maintain dark, nonstimulating environment
- Restrict visiting hours in acute stages
- Monitor I and O
- Position head of bed at 30–45°

Drug Therapy

Antibiotics, *e.g.,* penicillin, gentamicin, chloramphenicol

Antipyretics, *e.g.,* acetaminophen (Tylenol)

Nutrition Therapy

- Small, frequent feedings
- Fluid therapy: 3000 mL/24 hour

Client/Family Teaching

Teach client about:

Possibility of residual seizures
Medications (dose, effect, side-effect)

Evaluation

Treatment and client teaching are successful if client:

- Experiences no seizures or sensory or motor deficits
- Shows no further signs or symptoms of infection
- Is knowledgeable about condition and treatment

Multiple Sclerosis

Multiple sclerosis is a neurological demyelinating disease of the nervous system. It results in focal lesions in the brain and spinal cord.

Assessment

Health Status

- Episodic symptoms
- Fatigue

Visual Disturbances

- Diplopia
- Enlarged blind spot
- Nystagmus
- Optic neuritis

Motor Disturbances

- Weakness
- Spasticity
- Ataxia
- Tremors—intention tremors
- Staggering
- Paralysis
- Vertigo
- Dysarthria (difficult speech)
- Dysphagia (difficulty in swallowing)
- Urinary/bowel retention or incontinence

Personality/Emotional Disturbances

- Lapses in memory
- Emotional lability
- Depression
- Euphoria
- Impaired judgement/comprehension
- Difficulty conceptualizing
- Irritability

Sensory Disturbances

- Paresthesias (sensation of numbness)
- Loss of position sense
- Transient sensation of electric shocks (Lhermitte's sign)

Developmental Assessment

More females than males affected

Age group commonly affected is 20–40 years of age

Higher incidence in clients that contracted measles in childhood

Diagnostic Factors

EEG

CT scan

Examination of cerebrospinal fluid

Neurologic examination

Electromyography (EMG)

MRI

Psychosocial/Cultural Assessment

- Higher incidence in cold, damp climates

Nursing Plans and Interventions

Goals

- Precipitating and aggravating factors will be controlled
- Client will maintain highest possible level of independence
- Injury and infection will be prevented

Nursing Measures

- Administer medications and monitor for side-effects
- Reorganize environment to decrease intention tremors
- Encourage active and passive range of motion (ROM) exercise
- Provide bowel training
- Provide indwelling catheter care as appropriate
- Assist and support client to cope with chronic disease
- Assist with ADL as appropriate
- Identify factors precipitating exacerbations:
  Increased temperature
  Humid weather
  Intramuscular injections
  Fatigue
  Infections
  Hormonal changes

Drug Therapy

Steroids, adrenocorticotropic hormone (ACTH), prednisone to decrease inflammatory process; administer in morning with milk or meals to decrease gastric irritation

Muscle relaxants, *e.g.*, diazepam, to decrease spasticity; supportive treatment only

Nutrition Therapy

- Gluten-free diet, diet high in sunflower oil—controversial
- Diet high in bulk
- Dental soft diet if appropriate

Client/Family Teaching

Teach client about:

Avoiding fatigue, emotional stress, infections

Need for regular exercise, structured rest periods, good diet and adequate fluid intake

Medications: dose, effects, side-effects

Self-catheterization if appropriate

Importance of clutter-free environment to decrease intention tremors

Community resources

Evaluation

Treatment and client teaching are successful if client:

- Remains free from injury and infection
- Maintains stable weight
- Shows no muscle atrophy from disuse
- Is able to name medications and state dose, purpose, and side-effects, and explain exercise regimen
- Is knowledgeable about condition

Myasthenia Gravis

Myasthenia gravis is an autoimmune disorder of neuromuscular transmission, characterized by a decrease in acetylcholine or acetylcholine receptor sites.

Assessment

Health Status

- Weakness of voluntary muscles (become weaker with activity and improve with rest)
- Ptosis
- Diplopia
- "Snarly" smile
- Weak voice
- Nasal speech
- Dysphagia
- Close association with other autoimmune disorders, such as rheumatoid arthritis, lupus erythematosus, polymyositis, thyroid toxicosis

Developmental Assessment

Women under 40 years of age are 2–3 times more likely to be affected than men under 40

Women over 40 are also more likely to be affected than men over 40

Although not a hereditary disease, 15%–20% of infants born to a myasthenic mother have a transient case

Diagnostic Factors

Neurological examination
Tensilon test
Electromyogram
CT scan (for thymomas)
Thyroid studies

Nursing Plans and Interventions

Goals

- Client will not experience respiratory compromise
- Client will not experience myasthenic or cholinergic crisis
- Client will not suffer aspiration
- Client will cope effectively with changes in body image and self-concept

Nursing Measures

Monitor client for signs and symptoms of myasthenic crisis (not enough medication), including:

- Dyspnea, dysphagia, dysarthria
- Severe generalized weakness
- Increase in body secretions
- Apprehension
- Sudden marked increase in BP and pulse rate
- Absent cough reflex
- Urinary and fecal incontinence

Monitor client for signs and symptoms of cholinergic crisis (too much medication), including:

- Dyspnea, dysphagia, dysarthria
- Severe generalized weakness
- Increase in body secretions
- Apprehension
- Nausea, vomiting
- Abdominal cramps, diarrhea
- Muscle twitching
- Blurred vision
- Pallor

Medical/Surgical Treatment

Medication
Plasmapheresis
Surgery: thymectomy

Nursing Care

- Assess neurologic signs and symptoms (ptosis, swallowing ability, generalized muscle strength, vital capacity)
- Administer medications *exactly* on time (there is no half hour grace period)
- Plan client rest periods to avoid excessive fatigue
- Encourage independence but assist with ADLs as appropriate
- Ensure client avoids contact with people with infections

- If client will undergo a thymectomy, postoperative care is similar to general postoperative care but also includes frequent assessment of dressing, especially at back of neck, and for neck edema and crepitus
- If client requires ventilatory assistance due to respiratory failure, include frequent suctioning as appropriate, strict aseptic technique, consistent emotional support
- Ensure bed is in high-Fowler's position for eating or drinking, to decrease risk of aspiration

Drug Therapy

Anticholinesterase Medications, e.g., Pyridostigmine Bromide (Mestinon); Neostigmine (Prostigmin)

Inhibit the breakdown of acetylcholine

Administer *exactly* on time, even when npo

Monitor for crises

May be given with atropine (which may mask symptoms of impending crises)

Corticosteroids, e.g., Prednisone

Improve neuromuscular transmission

Administer with milk or meals in the morning

Monitor for side-effects

Nutrition Therapy

- Dental soft diet as appropriate for easy chewing
- May have nasogastric (NG) feedings in lieu of diet, due to dysphagia and potential for aspiration

Client/Family Teaching

Teach client about:

Stress management

Importance of seeking medical assistance when pregnant or with another illness (*e.g.*, infections)

Identifying activities, events that increase weakness

Avoiding extremes of temperature

Avoiding alcohol and caffeine

Medications: dose, purpose, side-effects, importance of taking medications on time and *never* skipping or changing dosage

Med-alert bracelet

Community and national support

Evaluation

Treatment and client teaching are successful if client:

- Remains free from crisis
- Has no respiratory or swallowing difficulties
- Is independent in ADL if appropriate
- Can name medication and state dose, purpose, side-effect
- Can state lifestyle adaptations necessary for independence
- Is willing to discuss chronic disease
- Is knowledgeable about disease

Parkinson's Disease

Parkinson's disease is a disorder of the extrapyramidal system (basal ganglia, thalamus, substantia nigra, red nucleus and the reticular formation), resulting from a deficiency or absence of the neurotransmitter dopamine. (Parkinsonian syndrome refers to symptoms mimicing Parkinson's disease but caused by medications or pathology).

Assessment

Health Status

- Involuntary tremors of hands, fingers, and head, aggravated by stress or fatigue
- Masklike facial expression
- Impaired voluntary movements
- Autonomic dysfunctions
- Depression
- Insomnia
- Rapid eye blinking
- Shiny, oily skin
- Muscle rigidity (cogwheel rigidity)

- Shuffling gait
- Akinesia (partial or complete loss of muscle movement)

Developmental Assessment

More males than females affected

Age group affected is usually people over 30

May be drug induced (long-term use of medications such as phenothiazines can produce parkinsonianlike symptoms

Diagnostic Factors

Neurological examination

Electromyography

Urine and cerebrospinal fluid studies for homovanillic acid (HVA, a metabolite of dopamine)

Observation of handwriting (cramped, small, irregular)

Nursing Plans and Interventions

Goals

- Client will achieve as much independence as possible
- Muscle contractures and atrophy will be prevented
- Skin integrity will be maintained
- Client will benefit from emotional support and understanding

Nursing Measures

- Assist with ADL as necessary
- Assist with exercises to lessen muscle rigidity
- Plan extra time for ADL so that client can maintain independence in self-care
- If client is incontinent, provide good hygiene and skin care
- If client is dysphagic, monitor diet consistency: food should be soft and easy to chew
- Monitor for side-effects of medication
- Encourage active and passive ROM exercises
- Ensure good oral hygiene
- Limit caffeine intake
- Prevent or limit alcohol consumption
- Monitor elimination patterns
- Encourage use of shoes, not slippers; encourage clutter-free room
- If client undergoes thalamotomy, nursing measures are same as for a client having neurosurgery

Drug Therapy

Levodopa (L-dopa)

Converted to dopamine in the brain

Administer with milk or meals to decrease gastric irritation

Monitor for orthostatic hypotension—change positions slowly

Carbidopa (Sinemet)

Used in conjunction with L-dopa because much of L-dopa is destroyed by gastric juices

Monitor for dyskinesia (defects in voluntary movement)

Monitor for orthostatic hypotension—change positions slowly

Anticholinergic Agents (e.g., *Benzotropine Mesylate*, [Cogentin], *Trihexyphenidyl Hydrochloride* [Artane])

Control drooling, rigidity, tremor

Suggest using hard candy, if possible, to promote salivation; anticholinergic drugs dry out mouth

Nutrition Therapy

- Dental soft diet as necessary
- Assist with feedings as necessary

Client/Family Teaching

Teach client about:

Medications: purpose, dose, side-effects (see drug therapy)

Community supports

Self-care assists, *e.g.*, Velcro fasteners instead of buttons; canes, walkers

Evaluation

Treatment and client teaching are successful if client:

- Maintains or increases level of independence with ADL
- Has decreasing or few episodes of emotional lability
- Can name medication and state dosage, effects, and side-effects
- Maintains skin integrity
- Remains free from injuries
- Is knowledgeable about disease and treatment

Larynx Impairment

Laryngeal Tumors

A laryngeal tumor is a neoplasm of the larynx that may involve only the glottic area (true vocal cords), or may extend to the supraglottic, subglottic or transglottic area. Ninety five percent of these neoplasms are composed of squamous cell carcinoma; others are composed of sarcomas and adenocarcinomas.

Assessment

Health Status

- Prolonged history of hoarseness (chronic laryngitis)
- Weight loss
- Inadequate nutritional intake
- Persistent cough
- Enlarged lymph nodes
- Aphonia (inability to speak)
- Painless lump in throat
- Pain on swallowing; burning pain in throat
- Dysphagia
- Dyspnea
- Foul breath

Developmental Assessment

Develops in middle to late adult years (ages 50–70) More males than females are affected, but the incidence of females being affected is increasing

Diagnostic Factors

Indirect laryngoscopy
Direct laryngoscopy
Biopsy
Tomography
Barium esophagogram

Psychosocial/Cultural Assessment

Associated with smoking, excessive alcohol intake, exposure to pollutants, occupational exposure to radiation, chronic infections

Nursing Plans and Interventions

Goals

- Client will experience decreased pain
- Client will increase nutritional intake
- Client will decrease or eliminate smoking or alcohol consumption

Nursing Measures

Preoperative Care

- Client may undergo partial or total laryngectomy or laryngofissure, so arrange visit by laryngectomee if possible
- Teach client about therapy, postoperative care, and loss of speech
- Ensure good oral hygiene
- Measure circumference of neck, assess gag reflex and coughing ability

Postoperative Care

- Suction as necessary
- Administer humidified oxygenated air
- Raise head of bed to a 30° angle
- Provide appropriate care for NG tube (decompresses stomach and prevents suture line contamination)
- Ensure good oral hygiene (*i.e.*, half strength hydrogen peroxide mouthwash every 2 hours)
- Assess for subcutaneous emphysema

- Support communication efforts, whether laryngeal, esophageal, or artificial speech, or surgical (prosthetic voice restoration)
- Provide appropriate care of wound drainage system (Hemovac)

General Considerations

- Liquefy secretions, and keep mucosa moist
- Offer foods that are easy to swallow
- Avoid offering acidic foods, to decrease pain
- Ensure good oral hygiene to relieve halitosis and prevent infection
- Assess for signs and symptoms of shock

Client/Family Teaching

Teach client to:

Recognize cancer warning signals

Use esophageal speech

Cover stoma when showering; keep shower head below level of neck

Use caution when washing hair

Avoid all water sports, if advised

Wear medic-alert bracelet

Suction and clean stoma

Practice good oral hygiene, including brushing tongue, palate, and inside of mouth

Seek medical attention for any respiratory tract infection

Avoid dusting powders after bathing

Avoid pollutants in environment, such as smoke, chemicals, hair spray

Evaluation

Treatment and client teaching are successful if client:

- Remains free of pain
- Can speak and has no difficulty swallowing
- Maintains weight and adequate nutrition
- Demonstrates proper technique for suctioning and cleaning laryngostoma
- Is knowledgeable about disease and treatment

Ear Impairment

Otosclerosis

Otosclerosis is a dystrophy of the temporal bone. It affects the bony labyrinth of the middle ear and causes a conductive hearing loss.

Assessment

Health Status

- Mild tinnitus
- Better hearing in a noisy environment
- Bilateral conductive hearing loss

Developmental Assessment

More females than males affected

Usually affects 15–45 year olds

Diagnostic Factors

Audiometry

Rinne test

Psychosocial/Cultural Assessment

- Hormonal changes, such as those associated with puberty, pregnancy, menopause, use of birth control pills, often exacerbate the disease
- More frequent in white population
- Increased rate of reoccurrence in black population

Nursing Plans and Interventions

Goals

- Injury will be prevented
- Client will be as comfortable as possible
- Client will not suffer further hearing loss
- Infection will be prevented

Nursing Measures

- Provide emotional support
- Assist with alternate forms of communication, *e.g.,* hearing aids, use of gestures
- Enforce smoking prohibition

Post-stapedectomy care includes:

- Assess for fever, vertigo, nausea, eye pain, headache
- Position client per physician's order (affected ear up or down)
- Explain that client must avoid blowing nose for 1 week
- Explain that client must avoid crowds or exposure to people with upper respiratory infection for 1 week

Drug Therapy

Antivertiginous agents, *e.g.* prochlorperazine (Compazine): side-effects include parkinsonianlike symptoms, postural hypotension, constipation

Client/Family Teaching

After surgery, teach client to:

Avoid sudden head movements

Call physician in case of changes in taste, or facial weakness

Postpone washing hair for 1–2 weeks

Avoid getting water into ear for 4 weeks

Avoid flying for 1 month

Teach client about:

Effects of smoking on ear

Importance of annual hearing tests

Medication: dosage, purpose, side-effect

Evaluation

Treatment and teaching are successful if client:

- Has maintained or restored hearing level
- Suffers no infection
- Suffers no injuries
- Does not smoke
- Is knowledgeable about condition and treatment

Meniere's Syndrome

Meniere's syndrome is a disorder of the labyrinth of the inner ear that results from an increased volume of endolymph.

Assessment

Health Status

- Alternating exacerbation and remission of signs and symptoms
- Dizziness
- Tinnitus
- Decreased hearing in affected ear
- Depression
- Nausea and vomiting, occurring especially with movement and head motion
- Headaches
- Vertigo
- Feeling of fullness in affected ear
- Ataxia during attack

Developmental Assessment

More females than males affected

Age group most commonly affected 40–60 year olds

Diagnostic Factors

Electronystagmography

Audiometry

Tuning fork test

Nursing Plans and Interventions

Goals

- Injury will be prevented
- Client will learn to manage own condition

Nursing Measures

- Provide emotional support
- Reduce stress
- Put side rails up, maintain bed in low position
- During attack, support head with pillows
- Administer medications as ordered
- Enforce smoking prohibition as appropriate
- Client may require assessments of drainage or signs and symptoms of infection following any surgical procedure on endolymph sac (shunting or decompressing)

Drug Therapy

Antivertiginous drugs, *e.g.*, dimenhydrinate (Dramamine), meclizine hydrochloride (Antivert), diphenhydramine hydrochloride (Benadryl)

Diuretics

Anticholinergics

Nutrition Therapy

- Salt-restricted or low-sodium diet
- Salt-free diet (Furstenberg diet)

Client/Family Teaching

Teach client about:

Smoking prohibition

Stress reduction strategies

Medications: dosage, purpose, side-effects

Dietary restrictions

Syndrome pathology and progression

Evaluation

Client teaching is successful if client:

- Copes positively and effectively with stress
- Avoids smoking
- Avoids injuries
- Is knowledgeable about condition and treatment

Eye Impairment

Glaucoma

Glaucoma results from an increase in intraocular pressure due to an imbalance between the production and outflow of aqueous humor. It results in atrophy of the optic nerve and loss of vision.

Assessment

Health Status

- Two types of glaucoma: acute or narrow angle, and chronic or closed angle (most common)
- Impaired peripheral vision
- Seeing halos or rainbows around lights
- Blind spots
- Poor night vision
- "Hard" eyeball
- Failure to perceive changes in color
- Decreased accommodation
- Periorbital discoloration
- Blurred vision

Developmental Assessment

Usually occurs after 40 years of age

May result from normal aging process

Most common form of blindness in United States

Diagnostic Factors

Visual fields test

Tonometry

Funduscopy

Psychosocial/Cultural Assessment

Most clients are elderly, and may require additional teaching and support services. The black population is more affected than the white population.

Nursing Plans and Interventions

Goals

- Client will suffer no further loss of vision
- Client will avoid injuries

Nursing Measures

- Administer prescribed eye medications
- Prevent client from performing Valsalva maneuver, because of increasing intraocular pressure
- Encourage routine eye examinations
- Depending on degree to which vision impaired, structure environment to prevent injury and promote independence: reduce clutter, increase lighting, avoid rearranging

furniture, arrange food on tray in consistent way (like time on a clock)
- Assist with ADL as appropriate but encourage independence

Medical/Surgical Treatment

Medication
Iridectomy
Trabeculoplasty
Trabeculectomy

Drug Therapy

Miotic eyedrops (pilocarpine): constrict pupil to enhance flow of aqueous humor; decrease amount of light and may increase risk of injury

β-adrenergic blockers, *e.g.,* timolol maleate (Timoptic)

Avoid administering any medication that dilates pupil (*e.g.,* atropine, antihistamines): may precipitate an attack and further damage the optic nerve

Client/Family Teaching

Client teaching may need to be creative, since many clients rely on vision to enhance learning. Teach client to:

Administer eye drops properly

Take medicines for lifetime

Wear medic-alert bracelet

Avoid over-the-counter cold remedies with antihistamines (may dilate pupil)

Understand medication dosage, purpose, side-effects

Avoid strenuous activities, constipation, and constrictive clothing around neck and waist

Provide for safety in home (*e.g.,* good lighting, especially all night in bathroom and on stairs; no clutter)

Call physician immediately in case of eye pain, sudden changes in vision, seeing halo around lights

Schedule routine eye examinations

Evaluation

Treatment and client teaching are successful if client:
- Suffers no further loss of vision
- Can self-administer eye medications properly
- Can name medications and state dosage, effects, side-effects
- Suffers no injuries
- Is knowledgeable about condition and treatment

Cataracts

Cataracts cause impaired vision due to opacity of the lens.

Assessment

Health Status
- Gradual, painless blurring of vision
- Monocular diplopia
- Gray or milky white appearance of pupil
- Irritation from glaring or bright lights

Developmental Assessment

Changes are due to normal aging process

Usually affects persons over 50 years of age

Cataracts may occur in an infant if its mother contracted rubella during first trimester of pregnancy

Clients with uncontrolled diabetes are prone to cataract formation

May be due to trauma

Diagnostic Factors

Ophthalmoscopy
Visual fields test
Funduscopy

Psychosocial/Cultural Assessment
- Elderly are primarily affected and may have need for additional teaching and support services

Nursing Plans and Interventions

Goals
- Client will avoid injury
- Client will not suffer further impaired vision
- If possible, client will have improved vision

Nursing Measures

Preoperative Care
- Instruct client not to touch affected eye
- Administer prescribed mydriatics or antibiotics
- Prevent client from performing Valsalva maneuver, or rapid eye movements
- Treat nausea and vomiting immediately
- Cut eyelashes (can use vaseline on scissors to avoid lashes falling into eye)

Postoperative Care
- Position client as ordered (on back or unoperative side)
- Assist with ADL if client has eyepatch or dark glasses and blurred vision
- Administer miotics or antibiotics as prescribed

Medical/Surgical Treatment

Medications
Cataract extraction (usually performed under local anesthetic and intraocular lens implantation)

Drug Therapy
Antibiotics (preventative measures)

Mydriatics (preoperatively): dilate pupil to facilitate operation; most commonly used mydriatic is atropine

Miotics (postoperatively): promote flow of aqueous humor; most commonly used miotic is pilocarpine

Client/Family Teaching
Teach client about:

Operative procedure (may be done on outpatient basis)

Postoperative self-care:
- Depth perception may be altered
- No reading for 24 hours
- No heavy work for 4–6 weeks
- No sexual relations for 1 week
- Wear sun glasses, (preferably wrap-around type), because of photosensitivity

Proper administration of eye medication

Medications: dosage, purpose, side-effects

Safety in home (no clutter, sufficient lighting in bathroom and stairs)

Importance of routine eye examinations

Evaluation
Treatment and client teaching are successful if client:
- Suffers no injuries
- Suffers no further loss of vision
- Has improved vision
- Suffers no infection
- Is knowledgeable about condition and treatment

Detached Retina

A detached retina results from separation of the retina from the choroid layer due to invasion of vitreous humor. It causes degeneration of the rods and cones and loss of vision.

Assessment

Health Status
- Shadow or "curtain" across eye
- Floating spots before eye
- Seeing flashes of light
- Blind spots
- Progressive loss of vision
- Blurred vision

Developmental Assessment

Normal aging changes may cause retina to detach from choroid

Higher incidence of retinal detachment among persons who play racket sports

Diagnostic Factors

Ophthalmoscopy
Visual acuity test
Visual fields test

Nursing Plans and Interventions

Goals

- Client will not suffer permanent loss of vision
- Client will be as comfortable as possible
- Client's anxiety will decrease
- Client will avoid injury

Nursing Measures

Preoperative Care

- Keep client in bed with eyes covered
- Maintain client's head in neutral position with retinal tear at lowest part of eye
- Administer prescribed sedatives and tranquilizers
- Provide emotional support

Postoperative Care

- Position client as ordered
- Maintain bedrest with eyes bandaged
- Apply cold compresses to reduce edema
- Prevent client from performing Valsalva manuever
- Promote safety (use side rails and place call bell within reach)
- Administer prescribed eye medications
- Provide emotional support

Medical/Surgical Treatment

Scleral buckle
Photocoagulation and laser beam treatment
Retinal cryotherapy

Drug Therapy (Preoperative and Postoperative)

Mydriatics (to dilate the pupil)
Cycloplegics (to paralyze ciliary muscle)
Steroids (to decrease intraocular pressure)
Antibiotics (to prevent infections)
Antiemetics
Analgesics and narcotics

Client/Family Teaching

Teach client to:

Contact physician if signs and symptoms of reoccurrence appear
Administer eye medication properly
Limit reading for 3 weeks
Avoid heavy lifting or sport activities for 4–6 weeks
Avoid sedentary work for 2 weeks
Have annual eye examinations

Evaluation

Treatment and client teaching are successful if client:

- Has improved or restored vision
- Suffers no injuries
- Suffers no infection
- Is knowledgeable about condition and treatment

Nose Impairment

Deviated Septum

A deviated septum protrudes into the nasal passage instead of maintaining its normal midline position.

Assessment

Health Status

- History of injury
- Postnasal drip
- Increased incidence of nasal obstruction with infections or allergies

Diagnostic Factors

Visual inspection
History of injury

Nursing Plans and Interventions

Goals
- Infection will be prevented
- Client will use enhanced nasal breathing

Nursing Measures

Postoperative Care
- Place in mid-Fowler's position
- Apply ice compresses to nose
- Monitor for signs and symptoms of nasal hemorrhage
- Assess for signs and symptoms of infection
- Provide frequent oral care
- Ensure client avoids blowing nose for 48 hours after packing is removed
- Ensure client avoids Valsalva manuever
- Expect to see tarry stools for several days postoperatively
- Provide emotional support for discolored and edematous face (lasts for 3–5 days)

Medical/Surgical Treatment
Submucosal resection (SMR)

Nasoseptoplasty

Drug Therapy
Antibiotics

Antihistamines to decrease nasal secretions

Nutrition Therapy
- Good fluid intake
- Client may be anorexic due to loss of smell: serve attractive and favorite foods

Client/Family Teaching
Teach client to:

Avoid Valsalva maneuver

Expect tarry stools for 2–4 days

Expect facial discoloration and edema 3–5 days

Maintain good oral care

Evaluation
Treatment and client teaching are successful if client:
- Suffers no infection
- Experiences increased ease of breathing

Skeletal Dysfunction

Fractures

A fracture is a break in the continuity of a bone.

Assessment

Health Status
General
- Signs and symptoms of fracture depend on type and location of fracture and extent of involvement of surrounding tissue
- Severe pain usually occurs immediately
- Point tenderness
- Edema at site of injury
- Ecchymosis at site of injury
- Muscle spasms
- Crepitation
- Paralysis
- Shock
- Deformity
- Impaired sensation
- Loss of normal function
- Abnormal mobility

Fractured Hip
- Affected hip abducted, externally rotated
- Affected leg shorter than unaffected leg
- Severe pain aggravated by movement
- Muscle spasms that intensify with movement
- Localized or peripheral edema
- Limited movement
- Temperature change in affected leg

Developmental Assessment

More common in elderly women because they are more likely to fall

May be caused primarily by degenerative or osteoporotic changes; women experience osteoporotic changes as result of menopause and have wider pelvis with tendency toward more hip deformities

Diagnostic Factors

X-rays
CT scans
Laboratory studies

Psychosocial/Cultural Assessment

- As dietary habits reduce calcium intake, incidence of fractures increases
- Clients on long-term steroid therapy more prone to pathological fractures

Nursing Plans and Interventions

Goals

- Client will not suffer complications
- Client will be as independent as possible
- Mobility will be restored

Nursing Measures

- Monitor vital signs frequently to assess for early signs and symptoms of infection
- Instruct client to turn, cough, breathe deeply every 2 hours
- Elevate injured part above level of heart if possible
- Administer prescribed narcotics and analgesics
- Apply ice packs to injured area as ordered
- Monitor I and O and regularity of bowel movements
- Use fracture pan as appropriate
- Encourage active ROM exercises on all unaffected extremities, isometric exercises on affected limb
- Use trapeze on bed as appropriate
- If or when limb is casted, support wet cast with pillows and handle with palms instead of fingers
- Inspect all areas of cast for drainage
- Assess for signs and symptoms of infection such as noxious odors, hot spots
- Assess distal extremities on affected limb
- Maintain alignment if affected extremity is in traction
- Assess for complications:
    Delayed union or nonunion of bones due to infections
    Disuse phenomenon
    Circulatory or nerve impairment
    Respiratory complications (pulmonary emboli)
    Infection
    Fat emboli
- Provide psychological support
- Provide good skin care in and around cast edges
- Maintain skin integrity on bony prominences

Postoperative Care (Internal Fixation or Hip Replacement)

- Assess for signs and symptoms of complications:
    Shock
    Hemorrhage
    Infection
    Paralytic ileus
    Fat emboli
    Thrombosis
    Hip dislocation
- Ensure client avoids acute flexion of operated hip
- Maintain internal rotation and extension—use trochanter rolls; may be in Buck's extension
- Turn client only with physician order
- Do not allow client to cross legs
- Encourage as much independence as appropriate

Drug Therapy

Prophylactic antibiotics
Muscle relaxants

Client/Family Teaching

Teach client to:

Use community supports
Use crutches if appropriate

Perform cast care

Not flex hip greater than 90°:
> Do not cross legs
> Do not flex hip when putting on shoes, socks
> Do not sit continuously for longer than 1 hour
> Do not sit in low, reclining or rocking chair
> Lie prone 30 minutes a day
> Place small pillow between knees when lying down

Perform prescribed exercises

Avoid driving for 6 weeks after surgery

Maintain safety in home (adequate lighting and caution on stairs)

Use slow, purposeful movements to gain balance upon rising

Evaluation

Treatment and client teaching is successful if client:

- Suffers no complications
- Is independent in ADL
- Has restored function
- Suffers no further injuries

Spinal Cord Injuries

Spinal cord injuries result from trauma to the spinal column. Destruction of gray matter and hemorrhage result from cord compression.

Assessment

Health Status

Below level of injury, client may experience:

- Decreased temperature control
- Decreased vasomotor tone
- Decreased sweating
- Decreased or absent reflexes
- Paralysis
- Paresia
- Urinary and fecal retention

Developmental Assessment

More males than females are injured

Usually affects persons 20–40 years of age

Diagnostic Factors

CT scan

Psychosocial/Cultural Assessment

Injuries usually result from car or motorcycle accidents, sports injury, or penetrating wounds (*e.g.,* gunshot).

Nursing Plans and Interventions

Goals

- Client will not suffer further cord injury
- Client will not experience respiratory difficulties
- Client will be as independent as possible
- Client will not experience complications

Nursing Measures

Acute Phase

- Assess neurologic and vital signs frequently
- Document location or absence of pain
- Assess respiratory status
- Assess muscle tone and activity
- Assess I and O
- Assess for spinal shock
- Enforce prescribed immobility (skeletal traction, tongs)
- Administer analgesics
- Encourage active/passive ROM exercises
- Provide adequate rest periods

Rehabilitative Phase

- Prevent complications of immobility
- Maintain skin integrity of bony prominences
- Perform measures described above
- Enforce daily bowel and bladder routine
- Teach self-catheterization
- Assess for signs and symptoms of autonomic dysreflexia: headache, increased blood pressure, bradycardia

- Monitor for possibility of paralytic ileus
- Provide sexual counseling
- Provide psychological and emotional support
- Refer client to home health agencies if appropriate

Drug Therapy

Corticosteroids to reduce cord edema

Antibiotics, prophylactically, if injury due to trauma

Stool softeners

Nutrition Therapy

- Diet high in bulk
- Prune juice
- Good fluid intake

Client/Family Teaching

Teach client about:

Self-catheterization

Transfer techniques

Aids to independence

Community supports

Skin assessments and skin care

Exercises as appropriate

Medications: dosage, purpose, side-effects

Evaluation

Treatment and client teaching are successful if client:

- Achieves maximum autonomy and independence
- Experiences no infection or complications
- Demonstrates positive acceptance of condition

Amputations

Amputation is removal of all or part of an extremity due to trauma or disease. Common etiologies are peripheral vascular disease, diabetes mellitus, arteriosclerosis, infection (*e.g.*, osteomyelitis), tumors, frostbite, and burns.

Assessment

Health Status

There are two types of surgical amputations: *open*, or *guillotine*, in which wound edges are left open so that purulent material may drain; and *closed*, or *flap*, in which the bone is cut shorter than the skin and muscles so that a flap can be created over the end of the stump.

Developmental Assessment

Amputations necessitated by disease (*e.g.*, peripheral vascular disease) usually affect elderly

Amputations necessitated by trauma usually affect men rather than women

Nursing Plans and Interventions

Goals

- Client will accept his or her condition
- Client will not suffer complications
- Client will be as independent as possible with ADL

Nursing Measures

Preoperative Care

- Provide foot board or cradles on bed as appropriate
- Elevate head of bed on shock blocks
- Administer prescribed narcotics and analgesics
- Provide preoperative teaching
- Openly discuss loss of body part
- If appropriate, maintain strength of extremity proximal to anticipated amputation through exercise

Postoperative Care

- Monitor vital signs, assess for signs and symptoms of shock, hemorrhage
- Maintain integrity of soft or rigid dressing
- Elevate affected limb
- Maintain proper body alignment
- Administer prescribed narcotics and analgesics

- If lower extremity amputated, have client in prone position for 30 minutes, 3–4 turns/day
- Use trochanter rolls as appropriate to maintain proper limb alignment
- When ordered, rewrap stump 4 times a day (to reduce edema and shape stump for prosthesis)
- Assist with active and passive ROM exercises
- Practice active listening and provide emotional support
- Have person with similar amputation visit client

Drug Therapy

Antibiotics (mainly used prophylactically)

Muscle relaxants to reduce spasms

Client/Family Teaching

Teach client about:

Stump bandaging

Exercises

Phantom-limb sensation/pain

Assistance with aids for ADL

Community support

Evaluation

Treatment and client teaching are successful if client demonstrates:

- No complications
- Positive acceptance of condition
- Independence in ADL

Joint Dysfunction

Osteoarthritis

Osteoarthritis is a nonsystemic disease of articular cartilage. It affects only joints and surrounding tissue. The joints become soft and rough due to enzyme digestion. Osteoarthritis is also called degenerative joint disease (DJD).

Assessment

Health Status

- Joint tenderness on palpation
- Crepitus on motion
- Presence of Heberden's nodes
- No inflammation
- Pain in movable weight-bearing joints, joints of hand
- Stiffness
- Decreased ROM

Developmental Assessment

More females than males affected

Usually affects persons 50–70 years of age

Associated with aging process

Diagnostic Factors

Serologic and synovial fluid examinations show no inflammatory changes

X-rays show narrowing of joint space and osteophyte formation

Psychosocial/Cultural Assessment

- Elderly clients are likely to have more difficulty coping with disease due to weaker support systems and decreased financial resources
- Clients that are obese are more prone to disease due to joint trauma

Nursing Plans and Interventions

Goals

- Client will experience decreased pain and swelling
- Client will increase activity and carry out ADL independently
- Client will decrease weight as appropriate

Nursing Measures

- Monitor pain and medicate as prescribed
- Provide hot/cold therapy as appropriate
- Structure periods of activity with periods of rest

- Encourage passive and active ROM activity
- Administer topical analgesic creams
- Monitor low-calorie dietary needs and refer for dietary consult as appropriate

Drug Therapy

Analgesics: aspirin, acetaminophen (Tylenol), propoxyphene hydrochloride (Darvon) to reduce pain; administer with milk or antacid to reduce gastric irritation

Nonsteroidal anti-inflammatory drugs (NSAID) such as ibuprofen (Motrin)

Nutrition Therapy

- Low-calorie, weight-reduction diet as appropriate
- Well-balanced diet

Client/Family Teaching

Teach client about:

Medications: purpose and side-effects

Pain reduction measures

Disease and activities that aggravate pain

Evaluation

Treatment and client teaching are successful if client:

- Experiences relief from pain
- Can state pain relief measures
- Can name medications and state dosage, route, purpose, side-effects
- Maintains weight at appropriate level
- Is knowledgeable about condition and treatment

Gout

Gout is a metabolic disorder caused by overproduction and accumulation of uric acid in the blood and by the deposition of uric crystals around and in joints and articular tissue.

Assessment

Health Status

- Extreme pain, swelling, and erythema in joints, especially great toe
- Signs and symptoms of inflammation may disappear during day but return at night
- Appearance of Tophi nodules
- May also have renal dysfunctions (albuminuria, renal calculi)
- May have gastrointestinal disturbances (anorexia, malaise)
- May exhibit tachycardia

Developmental Assessment

Genetic or familial tendency

Peak age of onset is 50–55 years of age

Higher incidence among males than among females

Diagnostic Factors

Serum studies

Synovial fluid examinations

X-rays of joints

Sedimentation rate measure

Psychosocial/Cultural Assessment

Higher incidence among alcoholics

Nursing Plans and Interventions

Goals

- Client will experience decrease in acute pain
- Client will not suffer reoccurrence
- Client will recognize and avoid precipitating factors
- Client will not suffer deformities

Nursing Measures

Acute Phase

- Promote complete bedrest
- Provide foot boards, cradles to decrease pressure on affected joints
- Apply hot or cold packs to decrease pain or inflammation
- Administer prescribed analgesics
- Assess for renal involvement: strain urine for presence of crystals; note flank pain
- Encourage good fluid intake
- Monitor I and O

Drug Therapy

NSAID, *e.g.*, naproxen (Naprosyn) and indomethacin (Indocin) for acute attacks

Drugs that enhance renal excretion of uric acid, *e.g.*, sulfinpyrazone (Anturane) and probenecid (Benemid)

Drugs that decrease production of uric acid: *e.g.*, allopurinol (Zyloprim)

Nutrition Therapy

- Low-fat, low-purine diet
- Increase fluid intake (2–3 L/day)
- Decrease consumption of kidney, liver, sweetbreads, red meats, beans, mushrooms
- Eliminate consumption of glandular meats, roe, shellfish, sardines, brain
- Include foods low in purine—vegetables (except legumes), eggs, cheese, nuts, gelatin

Client/Family Teaching

Teach client to:

Identify precipitating causes of attacks and attempt to control causes

Eliminate alcohol consumption

Understand medications: dosage, purpose, side-effects

Avoid using aspirin (counteracts uricosuric agents, *e.g.*, probenecid)

Follow low-calorie diet to lose weight, if appropriate—discourage fasting

Adhere to diet, medication regimen, increased fluid intake instructions

Evaluation

Client teaching is successful if:

- Pain is alleviated or decreased
- Activity is increased
- No deformities result
- Client is knowledgeable about disease and treatment

Rheumatoid Arthritis

Rheumatoid arthritis is a chronic systemic autoimmune disease of the joints that results from an inflammation of the synovial lining of the joints. The heart, lungs, bones, muscles, and eyes are also affected.

Assessment

Health Status

- Lymphadenopathy
- Peripheral neuropathy
- Fever
- Muscle atrophy
- Myositis
- Skin ulcers
- Weight loss
- Stiffness, redness, swellings, and warmth of affected joints
- Subcutaneous nodules (commonly found in subcutaneous area)
- Swan neck deformity and pain on movement
- Chronic effusions and nodules of lungs
- Pericarditis, cardiomyopathy, and cardiac valvular lesions
- Joint involvement, usually symmetric
- Joints most commonly involved are hands and feet

Developmental Assessment

More females affected than males; 2:1 or 3:1

Begins during years when career and family responsibilities are heaviest: 30–50 year old

Diagnostic Factors

Positive rheumatoid factor—"latex agglutination"

Increased sedimentation rate

Mild leukocytosis

Biopsy shows inflammatory changes in synovial tissue

X-rays show narrowing of joint space

Aspiration of synovial fluid shows increased turbidity and decreased viscosity

Psychosocial/Cultural Assessment

- Many "quack" remedies abound
- Common practice to wear copper bracelet

around affected joints—no scientific evidence that it helps

Nursing Plans and Interventions

Goals
- Inflammatory process will be controlled and client's pain will decrease
- Client will maintain functioning of all joints
- Client will not suffer deformities
- Client will be as mobile and independent as possible
- Client will cope positively with chronic disease
- Client will understand disease process and strategies to combat it

Nursing Measures
- For subacute or chronic pain, use heat to relieve stiffness and relax muscles
- For acute pain, use cold to prevent further edema and reduce stiffness
- Ensure client avoids joint positions that encourage contraction
- Encourage active and passive ROM activity
- Promote frequent changes of position
- Encourage wearing of shoes, not slippers
- Use resting splints
- Provide periods of activity as well as rest
- Use techniques of joint protection:
  - Use strongest joints (e.g., elbow, not wrist)
  - Maintain proper body alignment
  - Avoid twisting movements
- Evaluate for migratory joint involvement
- Monitor sedimentation rates
- Medicate client for pain prior to exercise and physical therapy
- Evaluate psychosocial aspects of client's condition: self-esteem, body image, depression
- Postoperatively from synovectomy, arthrotomy, or arthroplasty:
  - Maintain joint at rest for 3–5 days
  - Encourage passive ROM activity of affected joint when ordered
  - Encourage active ROM activity of affected joint 3–5 days postoperatively

Drug Therapy
Analgesics, salicylates: reduce inflammation and pain; administer with food or antacids to avoid gastric irritation

NSAID, e.g. indomethacin (Indocin), ibuprofen (Motrin), tolmetin sodium (Tolectin): inhibit inflammatory process

Steroids, e.g., prednisone: administer with food or antacid to prevent gastric irritation; administer only in morning; do not change dosage unless physician prescribes

Gold salts: suppress release of histamine prevent prostaglandin synthesis; suppress cellular immunity

Heavy metal antagonist (D-penicillamine): suppresses collagen formation

Nutrition Therapy
- Weight reduction if appropriate to decrease weight bearing on affected joints
- Well-balanced diet

Client/Family Teaching
Teach client about:

Purpose and side-effects of medication
Chronic disease
Joint protection and body alignment
Community supports
Importance of exercise or active ROM activity

Evaluation
Treatment and client teaching are successful if client:
- Feels relief from pain
- Experiences no further joint deformity or immobility
- Is able to perform active ROM exercises
- Is able to explain disease process and effects, dosage, and side-effects of medication

8

Nursing Care of the Client with Dysfunction of the Genitourinary and Reproductive Systems

Female Reproductive Problems

Uterine Fibroids or Uterine Leiomyomas

Uterine fibroids and leiomyomas are usually benign, slow-growing tumors of smooth muscle and connective tissue.

Assessment

Health Status

- Pain
- Low abdominal pressure
- Heavy or painful menstruation, irregular bleeding (menorrhagia)
- Backaches
- Constipation
- Dysmenorrhea (pain associated with menstruation)
- Enlarged, irregular uterus
- Urinary frequency
- Varicosities of lower extremities or vulva
- Anemia from heavy menstrual flow

Developmental Assessment

20%–25% of women over 30 develop this problem; more common in women who have never been pregnant

Tumor usually decreases in size after menopause

Diagnostic Factors

Pelvic examination

Pregnancy tests

Psychosocial/Cultural Assessment

- More common in black females

Nursing Plans and Interventions

Goals

- Client's childbearing ability will be preserved if possible
- Client will experience decrease in associated symptoms, *e.g.*, fatigue due to anemia

Nursing Measures

- Surgery usually performed only if symptoms severe

- See hysterectomy and endometriosis sections

Medical/Surgical Treatment

Myomectomy: removal of myoma or uterine tumor; performed if tumor interfered with maintaining a pregnancy

Hysterectomy: removal of uterus, no longer commonly used unless tumor enlarges to a 12-week gestation size or if excessive uterine bleeding is interfering with activities of daily living (ADL)

Drug Therapy

Vitamin B and iron therapy

Nutrition Therapy

- Foods high in iron
- High-fiber foods such as liver, oysters, clams, lean meat, leafy green vegetables, bran

Client/Family Teaching

Teach client to:

Report any changes in bleeding pattern to physician

Report heavy or prolonged menses to physician

Evaluation

Treatment and client teaching are successful if:

- Client can name medications and state dose, action, side-effects
- No further uterine bleeding occurs
- Client has increased energy levels
- Client's childbearing ability is preserved if appropriate
- Client is knowledgeable about condition and therapy

Uterine Prolapse

Uterine prolapse is marked downward displacement of the uterus.

1st degree: cervix remains in vagina
2nd degree: cervix protrudes from vaginal orifice
3rd degree: uterus protrudes from vaginal orifice

Assessment

Health Status

- Dysmenorrhea
- Chronic backache
- Pelvic pressure
- Easy fatigue
- Leukorrhea (white discharge from the vagina)
- Cervical ulcerations in 2nd and 3rd degree prolapse

Developmental Assessment

Condition may be due to:

Congenitally weak uterine ligaments
Strain of pregnancy (enlarging uterus)
Pelvic surgery
Adhesions following infections

Diagnostic Factors

History and physical examination
Pelvic examination

Nursing Plans and Interventions

Goals

- Client's pain will be reduced
- Client will be knowledgeable about condition
- Client's uterus will be restored to normal anatomic position or removed

Nursing Measures

- Encourage prescribed exercises utilizing gravity to restore uterus to normal position:
    "Monkey trot": walking on hands and feet with knees straight
    Knee-chest position
- Pessary must be removed at least once a day for cleaning by client, or by nurse if client is unable

Medical/Surgical Treatment

Hysterectomy

Insertion of pessary into vagina to treat uterine prolapse (also used for retroversion or cervical incompetence)

Exercises

Evaluation

Treatment and client teaching are successful if:

- Client experiences decreased pain
- Uterus returns to normal anatomic position
- Client is knowledgeable about condition and exercises
- Client is knowledgeable about need to remove and clean pessary if appropriate

Pelvic Inflammatory Disease and Salpingitis

Pelvic inflammatory disease (PID) is an infectious process involving the Fallopian tubes, ovaries, pelvic peritoneum, veins or connective tissue. Salpingitis is inflammation of the Fallopian tube and is the most common type.

Assessment

Health Status

Acute Phase
- Malaise
- Chills
- Fever
- Nausea and vomiting
- Tachycardia
- Severe lower abdominal pain
- Rebound tenderness
- Tender cervix
- Spotting, leukorrhea
- Dyspareunia (painful intercourse)
- Foul-smelling vaginal discharge

Chronic Phase (Due to Undiagnosed, Inadequately Treated, or Neglected PID)
- Low-grade fever
- Malaise
- Persistent abdominal aching
- Chronic low back pain
- Weight loss
- Enlarged, immobile adnexal muscle
- Retroverted uterus
- Menstrual disturbances

Developmental Assessment

May be complication of rupture of an adjacent structure (*e.g.,* appendix)

Infertility is common result

Diagnostic Factors

Rubin's test: tests patency of Fallopian tubes

Hysterosalpingogram: x-ray film of uterus and Fallopian tubes

Laparoscopy, culdoscopy

Serum cultures, vaginal smears

Sedimentation rate measures and white blood cell count

Psychosocial/Cultural Assessment
- May be complication of venereal disease (gonorrhea, chlamydia)
- May be complication of abortion
- Five times more common in women using intrauterine devices

Nursing Plans and Interventions

Goals
- Client will not suffer reoccurrence of PID
- Client's pain will be reduced
- Client will demonstrate positive coping regarding feelings about sexuality and reproduction

Nursing Measures
- Administer prescribed medications
- Promote bedrest (mid-Fowler's position)
- Provide hot water bottle or heating pad to lower abdomen to promote circulation and comfort
- Assess vaginal discharge (odor, amount, consistency, color)

- Monitor vital signs, especially temperature
- Assess level of pain
- Use active listening skills and provide emotional support
- Encourage sexual counseling if appropriate

Medical/Surgical Treatment

Salpingectomy

Pelvic exenteration: removal of all reproductive organs

Drug Therapy

Antibiotic therapy: cefoxitin, amoxicillin, penicillin

Probenecid: inhibits renal tubular excretion of organic compounds, such as antibiotics, thus increasing the time antibiotic remains in body

Client/Family Teaching

Teach client about:

Effects of PID on general health and reproductive functioning

Genital/rectal hygiene measures

Good handwashing techniques

Medications: dosage, effects, side-effects

Signs and symptoms requiring medical attention: return of original signs and symptoms or increased vaginal discharge

Evaluation

Treatment and client teaching are successful if client:

- Is able to name medication and state dosage, effects, side-effects
- Experiences no further complications
- Experiences no pain
- Employs positive coping mechanisms regarding sexuality and reproduction

Endometriosis

Endometriosis is the presence of functioning endometrial tissue outside the uterus. The problem results from a reflux of endometrial tissue into the pelvic cavity at the time of menstruation.

Assessment

Health Status

- Signs and symptoms are based on location of lesion or tissue (ovary is most common site of implantation of endometrial tissue)
- Dysmenorrhea
- Severe dyspareunia
- Sacral backache
- Infertility
- Menstrual abnormalities such as premenstrual spotting
- Pain (not always present)

Developmental Assessment

Difficult to discern because client may exhibit no signs or symptoms

Average age of those affected is 37–40 years

Diagnostic Factors

Laparoscopy (examination of abdominal cavity with a laparoscope)

Laparotomy (exploratory surgery through peritoneal cavity)

Biopsy

Psychosocial/Cultural Assessment

- Usually occurs in women who have delayed childbearing
- Higher incidence among women of higher socioeconomic status
- Uncommon among black women

Nursing Plans and Interventions

Goals

- Client's pain will be reduced
- Client will demonstrate positive coping with sexuality/reproductive issues (improved self-concept)
- Client will achieve pregnancy if desired or appropriate

- Client will not experience complications from surgery

Nursing Measures

- Administer prescribed medications
- Use active listening skills and provide emotional support (strong possibility of infertility)
- Provide appropriate counseling about childbearing (do not delay childbearing; risk of infertility increases as age increases)

Preoperative Care for Client Undergoing Total Hysterectomy and Bilateral Salpingo-Oophorectomy (TAH-BSO)

- Removal of Fallopian tubes and ovaries
- May be performed as either abdominal or vaginal surgery
- Provide emotional support (client may have feelings of loss and grief, or body image and self-conflict distress)
- Administer prescribed antiseptic vaginal douche

Postoperative Care

- Keep client npo until bowel sounds occur, then progress as tolerated
- Relieve flatulence by administering prescribed medications (simethicone) and encouraging prescribed exercises
- Administer prescribed analgesics or narcotics
- Assess for signs and symptoms of complications:
    - Hemorrhage (observe perineal pads for bright red blood; monitor blood pressure and pulse)
    - Pneumonia, bronchitis (encourage mobility and pulmonary exercises)
    - Infected wound sites (assess for foul-smelling vaginal or abdominal discharge)
    - Urinary tract infections (assess drainage for hematuria, encourage fluid intake)
    - Peritonitis (assess for abdominal pain, rigid abdomen, nausea, vomiting, and fever)
    - Thromboembolic conditions (antiembolic stockings should be worn; avoid positions that restrict venous return from legs; assess for rapid pulse, dyspnea, and chest pain)

Care for Client Receiving Blood Transfusions

- Take baseline vital signs immediately before administering blood
- Retake vital signs again in 15 minutes and then every hour until transfusion complete
- Maintain rate of infusion for first 15 minutes at no greater than 2 mL/min
- Most reactions occur within first 15 minutes of receiving blood or blood products
- Monitor client for fever, chills, pruritus (itching), change in vital signs (increased pulse, decreased blood pressure), pain (especially in flank area)
- In case of reaction, stop transfusion immediately; notify physician, keep vein open with normal saline; save unused blood and return to lab with proper notification

Medical/Surgical Treatment

Medications: analgesics or hormones
TAH-BSO

Drug Therapy

Antigonadotropin: synthetic androgen, *e.g.*, danazol; causes amenorrhea; side-effects include weight gain, acne, decrease in breast size, oily skin, deepening of voice; contraindicated for pregnant or breast-feeding women

High-dose birth control pills to shrink endometrial tissues

Client/Family Teaching

Teach client about:

Disease process and results of disease (infertility)

Importance of not delaying childbearing, if appropriate

Medications: dosage, effect, side-effects

Postoperative restrictions if applicable: no heavy lifting, no climbing stairs for 2–4 weeks; no sexual intercourse for 4–6 weeks

Evaluation

Treatment and client teaching are successful if client experiences:

- No complications from surgery
- Decreased pain
- Positive self-concept

Ovarian Cancer

Ovarian cancer is one of the leading causes of female deaths from cancer. More neoplasms come from the ovary than from any other reproductive organ. Ovarian cancer is difficult to detect; therefore the disease has frequently already spread when discovered.

Assessment

Health Status

- Enlarging abdominal girth
- Abdominal pain, pressure
- Nausea, vomiting
- Constipation
- Urinary frequency
- Abdominal or adnexal mass

Developmental Assessment

Can occur at any age, but greatest incidence is among women 40–60 years of age

Women at high risk include those who are infertile, nulliparous, or who have experienced early menopause (due to an ovarian imbalance)

Diagnostic Factors

Laparoscopy, laparotomy
History and physical examination

Psychosocial/Cultural Assessment

- Familial history predisposes
- Higher incidence in industrialized countries; a relationship may exist between exposure to chemical products and ovarian cancer
- Relationship between ovarian cancer and diet high in animal fat

Nursing Plans and Interventions

Goals

- Client will maintain positive self-concept
- Client will not suffer infection

Nursing Measures

- Practice active listening and provide emotional support
- Provide nursing measures for clients having radiation or chemotherapy (see testicular cancer section), postoperatively for abdominal hysterectomy, oophorectomy, salpingectomy
- Use aseptic technique when changing dressing
- Measure and record amount and character of drainage, if drainage device utilized
- Monitor I and O, vital signs
- Administer prescribed narcotics and analgesics
- Provide early ambulation to assist with peristalsis
- Prevent complications of immobility following surgery, by maintaining pulmonary hygiene and good circulation, and monitoring fluid and electrolyte imbalances

Drug Therapy

Narcotics and analgesics for pain, such as meperidine hydrochloride (Demerol) meperidine hydrochloride with phenergan, proproxyphene hydrochloride (Darvon)

Antibiotics, if appropriate, to prevent or treat infection

Antiflatulent medications such as Simethicone (Mylicon) to facilitate movement of flatus and to decrease pain

Client/Family Teaching

Teach client about:

Medications: dose, purpose, side-effects

Long-term therapy—radiation or chemotherapy

Prescribed postoperative restrictions on activity, including sexual activity

Evaluation

Treatment and client teaching are successful if client:

- Shows no signs and symptoms of infection
- Is pain free
- Maintains positive self-concept

Breast Cancer

Breast cancer is carcinoma of breast tissue, most commonly epithelial breast tissue. It is the most common cause of cancer deaths in women.

Assessment

Health Status

- Palpable lump, usually in upper outer quadrant of breast
- Unilateral increase in breast size; asymmetrical breast contour
- Dimpling of breast skin
- Nipple retraction, ulceration, or discharge
- Edema of breast causing an "orange peel" appearance
- Usually little if any pain
- Abnormal venous congestion in breast
- Metastasis to chest wall, lymph nodes, bone, liver, lung, brain

Developmental Assessment

Most often found in women over 50

Increased incidence in women ages 20–30

Family history of breast cancer increases risk

Increased risk if menses begin before age 14 or menopause occurs after age 55

Diagnostic Factors

Breast self-examination (BSE)
Mammography
Thermography
Ultrasoundography
Computerized tomography (CT) scan
Nuclear magnetic resonance imaging (MRI)
Breast biopsy

Psychosocial/Cultural Assessment

- Women who have never had children or who have delayed childbearing until after age 30 have increased risk
- Women who are overweight by 40% and who consume high-fat diets have increased risk
- More common in North America and Northern Europe than in Asia or Africa
- Questionable data on influence of breast-feeding or incidence among breast-feeding women—decreased or no risk

Nursing Plans and Interventions

Goals

- Client will preserve body integrity
- Client will demonstrate positive coping behaviors
- Client will not suffer infections

Nursing Measures

- Provide preoperative teaching about surgical procedures, routines, postoperative procedures, postoperative appearance of chest, drainage tubes, pain
- Engage client in preoperative discussions about feelings (loss, grief, fear)
- Administer prescribed analgesics and narcotics postoperatively
- Put pressure dressing on arm; elevate arm to help prevent edema
- Encourage passive range of motion (ROM) exercises to affected hand, wrist and elbow

- Ensure client does not abduct arm until wound is healed
- Measure and monitor character of drainage, if drainage device available, on each shift or as ordered
- Refer to support group, such as "Reach for Recovery"
- Practice active listening and provide emotional support

Medical/Surgical Treatment

Surgical measures include:

Lumpectomy: local excision of lump; research indicates that this combined with radiation may be as effective as radical mastectomy
Subcutaneous mastectomy: nipple and skin are left intact
Total mastectomy: all mammary tissue removed, muscles and axilla preserved
Radical mastectomy: all mammary tissue, muscles, axillary lymph nodes removed

Medical measures include:

Radiation therapy (radium implants in tumor)
Chemotherapy with agents such as cyclophosphamide, methotrexate, and fluorouracil

Uterine and Cervical Cancer

Uterine and cervical cancer refers to malignancy of the uterus or cervix.

Assessment

Health Status

- Abnormal vaginal discharge or bleeding
- Urinary frequency, if tumor large enough to put pressure on bladder
- Constipation, if tumor large enough to put pressure on colon

Developmental Assessment

Uterine cancer most common in postmenopausal women or those on prolonged estrogen therapy

Diagnostic Factors

Pap smear
Coloscopy
Punch biopsy
Cone biopsy

Psychosocial/Cultural Assessment

- Second most common tumor in women
- More common in women who were sexually active at an early age and who have children
- Type II herpesvirus associated with cervical cancer
- Incidence of cervical cancer higher in wives of uncircumcised men (especially with men demonstrating poor hygiene habits)

Nursing Plans and Interventions

Goals

- Client will demonstrate positive coping strategies to face diagnosis of cancer
- Client will preserve as much body integrity as possible
- Metastasis will be prevented

Nursing Measures

- For hysterectomy clients, see measures under endometriosis section

Radium Implant

- Ensure client has private room
- Enforce limited contact with caregivers and visitors (30 minutes per hour or per hospital policy)
- Permit no pregnant visitors or caregivers
- Enforce bedrest with limited movement to prevent dislodgement
- Provide care for indwelling Foley catheter to prevent dislodgement
- Treat all bowel and bladder discharges as contaminated
- If implant becomes dislodged, *do not touch*—call radiation therapy department immediately

- Provide emotional support and practice active listening
- Refer to support group through American Cancer Society
- Initiate discussions on feelings about sexuality and reproduction, if appropriate

Medical/Surgical Treatment

Simple hysterectomy

Radical hysterectomy with oophorectomy; salpingectomy

Radiation implants

Drug Therapy

For postoperative therapy for hysterectomy—see endometriosis section

Client/Family Teaching

Provide postoperative teaching to hysterectomy clients—see endometriosis section.
  Teach client about:

Radium implant (will be removed prior to leaving hospital)

Side-effects of radiation therapy: may develop adhesions; may have decreased vaginal lubrication and strictures; sexual intercourse recommended; if no sexual partner, special dilators available through radiation therapy department

Evaluation

Treatment and client teaching are successful if:

- Client displays positive coping behaviors (openly expressing feelings and thoughts to nurse, physician, or significant others)
- No metastasis to other body parts occurs

Male Reproductive Problems

Benign Prostatic Hypertrophy

Benign prostatic hypertrophy (BPH) is the most commonly occurring tumor of the prostate gland, and may be associated with an endocrine imbalance.

Assessment

Health Status

- Urinary stasis
- Urinary frequency (small amounts)
- Difficulty starting urinary stream
- Dribbling at end of micturition
- Distended bladder (may result from acute or chronic infections)
- Enlarged prostate identified by rectal examination
- Burning on urination
- Diminished force of urinary stream
- Decreased ability to maintain erection

Developmental Assessment

Incidence increases with age

Common health problem for men over age 50

Diagnostic Factors

Physical examination

Cystoscopy

Intravenous pyelogram (IVP)

Renal function studies

Complete blood count and electrolyte studies

Psychosocial/Cultural Assessment

- Acute urinary retention occurs more frequently after exposure to cold
- Consumption of spicy foods and alcohol may precipitate acute congestion of prostate

Nursing Plans and Interventions

Goals

- Client's pain will decrease
- Client will have restored urinary function
- Client will demonstrate positive coping behaviors
- Client will maintain normal sexual functioning

Nursing Measures
- Maintain asepsis and patency of indwelling Foley catheter
- Assess for bladder discomfort, distension
- Maintain fluid intake between 2500–3000 mL/24 hours or as ordered
- Monitor I and O
- Monitor for hematuria

Preoperative Care

Teach client that after surgery, he must:

Avoid attempting to void around catheter

Avoid straining during bowel movement

Practice perineal exercises to decrease incontinence

Recognize possibility of postoperative impotence

Postoperative Care
- Administer prescribed analgesics or narcotics, and antispasmodics and laxatives
- Maintain continuous bladder irrigation as ordered
- Monitor urine for hematuria, blood clots, pieces of tissue
- Avoid taking rectal temperature, using rectal tubes, and administering enemas
- Assist with active and passive ROM activity; instruct client to turn, cough, and breathe deeply at regular intervals; provide antiembolic stockings
- Ensure client avoids vigorous coughing
- Assist with perineal exercises
- Assist with early ambulation if possible
- Monitor for complications of surgery, including:
    Hemorrhage
    Water intoxication from irrigating fluid (monitor serum sodium for hyponatremia and monitor for signs and symptoms of circulatory overload)
    Urinary obstruction
    Cystitis
    Pyelonephritis
    Renal failure

Medical/Surgical Treatment

Surgical prostatectomy: transurethral (TUR), suprapubic, retropubic, or perineal

Medical: urinary antiseptics with prostatic massage, or encouraging sexual intercourse to relieve congestion

Nutrition Therapy

- Foods high in fiber to promote peristalsis
- High-acid food and fluids such as tomatoes or cranberry juice to keep urine acid

Drug Therapy

Belladonna and opium (B and O) suppositories for bladder spasms

Androgen therapy (conservative treatment modality)

Client/Family Teaching

Teach client about:

Perineal exercises

Good hygiene

Avoiding vigorous coughing, straining at stool

Avoiding heavy lifting for 3 weeks after surgery

Abstaining from sexual activity for at least 4 weeks

Continuing high fluid intake after discharge

Signs and symptoms of infection, developing urethral strictures, and obstructions

Evaluation

Treatment and client teaching are successful if:

- At discharge, client is free from pain
- Client has no alterations in urinary patterns
- Client displays positive coping behaviors (openly discusses feelings and thoughts about procedure and sexual/reproductive implications)
- Client is able to explain necessary temporary changes in lifestyle

Cancer of the Prostate

Cancer of the prostate is a neoplasm of the prostate gland. It is the second most common cancer affecting males, and the third most common cause of death for men from cancer. Cancer of the prostate may occur simultaneously with prostatic hypertrophy.

Assessment

Health Status

- Symptoms of urethral obstruction: urinary retention, stasis; difficulty initiating stream; urinary tract infections
- Metastasis is common—symptoms include bone pain, low back pain radiating down legs, weight loss, anemia
- Hematuria
- Enlarged prostate (hard nodule)
- Blood in ejaculate

Developmental Assessment

Incidence is highest among males 50–70 years of age
May have genetic tendency
May be caused by hormonal changes
The younger the client, the more lethal the disease

Diagnostic Factors

Cystoscopy
IVP
Ultrasound
CT scan
Biopsy

Psychosocial/Cultural Assessment

- Higher incidence among blacks than among whites
- Higher incidence among males taking androgenic hormones ("muscle building steroids")
- Environmental factors may have role in etiology (*e.g.*, industrial exposure to cadmium)
- Gonorrhea increases chance of developing prostate cancer

Nursing Plans and Interventions

Goals

- Client will maintain normal elimination patterns
- Client will maintain normal sexual functioning
- Client will maintain positive self-concept
- Client's pain will decrease

Nursing Measures

- Encourage use of sperm bank prior to therapy, if appropriate
- Monitor I and O
- For postoperative prostatectomy clients, use aseptic technique to care for indwelling catheter
- Maintain catheter patency (irrigate catheter as ordered)
- Promote perineal exercises 1–2 days postoperatively
- Care for fecal incontinence if necessary
- Provide active listening, support, and encouragement
- Assess for return of voluntary urinary control
- Intermittent catheterization may be necessary
- Administer prescribed antiandrogen therapy (*e.g.*, estrogen)
- Provide nursing care for client receiving chemotherapy or radiation therapy (see cancer of testes section)
- Client may be candidate for penile prosthesis
- Encourage use of antiembolic stockings (increased incidence of thrombophlebitis)

Drug Therapy

Estrogen for regression of symptoms; side-effects include gynecomastia, feminization, ankle edema, decreased libido

Diuretics such as furosemide (Lasix) to help control edema (monitor electrolytes, especially potassium)

Nutrition Therapy

- Low-salt diet to assist in edema control
- Diet including food from all four food groups; adequate caloric intake

Client/Family Teaching

Teach client about:

Medications: dose, purpose, side-effect
Nutrition therapy
Long-term therapy (radiation, chemotherapy)

Evaluation

Treatment and client teaching are successful if:

- Urinary and bowel elimination patterns are normal
- Client maintains positive self-concept
- Client retains normal potency or positively copes with impotency (approximately 30% of clients suffer impotency)

Cancer of the Testes

Cancer of the testes arises from germ cell epithelium of the testis. There are two types, seminomas and nonseminomas.

Assessment

Health Status

- Painless lump on testes
- Scrotum maintains shape unless tumor is grossly enlarged
- Heaviness in groin area
- Abdominal and inguinal aching
- Frequent sites of metastasis are supraclavicular area, abdomen, lung
- May have gynecomastia

Developmental Assessment

Affects men ages 15–40 (leading cause of cancer in that age group)

Diagnostic Factors

Radioimmunoassay: increased human chorionic gonadotropin (HCG)
Ultrasound
Transillumination
Biopsy is contraindicated

Psychosocial/Cultural Assessment

- Incidence higher among whites than among blacks
- Incidence higher among men with history of cryptorchidism

Nursing Plans and Interventions

Goals

- Client will maintain sexual functioning
- Client will not suffer complications of chemotherapy or radiation therapy
- Client will demonstrate positive adaptation to body image change

Nursing Measures

- Practice active, supportive listening

Nursing Care for Clients Receiving Chemotherapy or Radiation Therapy

- Administer prescribed antiemetics
- Provide rest periods throughout day
- Prevent infection
- Maintain good oral and body hygiene
- Monitor fluid status, I and O
- Monitor laboratory values, especially white blood cell counts and electrolytes
- Maintain skin integrity (avoid soaps, creams, heat applications)
- Prevent traumas that can lead to hemorrhaging

- Do not offer spicy foods; provide frequent mouth care to help relieve stomatitis
- Have client gargle with lidocaine viscous to relieve pain of stomatitis
- Encourage use of hair piece if client experiences alopecia

Postoperative Care for Orchiectomy Client
- Promote early ambulation
- Administer prescribed analgesics
- Apply ice pack to scrotum for 24 hours
- Provide psychological support

Drug Therapy

For client receiving chemotherapy, depending on stage of testicular cancer, vinblastine, cisplatin, bleomycin, methotrexate, vinca-leukoblastine (Vincristine), actinomycin

Antiemetics to help decrease chemotherapy-induced nausea and vomiting

Client/Family Teaching

Teach client about:

Testicular self-examination for other testicle

Medications: dose, purpose, side-effects

Skin care

Potential for infection (chemotherapy or radiation therapy), and signs and symptoms

Evaluation

Treatment and client teaching are successful if client maintains:

- Positive self-concept
- Sexual functioning (erectile ability)
- Skin intact without burns, lesions, redness

Sexually Transmitted Diseases

Syphilis

Syphilis is an infectious, chronic venereal disease, characterized by tissue or organ lesions caused by a spirochete (*Treponema pallidum*). It is transmitted by direct contact between humans and freshly contaminated material. The organism may enter any broken area of skin or mucous membrane.

Assessment

Health Status

Syphilis is classified in three stages.

Primary Stage
- Painless chancre, appearing as a papule, vesicle or ulcer on penis, lips, labia, oral cavity, anus
- Chancre usually located at point of entry of spirochete, 9–90 days after sexual contact
- In female, chancre can go unnoticed on cervix or vagina, but is usually on vulva
- Enlarged lymph nodes occur approximately 2 weeks after appearance of chancre
- Chancre will heal by itself in 1–5 weeks

Secondary Stage
- Systemic symptoms appear: headache, fever, malaise, generalized nonpruritic skin rash, nausea, constipation, anorexia, alopecia, pain in long bones
- Enlargement and induration of lymph nodes
- Without treatment, symptoms disappear in 2–8 weeks

Tertiary Stage (May Develop Soon After Initial Infection, or Over 20 Years Later)
- Skin, muscles, digestive organs, liver, lungs, eyes, and endocrine glands are involved
- Cardiovascular organs (heart and blood vessels) are affected
- Central nervous system is involved: possible paresis, paralysis, and various types of psychosis

Developmental Assessment

May be transmitted from mother to fetus via placenta after 4th month

Most frequently seen in adolescents and young adults

Diagnostic Factors

Dark field microscopic examination

Serology tests: Venereal Disease Research Laboratory test (VDRL), rapid plasma reagin test

Lumbar puncture

Psychosocial/Cultural Assessment

- More prevalent in urban areas
- Males infected more than females
- Incidence increasing, especially among clients with acquired immunodeficiency syndrome (AIDS)

Nursing Plans and Interventions

Goals

- Client will not suffer further transmission of disease
- Sexual partners of client will be contacted and treated
- Lesions will not be infected
- Client will demonstrate positive coping behaviors

Nursing Measures

- Administer prescribed IV penicillin
- Demonstrate positive attitude, and provide active listening and emotional support
- Refer to public health agency
- Use caution when handling laboratory specimens

Drug Therapy

Penicillin is drug of choice, IV or IM; oral penicillin has questionable effects

Tetracycline or erythromycin can be used if client allergic to penicillin

Client/Family Teaching

Teach client about:

Course of illness

Rationale for antibiotic therapy

Importance of finding and notifying sexual contacts

Importance of repeated serology examinations (monthly for 1 year, then every 3 months until results negative)

Prevention: good hygiene after sexual activity where applicable, and for oral cavity, anus, pelvic areas

Importance of avoiding sexual contact until antibiotic therapy is completed

Evaluation

Client teaching is successful if:

- Recurring signs of disease are treated promptly
- Client's sexual contacts are made known to appropriate public health officials
- Client can explain disease progression, safe sexual practices, good hygiene practices

Gonorrhea

Gonorrhea is the most common infectious disease in the United States. It is a venereal disease characterized by inflammation of the genital mucous membranes due to invasion by Neisseria gonorrhoeae (a gram-negative diplococcus). One of its slang names is "the clap."

Assessment

Health Status

- Purulent, greenish yellow discharge from cervix or penis
- Rectal discharge
- Inflamed Bartholin's ducts and Skene's glands
- Painful or frequent urination
- *Female:* acute pelvic inflammatory disease
- *Male:* prostatitis, epididymitis
- With acute infection, 60% of women may be asymptomatic; males also frequently asymptomatic

Developmental Assessment

Infants' eyes may be exposed to gonorrhea bacteria during birth process—they are given silver nitrate prophylactically

Age group at highest risk is 20–24 years of age

Diagnostic Factors

Gram stain of urethral discharge

Organism culture from cervical, urethral secretions, rectum, throat

Serological studies to rule out syphilis and other venereal diseases (treatment of gonorrhea may mask signs and symptoms of other venereal diseases, especially syphilis)

Psychosocial/Cultural Assessment

- Transmitted by sexual contact
- Homosexual men can harbor the organism in mouth as well as rectum
- High reinfection rate

Nursing Plans and Interventions

Goals

- Client will not suffer further transmission of disease
- Client will not experience problems with sexuality, reproduction, or self-esteem
- Sexual partners of client will be contacted and treated
- Client will demonstrate positive coping behaviors

Nursing Measures

- Administer prescribed antibiotics
- Apply moist heat, give Sitz baths
- Wear gloves when obtaining specimens

Monitor for complications, including:

- *Female:* acute or chronic salpingitis, pelvic inflammatory disease, infertility due to tubal occlusion
- *Male:* Prostatitis, epididymitis

Drug Therapy

Penicillin is drug of choice, but many penicillin-resistant strains exist

For resistant organisms, IM spectinomycin or cefoxitin

Client/Family Teaching

Teach client about:

Prevention: using condoms and other safe sexual practices

Good hygiene

Necessity of contacting sexual partners for treatment

Importance of abstaining from sexual contact until drug therapy completed

Evaluation

Treatment and client teaching are successful if:

- Client can discuss sexual and reproductive issues with nurse, physician, or significant others
- Appropriate public health officials have been notified

Genital Herpes

Genital herpes is an incurable sexually transmitted disease of the genital region, usually caused by an infection by herpes simplex type II. Herpes genitalis is not a reportable disease. It is a lifelong disease that cannot be cured, only controlled.

Assessment

Health Status

- Appearance of painful vesicles or ulcers in genital region
- Fever, malaise
- Inguinal node enlargement
- Secondary infections can reoccur every few weeks or once or twice a year, with no lymphadenopathy
- Pain, itching of lesions

Developmental Assessment

Usually affects persons 15–30 years of age

Can cause serious complications or fatal infection to newborns

Reoccurrence more frequent among men

Diagnostic Factors

Pap smear

Microbiological smears

History and physical examination

Psychosocial/Cultural Assessment

- Disease transmitted when lesions present
- Women infected in early stages of pregnancy have increased chance of miscarriage
- Cesarean delivery usually necessary to prevent endangering fetus
- Genital herpes associated with cervical cancer

Nursing Plans and Interventions

Goals

- Client will not suffer reoccurrence (up to 75% have at least one reoccurrence)
- Secondary infections will be prevented
- Further spread of disease will be prevented

Nursing Measures

- Administer prescribed antiviral agents
- Administer alcohol or other drying agents to dry lesions, then dust with corn starch
- Administer prescribed analgesics or sedatives
- Practice active listening without judgment
- Help client accept chronicity of disease
- Use gloves when coming into contact with exudate

Drug Therapy

Antiviral agent (*e.g.*, acyclovir) to reduce duration of attacks (does not cure)

Burow's solution or hydrogen peroxide to cleanse lesions

Client/Family Teaching

Teach client to:

Refrain from sexual activity when lesions present

Seek good prenatal care if pregnant

Notify sexual partner(s)

Understand medication: dosage, purpose, side-effects

Practice good hygiene

Recognize predisposing factors:
    Fever
    Emotional upsets
    Premenstrual states
    Overexposure to heat and sunshine

Evaluation

Treatment and client teaching are successful if:

- Reoccurrences are less frequent
- No secondary infection occurs

Chlamydia

Chlamydia is one of the most common sexually transmitted diseases. This organism is the major cause of nongonococcal urethritis. Symptoms are those of urethral inflammation. It may cause acute salpingitis or pelvic inflammatory disease (PID).

Assessment

Health Status

- Dysuria
- Thin, watery discharge initially; later thick, white, creamy discharge from urethra or vagina
- May also have gonococcal infection
- May be asymptomatic
- Lower abdominal pain
- Testicular pain
- Rectal pain

Developmental Assessment

Greatest incidence among persons less than 20 years of age

Infections can be transmitted to infants during delivery, causing pneumonia or conjunctivitis

Diagnostic Factors

Gram stain and culture

Direct fluorescent antibody test

Enzyme immunoassay test

Psychosocial/Cultural Assessment

- 30%–40% of cases reoccur within 6 weeks
- More prevalent among heterosexual men than among homosexual men

Nursing Plans and Interventions

Goals

- Infection will be eradicated
- Reoccurrence will be prevented
- Complications will be prevented

Nursing Measures

- Administer prescribed antibiotics
- Practice active, nonjudgmental listening

Drug Therapy

Oral tetracycline or erythromycin for 7–10 days

Administer tetracycline when client has empty stomach; client may experience photosensitivity; females should avoid becoming pregnant while taking tetracycline

Client/Family Teaching

Teach client:

Dose, purpose, side-effects of medication

Importance of limiting sexual partners to help control spread of disease

To use condom and spermicide

Importance of avoiding intercourse for 1 month after treatment (reoccurrence is common)

Necessity of taking medication prescribed length of time (reoccurrence and complications—epididymitis, proctitis, pelvic inflammatory disease, endometritis—likely if untreated)

To avoid alcohol during treatment phase

Necessity of notifying sexual contacts for medical evaluation and treatment

Evaluation

Treatment and client teaching are successful if:

- Infection is eradicated and does not recur
- No complications result

Acquired Immunodeficiency Syndrome (AIDS)

Acquired immunodeficiency syndrome (AIDS) is characterized by a breakdown or defect in the body's cellular immune system. It is caused by a T-cell lymphotropic virus (HIV III, and possibly HIV II). AIDS-related complex (ARC) is a less severe variation of the syndrome. It exists when at least two defined symptoms of immunodeficiency have been diagnosed and two abnormal laboratory values have been reported.

Assessment

Health Status

- Fever of at least 100°F
- Lymphadenopathy
- Diarrhea
- Night sweats
- Fatigue or chronic fatigue
- Weight loss
- Persistent cough
- Anorexia
- Client bruises easily
- Unexplained bleeding
- Arthralgias
- Myalgias
- High risk for opportunistic infections, including:
    Cytomegalovirus (CMV)
    Pneumocystis carinii pneumonia (PCP)
    Mycobacteria
    Herpes simplex virus (HSV)
    Cryptococcal disease
    Toxoplasmosis
    Cryptosporiodosis

Table 8-1. Recommendations for Blood and Body Fluid Precautions (Centers for Disease Control)

- All health care workers should wear gloves to prevent skin from touching blood and body fluids.
- Gloves should be changed after contact with each client.
- Masks and protective eye and face wear should be worn if there is a possibility of contact between droplets of blood or body fluids and mucous membranes of eyes, nose or mouth.
- Gowns should be worn if the client's blood or body fluid is likely to come in contact with the health care worker.
- Hands or other skin surfaces should be washed immediately if contaminated with blood or body fluids.
- Hands should be washed immediately after gloves are removed.
- Needles should not be recapped.
- Contaminated needles and syringes should be placed in a puncture-resistant container promptly after use.
- If the client needs mouth-to-mouth resuscitation, mouth pieces and other ventilatory equipment should be available (even though saliva has not been implicated in transmission of the virus).
- Any health care worker who has a dermatologic condition that involves weeping sores or exudates should refrain from direct client care.
- Pregnant health care workers are especially cautioned to adhere to these precautions.
- The above blood and body fluid precautions should be implemented when working with *all* patients.

Adapted from Centers for Disease Control: Recommendations for prevention of HIV transmission in health-care settings. MMWR: Vol 36, Suppl 2S, 1987

Kaposi's sarcoma
Histoplasmosis

Developmental Assessment

Infants may acquire the disease *in utero* from an infected mother, or from breast milk of an infected mother.

Diagnostic Factors

Complete blood count

Skin tests

Repeated enzyme immunoassay (EIA); tests for human T-cell lymphotrophic virus type III (HTLV III)

Psychosocial/Cultural Assessment

- Many groups are at risk to contract AIDS
- Groups at highest risk are homosexual and bisexual men with multiple sexual partners
- Other high-risk groups include IV drug users, hemophiliacs, Haitians, and Haitian immigrants
- Transmitted via bodily secretions, such as semen, tears, saliva, breast milk, blood, and blood products
- Mortality is higher among females than among males, and is higher among blacks and Hispanics than among whites

Nursing Plans and Interventions

Goals

- Further transmission of the disease will be prevented
- Client's risk of opportunistic infection will be reduced
- Client will demonstrate positive coping
- Client's fear and anxiety will be reduced
- Client will be as comfortable as possible

Nursing Measures

- Assess for signs and symptoms of anxiety
- Assess current coping strategies
- Initiate teaching about cause and treatments for disease process at level appropriate for client
- Encourage nonjudgmental attitude on the part of all members of health care team
- Use active listening communication skills
- Encourage support group participation as appropriate
- Promote social interaction as appropriate
- Support client experiencing anticipatory grief
- Maintain blood and body fluid precautions (see Table 8-1)
- Assess for signs and symptoms of dehydration
- Assess respiratory system for changes in breath sounds, tachypnea, dyspnea
- Provide for rest periods, oxygen, and humidification as necessary
- Assess skin for breaks in integrity and for hydration status
- Monitor nutritional status and weight daily
- Monitor elimination patterns (diarrhea is common)
- Encourage good hygiene habits, especially toileting
- Assess for signs and symptoms of infection, such as increased temperature, chills, areas of redness and warmth
- Encourage fluid intake of at least 1500 mL/day to prevent dehydration and urinary tract infections
- Avoid client contact by persons with active infectious processes (such as a cold)
- Provide good oral care, especially when oral lesions present
- Provide anal care (washing, soothing ointments) for discomfort
- Encourage activity and self care as appropriate

Drug Therapy

Symptomatic and supportive drug therapy such as analgesics, antibiotics, antifungal agents

Gamma globulin therapy (purified concentrated solution of antibodies)

Interferon and interleukin-2

Ribavirin and azidothymidine (antiviral agents)

Nutrition Therapy

- Frequent high-calorie nutritional supplements
- May require dental soft diet due to mouth lesions

Client/Family Teaching

Teach client about:

Safe sexual practices, such as abstinence, use of condoms, and avoiding practices that injure mucous membranes

Good hygiene practices

Necessity of treating or testing sexual contacts

Importance of avoiding persons with acute infectious processes

Well-balanced diet with adequate fluid intake

Necessity of frequent medical check-ups

Avoiding donating blood or organs

Avoiding sharing articles that may become contaminated with blood, such as toothbrushes or razors

Necessity of notifying health care professionals of positive antibody status

Mode of transmission of virus
Medical therapy and drug regimen

Evaluation

Treatment and client teaching are successful if client:

- Remains free from infection
- Can explain safe sexual practices
- Demonstrates positive coping behaviors
- Maintains stable weight
- Can explain methods to protect others and self from infection

Renal Dysfunction

Glomerulonephritis

Glomerulonephritis is an inflammatory process that destroys the glomeruli and ultimately the nephron of the kidneys. It may be acute, subacute, or chronic.

Assessment

Health Status

- History of streptococcal infection, such as streptococcal sore throat or impetigo
- Visual disturbances
- Anorexia, weakness, nausea, headaches, increased blood pressure, dizziness, increased temperature
- Palpable kidneys
- Periorbital edema
- Papilledema or retinal hemorrhage
- Hematuria, coffee colored urine

Developmental Assessment

More common in children and young adults
More common in males than in females
May be associated with lupus, erythematosus, hypertension, endocarditis, diabetes mellitus, disseminated intravascular coagulation (DIC)

Diagnostic Factors

IVP or retrograde pyelograms
ASO titer (antistreptolysin) and C-reactive protein (CRP)
Serum studies, especially electrolytes, hematocrit, hemoglobin, blood urea nitrogen (BUN)
Renal function studies
Urinalysis for hematuria, protein urea

Psychosocial/Cultural Assessment

- May be associated with lower economic status

Nursing Plans and Interventions

Goals

- Kidney functioning will be preserved
- Client will not suffer hypertension
- Client will not experience cardiopulmonary complications
- Client will learn good health practices

Nursing Measures

- Administer antibiotics, diuretics, antihypertensives as prescribed
- Follow seizure precautions (due to uremia)
- Enforce bed rest
- Monitor I and O
- Monitor daily weight
- Monitor vital signs, especially blood pressure, every 4 hours
- Encourage active/passive ROM exercise; reposition every 2 hours
- Provide skin care and skin assessments (edema predisposes to breakdown)
- Provide oral hygiene
- For indwelling Foley catheter, use aseptic technique
- Prevent exposure to any other infection
- Reduce dietary protein
- Encourage many diversional activities to prevent boredom

Drug Therapy

Antibiotics, including penicillin to eradicate remaining β-hemolytic streptococcus

Antihypertensives

Diuretic therapy

Nutrition Therapy

- Foods normal in carbohydrates and fats but low in protein (catabolism of protein increases BUN)
- Limited sodium and potassium (no carbonated beverages, junk food, bacon, pickles, canned foods)
- Fluids may be restricted to 1000–1500 mL/24 hours

Client/Family Teaching

Teach client about:

Prompt attention to infectious processes, especially sore throat

Avoiding overexcitation and drafty environments

Diet restrictions

Need for tutor (as appropriate) due to prolonged convalescence

Necessity of adequate rest

Necessity of taking medications as prescribed

Recovery period (may be as long as 2 years)

Evaluation

Treatment and client teaching are successful if:

- Client can name medications and state dosage, purpose, side-effects
- Vital signs remain within normal limits and no cardiopulmonary complications occur
- No further renal damage occurs (all test results remain within normal limits)

Renal Calculi

Renal calculi are stones in the kidney. The condition is also called nephrolithiasis. Calculi are commonly composed of calcium salts.

Assessment

Health Status

- Pain, usually flank, may be mild to excruciating, depending on location of stone
- Ureteral spasms (also result in pain)
- Nausea, vomiting
- Hematuria
- May have chills, fever

Developmental Assessment

Men more frequently affected than women

Genetic defect may predispose to stone formation

Diagnostic Factors

Kidney, ureter, bladder (KUB) x-rays

CT scans

Cystoscopy

Test for etiology of stone formations: gout, hyperparathyroidism, excess medication (antacids, vitamin C, steroids), excess of certain foods (milk)

Psychosocial/Cultural Assessment

- Usually occur within same family
- Rare in black people
- High incidence of reoccurrence

Nursing Plans and Interventions

Goals

- Client's pain will be reduced
- Condition will not recur
- Client will not experience complications, such as fluid and electrolyte imbalances or urinary or kidney damage

Nursing Measures

- Administer prescribed narcotics to control pain
- Administer prescribed antispasmodics, antibiotics
- Monitor I and O

- Encourage high fluid intake (3–4 L) as appropriate
- Provide emotional support for client undergoing treatments
- Strain all urine through a fine mesh gauze

Medical/Surgical Treatment

Ultrasound vibrations to break down stones

Lithotripsy (shock waves through water to break down stones): extracorporeal shock wave or percutaneous

Ureterolithotomy

Litholapaxy

Drug Therapy

Antibiotics to eradicate infection

Antispasmodics

Narcotics: client may use patient-controlled analgesia (PCA) pump; may receive fairly high doses of morphine (monitor for respiratory depression)

Allopurinol if client has uric acid stones (see gout section)

Phosphates if client has calcium stones

Nutrition Therapy

- High fluid volume intake
- If stone composed of uric acid, diet low in purines (see gout section)
- If stone composed of calcium, questionable whether diet should be low in calcium
- Cranberry juice, eggs, cheese, prunes, plums, to promote acid urine

Client/Family Teaching

Teach client about:

Medication: dosage, purpose, side-effects

Nutritional restrictions as applicable

Need for frequent medical checkups

Avoiding situations that promote urinary stasis (such as long periods of inactivity)

Evaluation

Treatment and client teaching are successful if client:

- Suffers no further pain
- Experiences no complications of therapy
- Can explain signs and symptoms of calculi and necessary therapy
- Can explain prevention measures
- Can state the name, effect, dosage, and side-effects of all medications

Renal Tumor

A renal tumor, or malignant tumor of the kidneys, is usually an adenocarcinoma or hypernephroma. They usually develop in the pole of a single kidney and have a capsule.

Assessment

Health Status

- Gross hematuria
- Dull flank pain
- Nausea, vomiting
- Weakness, loss of weight, bone pain
- Frequent sites for metastasis are liver, lungs, long bones, other kidney
- Alterations in urinary output
- Polycythemia

Developmental Assessment

Men more often affected than women

Usually affects persons 50–60 years old

Diagnostic Factors

IVP

CT scan

Urinalysis

Renal function studies

Renal biopsy

Nursing Plans and Interventions

Goals

- Client will maintain optimal kidney functioning
- Client will remain free from infection

Nursing Measures

Preoperative Care for Nephrectomy Client

- Avoid administering nephrotoxic drugs
- Monitor I and O
- Assess for signs and symptoms of acute renal failure
- Teach client about splinting, coughing, deep breathing

Postoperative Care

- Monitor vital signs, especially temperature (may suggest onset of complications)
- Prevent pulmonary complications due to incision in accessory muscles (strongly encourage deep breathing, coughing, ambulation as soon as possible after surgery)
- Administer prescribed pain medications
- Assist with incentive spirometry as indicated
- If client has chest tube(s), maintain patency of system, and measure drainage every shift
- Assess for bowel sounds (paralytic ileus is common complication)
- Use aseptic technique for wound care
- Monitor I and O
- Monitor laboratory studies, serum creatinine level, BUN, electrolytes, urine specific gravity
- Monitor daily weight
- Monitor for signs and symptoms of adrenal insufficiency
    - Decreased blood pressure due to hypovolemia
    - Nausea, vomiting, diarrhea, anorexia
    - Possible hypoglycemia

Medical/Surgical Treatment

Radical nephrectomy: removal of kidney, adrenal gland, surrounding lymph nodes
Partial nephrectomy

Client/Family Teaching

Teach client to:

Avoid contact sports
Avoid urinary tract infections (proper hygiene, adequate fluid intake)
Avoid heavy lifting or other strenuous activities for 6–8 weeks postoperatively
Follow well-balanced diet
Understand that he or she can live with one kidney

Evaluation

Treatment and client teaching are successful if:

- Remaining kidney functions at optimal level
- No complications related to surgery result
- No signs and symptoms of infections occur

Acute Renal Failure

Acute renal failure involves sudden severe reduction of renal function. The accumulation of metabolic waste products and electrolyte and fluid imbalances result from severe ischemia related to trauma, obstruction, toxic substances, or glomerulonephritis.

There are three periods of acute failure: the *oliguric* phase usually lasts 10–12 days and is characterized by urine output less than 400 mL/24 hours, hematuria, nausea, lethargy, elevated potassium, BUN, magnesium, and uric acid levels. The *diuretic* phase usually lasts 7–10 days and is characterized by gradual increase in urinary output (output depends on degree of "fluid overload" from oliguric phase). Renal function remains abnormal. The *recovery* phase lasts a few months to 1 year. Renal function is gradually restored but may never return to its pre-failure state (may always have some residual damage).

Assessment

Health Status

- Oliguria (less than 400 mL/24 hour) common in early stage, or anuria (rare)
- Drowsiness, weakness, twitching, confusion, itchy skin, mental irritability, altered thought processes (all due to uremia)

- Halitosis, urinous breath, muscle twitching, anorexia, nausea, vomiting, diarrhea or constipation (all potentially due to metabolic acidosis); increased potassium
- Hypertension, rales, weight gain, pitting edema due to fluid overload, pale skin
- Bruising, oozing of blood, decreased hemoglobin and hematocrit due to increased capillary fragility, decreased platelet adhesiveness, or diminished synthesis of erythropoietin

Developmental Assessment

Greatest incidence among persons who have experienced major trauma, extensive burns, extensive loss of blood, or severe myocardial infarction

High incidence among persons taking nephrotoxic drugs or ingesting nephrotoxic substances

Diagnostic Factors

IVP

Renal arteriography

Electrocardiogram (ECG)

Blood studies: BUN, creatinine, electrolytes, arterial blood gases, Hct and Hgb, WBC, coagulation studies

Urine studies: creatinine clearance, urine electrolytes, urea nitrogen

Nursing Plans and Interventions

Goals

- Renal functioning will be restored
- Further renal damage will be prevented
- Other system involvement and damage will be prevented
- Client will comply with long-term medical regimen

Nursing Measures

- Monitor vital signs, neurologic signs, mental status
- Monitor laboratory values, especially BUN and electrolytes
- Maintain strict I and O to monitor fluid status (fluid overload may result in congestive heart failure, pulmonary edema, hypertension)
- Monitor daily weight
- Measure urine specific gravity
- Administer prescribed diuretics
- In oliguric phase, may administer sodium polystyrene (Kayexalate) enemas to decrease very high potassium levels; assess for dysrhythmias; fluids may be restricted—allow client some responsibility for deciding when to take restricted fluids; provide good oral hygiene
- In diuretic phase, potassium may drop to very low levels, fluid rate may increase: may administer potassium supplements
- Monitor diet and nutrition therapy
- Prevent pulmonary complications: keep airway patent; change position every 2 hours; encourage coughing and deep breathing; monitor respiratory status
- Prevent complications of immobility: encourage active and passive ROM exercise, assess skin integrity
- Alleviate pruritus by bathing frequently with bland soap and applying topical ointments
- Prevent infection: use aseptic technique with Foley catheters, IVs, wounds; arrange for private room if possible; prevent contact with people with active infectious process
- Prevent complications of capillary fragility and anemia: prevent unnecessary trauma, avoid intramuscular injections if possible, keep fingernails short, use soft toothbrush, prevent overexertion, provide frequent rest periods, prevent constipation
- Monitor need for dialysis (peritoneal or hemodialysis); see interventions in chronic renal failure section
- Provide emotional support, employ active listening

- Provide sexual counseling if necessary
- Administer prescribed blood products

Drug Therapy

Potassium supplements, sodium supplements

Antihypertensives

Diuretics

Cardiac glycosides, such as digoxin

Vitamins

Aluminum hydroxide (Amphojel) (to bind phosphorus)

Avoid drugs that contain potassium, such as potassium penicillin

Avoid administering any drug that is nephrotoxic

Nutrition Therapy

- Low-protein diet, but not low enough to cause negative nitrogen balance
- Low-carbohydrate diet but not low enough to cause gluconeogenesis from body protein or to produce ketones from fat metabolism
- Foods low in potassium while client in oliguric phase
- Avoid offering salt substitutes (low in sodium but high in potassium)

Client/Family Teaching

Teach client about:

Dietary regimen: allowances, restrictions

Medications: dosage, purpose, side-effects

Signs and symptoms of infection: fluid overload or retention, hypertension

Need for continual medical supervision

Evaluation

Treatment and client teaching are successful if:

- Client has acceptable renal functioning
- No other body system has been damaged
- Client understands and follows medical regimen

Chronic Renal Failure

Chronic renal failure (CRF) is progressive irreversible destruction of renal tissues, resulting in minimal renal functioning. CRF may result from unresolved acute renal failure or it may occur insidiously.

Assessment

Health Status

- See acute renal failure section for most signs and symptoms
- Possible "uremic frost" (skin discoloration due to deposit of uric acid crystals in skin)
- Frothy urine

Diagnostic Factors

See acute renal failure section

Nursing Plans and Interventions

Goals

- Remaining renal functioning will be preserved
- Further renal compromise will be prevented
- Other body system damage will be prevented
- Client's quality of life will improve as appropriate

Nursing Measures

- See acute renal failure section
- See measures listed below pertaining to medical treatment
- Maintain strict restriction of dietary sodium and potassium in oliguric or anuric phase
- Monitor fluid restrictions
- Administer prescribed diuretics
- Provide emotional support and active listening to help client cope with chronic disease, loss of functioning body part

Medical/Surgical Treatment

Peritoneal dialysis interventions are usually performed while a CRF client is being evaluated for hemodialysis or kidney transplant.

Peritoneal Dialysis: Nursing Care
- Provide emotional support, create open, trusting atmosphere to help allay client's fears
- Ensure client voids prior to insertion of trochanter
- Monitor baseline vital signs and weight
- During procedure, observe fluid output for blood and for colors other than pale yellow
- Maintain strict monitoring of I and O
- Monitor vital signs frequently during procedure
- Monitor for signs and symptoms of hypotension, infection, hyponatremia, hypovolemia, peritonitis
- Provide diversional activities
- Have bedpan or commode ready in case client has diarrhea while undergoing dialysis

Continuous ambulatory peritoneal dialysis (CAPD) allows the client greater freedom and independence than hemodialysis or conventional peritoneal dialysis. The dialysate is drained 4 times a day, 7 days a week; exchanges occur every 4–5 hours and at bed time. Some clients prefer to undergo CAPD than to be machine dependent.

Providing nursing care for clients undergoing *hemodialysis* and renal transplantation requires special training, but brief, general guidelines are presented below.

Hemodialysis: Nursing Care
- Monitor baseline vital signs and weight
- Maintain aseptic technique, especially around shunt
- Monitor shunt site for signs and symptoms of infection; assess for thrill and bruit
- Monitor I and O
- Monitor for signs and symptoms of depression (common with dialysis clients)
- Refer client to support agencies
- Assist client to cope with chronic disease, machine dependency
- Monitor for complications of long-term therapy:
   Noncompliance
   Osteodystrophy
   Peripheral neuropathies
   Obstruction of shunts
   Sexual/reproductive dysfunctions

Renal Transplantation: Preoperative Nursing Care
- Teach client about procedures, postoperative period, and discharge plans
- Provide emotional support

Renal Transplantation: Postoperative Nursing Care
- Protective isolation due to immunosuppressive drugs
- Maintain strict monitoring of I and O
- Monitor vital signs frequently
- Monitor daily weight
- Prevent complications of immobility (see acute renal failure section)
- Prevent infection (see acute renal failure section)
- Monitor for signs and symptoms of rejection: anorexia, malaise, decreased urinary output, fever, edema, increased BUN, creatinine, hypertension, weight gain

Drug Therapy

Corticosteroids to suppress immune system to decrease rejection of transplanted organ—azathioprine, cyclophosphamide, cyclosporine (one of the most commonly used immunosuppressive drugs, however, major side-effect is nephrotoxicity)

Nutrition Therapy

See acute renal failure section

Client/Family Teaching

See acute renal failure section

Cystitis

Cystitis is inflammation of the wall of the bladder. It may be primary or result from an infectious process elsewhere in the urinary tract.

Assessment

Health Status

- Fever
- Suprapubic pain
- Cloudy urine
- Burning on urination
- Hematuria
- Foul-smelling urine

Developmental Assessment

Frequently occurs in school-age girls, due to intentional withholding of urine

May occur in males due to enlarged prostate

Diagnostic Factors

History and physical examination

Urinalysis

Urine culture and sensitivity test

Psychosocial/Cultural Assessment

- Incidence is greater among females than among males
- May result from vaginal trauma (often occurs 36–72 hours after intercourse)
- May result from anal to vaginal contamination

Nursing Plans and Interventions

Goals

- Client's pain will be reduced or eradicated
- Further infection will be prevented
- Reoccurrence will be prevented

Nursing Measures

- Monitor I and O
- Monitor vital signs, especially temperature, every 4 hours
- Encourage warm Sitz baths, tub baths
- Administer prescribed analgesics, antibiotics
- Encourage proper hygiene
- Monitor for complications: chronic cystitis, calculi, pyelonephritis, septicemia
- Practice active listening and provide emotional support
- Encourage adequate fluid intake

Drug Therapy

Antibiotic therapy appropriate for causative organism

Phenazopyridine hydrochloride (Pyridium) for symptomatic relief of bladder pain (turns urine orange red color)

Nutrition Therapy

- Avoid offering carbonated beverages
- Encourage an acid/ash diet: meats, eggs, cheese, cranberries

Client/Family Teaching

Teach client about hygiene practices, including:

Voiding after sexual intercourse

Cleansing anal area after bowel movement (wipe front to back)

Wearing cotton instead of nylon or polyester underwear

Avoiding perfumed powders, bubble baths

Rinsing clothes following wash if using bleach or harsh soap powders

Teach client about:

Medications: dosage, purpose, side-effects

Disease and causes

Evaluation

Treatment and client teaching are successful if client is:

- Free of pain and symptoms of infection
- Knowledgeable about hygiene and preventative measures

Bladder Tumors and Neoplasms

Bladder tumors and neoplasms are the most common tumors of the genitourinary tract. They usually involve the bladder neck and ureteral orifices.

Assessment

Health Status
- Painless intermittent hematuria
- Dysuria
- Intermittent anuria, polyuria
- Signs and symptoms of infection: temperature, burning upon urination, frequency, urgency
- May have decrease in force of urinary stream
- Common metastasis sites are tissue surrounding bladder and tissues supplied by bladder lymph nodes

Developmental Assessment

2–3 times more common in males than in females

Occurs most often between ages 50–70

Diagnostic Factors

Cystogram

Urine studies

Psychosocial/Cultural Assessment
- Relationship with smoking
- Relationship with exposure to industrial chemicals
- Coffee and artificial sweeteners may be etiologic factors

Nursing Plans and Interventions

Goals
- Patency of urinary tract will be maintained
- Client will maintain normal kidney function
- Client will remain free from infection
- Client will accept change in body image, if appropriate

Nursing Measures

Preoperative Care
- For radical cystectomy, help client prepare mentally for urinary diversion—possibilities include:
  - Ureteroileal conduit
  - Colon conduit
  - Ureterosigmoidostomy and ureteroileosigmoidostomy
  - Ureterostomy
  - Continent vesicostomy
- Monitor I and O
- Monitor daily weight
- Provide preoperative teaching: turning, coughing, and deep breathing

Postoperative Care
- Monitor vital signs as ordered
- Assist with leg exercises and early ambulation to promote venous return
- Monitor I and O
- Monitor daily weight
- Specific nursing care depends on type of urinary diversion, but general guidelines include:
  - Provide good skin care
  - Control odor: avoid offering foods that give urine strong odor (*e.g.*, tomatoes, asparagus)
  - Refer to ostomy association
  - Provide emotional support while client experiences alteration in body image

Medical/Surgical Treatment

Chemotherapeutic agents such as 5-fluorouracil, methotrexate, bleomycin

Partial or radical cystectomy

Urinary diversions may be necessary

External cobalt radiation to retard tumor growth

Nutrition Therapy (If Conduit to Intestines Possible)

- Avoid offering foods that produce strong odor in urine (*e.g.*, tomatoes, asparagus)

- Avoid offering gas-producing foods such as beans, cabbage, brussel sprouts, prunes, raisins

Client/Family Teaching

Teach client about:

Skin and stoma care (if applicable)

Necessity of adequate nutrition and fluid intake, and dietary restrictions (if applicable)

Avoiding use of enemas, laxatives, if client has diversion to intestines

Evaluation

Treatment and client teaching are successful if:

- Urinary tract remains patent
- Kidney function remains normal
- Client accepts new image incorporating alteration in elimination
- Client is free from infection

Bibliography for Unit II
Care of the Adult Client

Alderman C: AIDS: Blazing the trail. Nurs Times 83: 33–34, 1987

Armstrong M et al: McGraw-Hill Handbook of Clinical Nursing. New York, McGraw-Hill, 1979

Atwell B: Sex and the cancer patient, an unspoken concern. Patient Educ Counsel 5:123–126, 1984

Bates P: Three post-op perils of prostate surgery. RN 47:40–43, 1984

Bennett J: What we know about AIDS, Part 1. Am J Nurs 86:1016–1021, 1986

Benz C: Chronic renal failure and the common denominator theory: A practical application. Nephrol Nurs 4:4,6,10, 1982

Bergstein J: Hematuria in the young. Emerg Med 18: 20–24,29,33–34, 1986

Birdsall C: How do you manage peritoneal dialysis? Am J Nurs 86:592,596, 1986

Brunner L, Suddarth, D: The Lippincott Manual of Nursing Practice, 4th ed. Philadelphia, JB Lippincott, 1986

Clark N et al: Prostatectomy: A guide to answering your patient's unspoken questions . . . a patient teaching aid. Nurs 14:48–51, 1984

Coleman E: When the kidneys fail. RN 49:28–38, 1986

Crawford E: Diagnosis and management of prostate cancer. Hosp Pract 21:159–163,167–168,171–172, 1986

Datta P: Carcinoma of the urinary bladder. Nurs Times 80:24–26, 1984

DeBrow M: AIDS—No easy answers. Imprint 34: 33–35, 1987

Dugan K: The bleak outlook on ovarian cancer. Am J Nurs 85:144–147, 1985

Earle D: Poststreptococcal acute glomerulonephritis. Hosp Pract 20:84e–j,84o–p,84u, 1985

Emmons J: Towards control of chlamydial infections. Nurs Pract 10:21–22, 1985

Farrel B: AIDS patients: Values in conflict. Crit Care Nurs Quart 10:74–85, 1987

Faulkenberry J: Cancer in women: A case for cancer prevention and early detection. Dim Onc Nurs 1:4–7, 1985

Garner C et al: Endometriosis. J Obstet Gynecol Neonat Nurs 14:10s–20s, 1985

Glover E: Herpes: Removing fact from fiction. Health Ed 15:6–10, 1984

Harum A: Renal nutrition for the renal nurse. Am Nephrol Nurs Assoc 11:38–44, 1984

Hudson E et al: Screening hospital patients for uterine cervical cancer. J Clin Pathol 36:611–615, 1983

Johnson D: Pathophysiology of renal failure. Crit Care Nurs 5:18,20, 1985

Klug R: AIDS beyond the hospital: Children with AIDS. Am J Nurs 86:1126–1132, 1986

Kniesl C, Ames S: Adult Health Nursing: A Biopsychosocial Approach. Menlo Park, CA, Addison-Wesley, 1986

Larson E: Epidemiologic correlates of breast, endometrial, and ovarian cancers. Cancer Nurs 6: 295–301, 1983

Lewis S, Collier I: Medical-Surgical Nursing: Assessment and Management of Clinical Problems, 2nd ed. New York, McGraw-Hill, 1987

Loricks A: Chlamydia—An unheralded epidemic. Am J Nurs 87:920–922, 1987

Luckmann J, Sorensen K: Medical-Surgical Nursing: A Psychophysiologic Approach, 3rd ed. Philadelphia, WB Saunders, 1987

Mast M: Primary care of the mastectomy patient. Nurs Pract 9:30,32, 1984

Matje D: Stress and cancer: A review of the literature. Cancer Nurs 7:399–404, 1984

McCormick A et al: RN master care plan: The patient in acute renal failure. RN 49:35–37, 1986

Miles P: Sexually transmitted diseases. J Gynecol Nurs 13:102s–124s, 1984

Mishell D: Putting a stop to salpingitis. Emerg Med 16:22–25,28–30,32, 1984

Morbidity and Mortality Weekly Report No. 36. Supplement revision of the CDC surveillance case definition for acquired immune deficiency syndrome. Atlanta, Centers for Disease Control, 1987

Phipps W, Long B, Woods N. Medical-Surgical Nursing: Concepts and Clinical Practice, 3rd ed. St. Louis, CV Mosby, 1987

Pullman T et al: Pathophysiology of chronic renal failure. Clin Symp 36:3–32, 1984

Robertson C et al: Overview of ovarian cancer. Dim Onc Nurs 1:11–13, 1985

Ruge C: Shock (wave) treatment for kidney stones. Am J Nurs 86:400–401, 1986

Sandellas J: Cancer prevention and detection: Testicular cancer. Cancer Nurs 6:468–486, 1983

Stark J: Combating acute tubular necrosis. Nurs Life 5:33–40, 1985

Sublett P: Cystitis: A woman's woe. Am Urolog Assoc Allied J 6:4–5, 1986

Torrington J: Pelvic inflammatory disease. J Obstet Gynecol Neonatal Nurs 14:21s–31s, 1985

Whittaker A: Acute renal dysfunction: Assessment of patients at risk. Focus Crit Care 12:12–17, 1985

Zschoche D (ed): Mosby's Comprehensive Review of Critical Care. St. Louis, CV Mosby, 1986

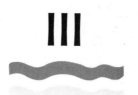

Care of the Client During Childbearing

9

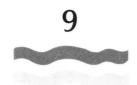

Nursing Care During the Antepartal Period

The Client with a Normal Pregnancy

Physiological Adaptations of the Conceptus (Stage of Human Prenatal Development)

Ovum. The ovum develops during the period from conception until primary villi appear. It begins 4 weeks after the woman's last menstrual period (LMP) and lasts about 12–14 days. By the end of this period, implantation is complete.

Embryo. The embryo stage lasts from the ovum stage to 8 weeks (10 weeks since LMP). All principle organ systems are established during this period. The conceptus is most vulnerable to environmental agents (*e.g.*, viruses, drugs, radiation, infection) during this period—exposure can result in major congenital anomalies.

Fetus. The conceptus is called a fetus from the end of the embryo stage until delivery. The fetus is less vulnerable than the embryo to teratogenic agents, but such agents may interrupt normal functional development.

Maternal Physiological Adaptations

Subjective Changes

- Amenorrhea: majority of women have no periodic bleeding after conception; 20% have spotting
- Nausea and vomiting: 50%–75% experience "morning sickness"; however, problem can persist all day; lasts 8–12 weeks
    Interventions: suggest consuming dry carbohydrate before arising, and remaining in bed until nausea subsides; clear liquids, 5–6 small meals per day
- Breast changes: sensations vary from mild tingling to frank pain due to hormone stimulation
- Urinary frequency: bladder irritability perhaps due to hormones; nocturia, frequency, and urgency are present first and third trimesters due to pressure of fetus on bladder
    Interventions: teach client Kegel's exercises to strengthen perineal muscles (tightening and relaxing); limit fluid intake before bedtime
- Fatigue: occurs in early pregnancy and third trimester and is of unexplained etiology
    Interventions: provide reassurance, rest, good nutrition

Table 9-1. Definitions in Maternity Care

Gravida: Number of pregnancies

Parity: Number of pregnancies that reached viability (fetal weight of at least 601 g and gestation of at least 24 weeks); *example:* 6 pregnancies, 1 abortion, 1 set of twins = G6P5

Expected date of confinement (EDC): According to Nägele's rule, count back 3 months from LMP and add 7 days; *example:* LMP of June 23 = March 23 + 7 days = EDC March 30

- Constipation: appears early and may persist throughout pregnancy; influenced by increased levels of progesterone
    Interventions: monitor fluids and diet and teach relaxation techniques
- Weight gain: rapid weight gain not associated with early pregnancy; some women experience weight loss; for normal, healthy women of normal height and weight with one fetus, normal weight gain is 22–32 pounds—2–4 pounds during first trimester, 1 pound/week second and third trimesters; obesity presents a problem, but pregnancy is not time to diet—good nutrition is necessary for fetal growth and development
- Quickening ("feeling life"): first recognition of fetal movements; for multipara, 14th–16th week, for primipara, 18th week or later

Objective Changes and Diagnosis of Pregnancy

Pregnancy Tests

- Immunologic assays for human chorionic gonadotropin (HCG), which is secreted from time of implantation and can be detected in urine 42 days after LMP
- Radioimmunoassay is so accurate it is regarded as diagnostic as early as 5th week, but it is not readily available
- Ultrasonography has successfully identified embryo as early as 6th week, but is most accurate after 3rd month

Pelvic Changes

- Chadwick's sign: bluish discoloration of vaginal walls appearing as early as 6th week
- Leukorrhea: white, mucoid vaginal discharge that increases in amount as pregnancy progresses

Integumentary Changes

- Increased pigmentation
- Chloasma ("mask of pregnancy"): appears after 16th week—stay out of sun
- Linea nigra: line from symphysis pubis to umbilicus, appearing around 3rd month
- Striae gravidarum: stretch marks that usually appear in second half of pregnancy

Fetal Heart Tones (FHT)

- Detected with electronic devices 10th–12th week, with fetoscope 17th–18th week

Palpable Uterine Enlargement

- Fetal movements palpable 18th–24th week
- Fetal outline palpable after 24th week
- Fundal height measurement provides gross estimation of duration of pregnancy to validate expected date of confinement (EDC); identification of intrauterine growth retardation; indication of multiple gestation; evidence of polyhydramnios

Braxton-Hicks Contractions

Occasional, intermittent contractions, usually not painful

Common Discomforts

- Nausea and vomiting (see subjective changes)
- Urinary frequency and urgency (see subjective changes)
- Heartburn: caused by effects of progesterone, enlarged uterus, and tension
    Interventions: Encourage client to limit gas-producing and fatty foods, eat small meals, and maintain good posture
- Constipation (see subjective changes)

- Leg cramps: caused by calcium-phosphorous imbalance
  Interventions: correct imbalance by diet with adequate calcium, having client stretch affected muscle by standing up and leaning forward, dorsiflexing foot
- Backache
  Interventions: teach good posture and body mechanics; importance of avoiding fatigue, wearing shoes with heels no greater than 2 inches, using firm mattress; pelvic rock exercise—rocking pelvis back and forth
- Hemorrhoids: causes include increased pressure from uterus, restricting venous return from legs
  Interventions: teach client to avoid constipation, perform Kegel's exercise

Health Promotion Needs

Prenatal Care

During the woman's initial physician consultation, many assessments are performed, including the following laboratory tests: Pap smear, culture for gonorrhea, test for syphilis, blood type and Rh, hemoglobin and hematocrit, and rubella titer measurement.

Return visits include assessment of the woman's health status and the progress of the pregnancy. Leopold's maneuvers are performed to determine fetal presentation, position, and presenting part. Fundal height is measured at each visit to determine normal growth and validate EDC. Lack of growth may indicate intrauterine growth retardation. Excessive growth may indicate multiple gestation or polyhydramnios.

Rest and Activity

The client's employment will be discussed at the first prenatal visit. Continuation of employment will depend on the amount of physical activity and any hazards involved in her job.

Moderate exercise is encouraged but exercise to the point of exhaustion or fatigue is discouraged because it will compromise the amount of oxygen available to the fetus. Rest is important for the welfare of mother and baby.

Air travel is recommended for long distances, and use of seat belts is recommended for car travel.

Use of Drugs

The teratogenicity of many drugs is unknown. Use of all drugs, including aspirin, should be limited. The client should be encouraged to consult a physician before taking any drug.

Smoking 1 pack or more per day increases the client's risk of delivering a small-for-gestational age baby, and increases the risk of perinatal mortality.

Drinking alcoholic beverages during pregnancy can result in fetal alcohol syndrome. An occasional drink appears to be permissible.

Nutritional Care

- Increase in protein, vitamins, and minerals is necessary during pregnancy to meet fetus' needs
- The client who is a *vegetarian* should select a variety of plant foods, *e.g.*, grains, legumes, nuts, and seeds, to obtain complete proteins
- There is an increased need for sodium during pregnancy. Routine restriction of sodium for clients with pregnancy-induced hypertension is discouraged; however, for clients with chronic hypertension, foods high in sodium, *e.g.*, pretzels, potato chips, soft drinks, canned or processed foods, should be restricted
- *Iron and folic acid supplements* are necessary to meet needs of mother and fetus: hemodilution occurs as the mother's blood volume increases, and iron is stored in the fetal liver during last half of pregnancy

Fetal Assessment

- Estriol test for fetal well-being: estriol level in maternal urine (24-hour specimen) reflects condition of fetoplacental unit: level decreases in case of failing pregnancy, anencephaly, fetal death, dysmaturity, pregnancy-induced hypertension (PIH), complicated diabetes

    Nursing measures: give instructions, explanations, and emotional support

- Amniocentesis (after 14th week gestation)

    Indications: mainly for prenatal diagnosis of genetic problems and determination of gestational age in last trimester; a lecithin/sphingomyelin (L/S) ratio indicates fetal lung maturity

    Ultrasound is used to visualize location of placental unit, to avoid inserting needle at placental site

    Complications are few; the mother should report any cramping or bleeding after procedure

    Nursing measures: give instructions, explanations, and emotional support

- Nonstress test for fetal well-being: FHR acceleration in response to fetal movement is desired outcome; routine test for high-risk mothers beginning around 34th week; high-risk pregnancy can continue when tests conducted once or twice a week are reactive; contraction stress test determines whether fetus can withstand decreased oxygen during contractions

    Nursing measures: give instructions, explanations, and emotional support

- Ultrasound: used for confirming gestational age and fetal growth, identifying structural defects and placental position; preparation includes full bladder to aid in visualization

    Nursing measures: give instructions, explanations, and emotional support

Developmental Tasks of the Expanding Family

Parents' Tasks

First Trimester

- Accept pregnancy (both parents)
- Father must cope with his own psychosomatic symptoms such as nausea, lassitude, aches, and pains, if present
- May confront increased concern for economic security

Second Trimester

- Mother becomes introspective, focusing attention on self and baby; father may feel ambivalent and jealous
- Both adjust to changing self-concepts and changing relationships with family members

Third Trimester

- Both prepare for labor, delivery, and parenthood

Interventions

- Encourage father to take active role during pregnancy
- Assist couple to keep lines of communication open

Siblings' Tasks

- 1-year-old child: unaware of changes
- 2-year-old child: notices changes
- 3 or 4-year-old child: notices changes, may listen to FHR, feel baby kick
- School-age child: takes a more clinical interest in "how's" and "whys"
- Early adolescent: may find change difficult to accept, or believe parents "too old"

Preparation for Childbirth

Childbirth Education (CBE)

- *Goals:* helpful sharing of fears and concerns with other couples or parents-to-be; support through labor and delivery by husband or significant other if applicable
- *Content:* exercises to prepare body for labor and delivery, breathing techniques, relaxation techniques, including effleurage and sacral pressure for back pain, methods to alleviate pain

Signs of Impending Labor (True and False Labor)

Uterine Contractions
- True labor: regular contractions in lower back, radiating to front, intensified by walking—nullipara should go to the hospital when contractions are regular and 5 minutes apart; multipara should go to the hospital when contractions are regular and 10 minutes apart
- False labor: irregular contractions in abdomen

Rupture of Membranes (ROM)
- If occurs at home, client should call physician
- Fern test or ph determination verifies ROM: in ph determination, nitrazine paper turns blue if amniotic fluid is present (alkaline)

Bloody Show (Mucous Plug)
- Show usually present in true labor but not in false

Dilation of Cervix
- In false labor, no change; in true labor, becomes effaced and dilates progressively

The High Risk Prenatal Client

Epidemiological and Other Risk Factors for Mother and Fetus

Age
- 16 and under: risk due to immature bodies and psychosocial factors (noncompliance with medical instructions may result in premature labor, PIH, anemia)
- Over 35: increased incidence of Down's syndrome and chromosomal abnormalities; amniocentesis is offered in early pregnancy

Economic Status and Education
- Premature birth and birth of low birth weight infant more likely when parents have limited income and when mother has grade school rather than college education

Marital Status
- Lack of support systems and insufficient income frequently are problems when mother unmarried

Multiparity
- Grand multiparas (5 or more pregnancies) are more likely to have complications, such as hemorrhage and dystocia

Multiple Pregnancy
- May be surmised if rapid uterine growth occurs
- Diagnosed by ultrasound, hearing two heart beats, increased HCG
- Complications: maternal anemia; preterm birth; postpartum hemorrhage; parents' coping mechanisms may be overwhelmed with care of two or more infants; exhaustion; increased financial expense

Infertility
- Crisis for couple: both partners should have evaluative work-up to identify problem or problems; any pregnancy and its outcome are of supreme importance to couple
- Treatment methods widely discussed in media include artificial insemination, in vitro fertilization, and surrogate motherhood; in cases of anovulation, endocrine therapy with clomiphene citrate (Clomid) or menotropins (Pergonal) to achieve ovulation is news when multiple pregnancies result from overstimulation of ovaries

Preexisting Medical Conditions as Risk Factors for Mother and Fetus

Diabetes
- Physiological need for insulin increases during pregnancy; if pancreas is not able to meet needs, gestational diabetes develops

- Control is of utmost importance for the insulin-dependent diabetic during pregnancy
- Ketoacidosis in the mother is a dire situation for fetus because carbon dioxide and oxygen exchange does not occur at the placenta; fetus may become asphyxiated and die
- Insulin requirements decrease during first trimester and increase during second and third trimester; dosage based on blood glucose determinations (glucose in urine is not accurate assessment due to decreased renal threshold for sugar during pregnancy)
- Babies usually delivered early to prevent stillbirth or cephalopelvic disproportion

Cardiovascular Disease

- Pregnancy strains cardiovascular system—in the presence of cardiac disease, cardiac decompensation can occur

Outcomes

- Clients with classes I (no limit of activity) and II (slight limitation of activity) heart disease may, with careful monitoring, enjoy normal pregnancy and delivery
- Clients with class III (considerable limitation of activity) usually avoid complications if required bedrest is maintained
- Incidence of morbidity and mortality increases with class IV (unable to undertake any physical activity without discomfort)

Interventions

- Prenatal period: provide iron supplements, rest, adequate nutrition
- During labor: administer generous amount of oxygen; administer antibiotics to prevent subacute bacterial endocarditis; prevent exhaustion
- Postpartum: period immediately after delivery is hazardous for client with cardiac disease, due to rapid increase of cardiac output; watch for cardiac decompensation, provide for rest and progressive ambulation

Iron-deficiency Anemia

- Most common medical disorder of pregnancy
- Hemoglobin and hematocrit are assessed periodically, especially in 32d–34th weeks when hemodilution occurs as result of increased blood volume
- Increased risk of hemorrhage, premature or small-for-gestational age baby, anomalies
- Interventions: provide oral iron and vitamin C supplements

Complications of Pregnancy

Hyperemesis Gravidarum

- Exaggerated nausea and vomiting
- Interventions: hospitalization; administer parenteral fluids for 48 hours; administer sedatives; provide dry diet in six small daily feedings with clear liquids 1 hour later, and monitor carefully; encourage client to discuss feelings; refer for psychotherapy

Pregnancy-induced Hypertension (PIH)

- 3 cardinal signs occur after 20th week: elevated BP, edema, proteinuria
- Preeclampsia and eclampsia are types of PIH
- Mild preeclampsia: systolic pressure elevated 30 mmHg, diastolic pressure elevated 15 mmHg
- Severe preeclampsia: BP 160/110, protein +3 or +4
- Other signs and symptoms: headache, visual problems, hyperreflexia, clonus, epigastric pain
- Eclampsia: severe preeclampsia plus seizures
- Interventions: assess vital signs frequently (circulatory collapse may occur); assess for proteinuria and reflexes; provide quiet environment; administer magnesium sulfate (CNS depressant) as ordered—repeat dose

only if respirations are 12–14 breaths/minute or more, urine output is 25 mL/hr, and reflexes are present

Bleeding Disorders

Hemorrhage

- Disseminated intravascular coagulation (DIC), a pathologic form of clotting due to hemorrhage and other factors, may result
- Hemorrhagic disorders are medical emergencies that require expert teamwork to minimize effects and prevent DIC
- Treatment for DIC is whole blood and whole blood components such as cryoprecipitate, platelets, fresh frozen plasma

Abortion

- Early: before 16 weeks gestation
- Late: 16–24 weeks gestation
- Types: threatened (intervention: provide bedrest, prevent stress); inevitable (intervention: dilation and curettage); incomplete (intervention: D & C); complete; missed
- Providing psychological support is important

Ectopic Pregnancy

- Fetus is implanted outside uterine cavity
- Client complains of unilateral pain over mass
- Assess for hemorrhage, shock, referred shoulder pain
- Major problem is hemorrhage; usually managed by laparotomy with excision of fallopian tube

Hydatidiform Mole

- Developmental anomaly of placenta; signs and symptoms noticeable around 12th week of gestation
- Assess for uterus larger than expected for gestation, excessive nausea and vomiting, brownish red vaginal discharge, symptoms of PIH, elevated HCG titers, absence of FHR
- Management: evacuation of uterus; periodic HCG titers (continued high titers indicate possible choriocarcinoma); birth control pills advised to prevent pregnancy

Placenta Previa

- Placenta is implanted in lower uterine segment and impedes descent of fetus
- Types: complete or total (completely occludes cervical os), partial, marginal, and low-lying
- Client experiences painless bright red uterine bleeding in third trimester
- Management includes bedrest until fetal lungs are mature or client goes into labor; delivery may be vaginal or cesarean (cesarean for greater than 30% placenta previa or in case of excessive bleeding)

Abruptio Placentae

- Premature separation of placenta after the 20th week; more likely when client is hypertensive or a multipara
- Client experiences small to moderate amount of dark red bleeding; may be accompanied by hypovolemia, shock, uterine hypertonicity, and pain
- Management includes delivery of fetus, blood replacement

Infections

Urinary Tract Infections

- Asymptomatic bacteriuria occurs in small percentage of pregnant women; may result in cystitis or pyelonephritis
- Premature labor and delivery more likely

Sexually Transmitted Diseases (STD)

- Moniliasis: assess for thick, curdy, white, vaginal discharge that may be malodorous, and for vulvar pruritus; interventions include providing nystatin (Mycostatin) vaginal suppositories and instructing client to

- abstain from intercourse until cured or treat sexual partner
- Gonorrhea: culture is done at client's first prenatal visit; if positive, treatment usually is oral ampicillin. If organism is present at delivery, newborn may be blind unless treated with silver nitrate or penicillin
- Chlamydia: presently the most common vaginal infection; may also cause blindness in the newborn; symptoms similar to gonorrhea—treated with erythromycin
- Syphilis: test is performed at first prenatal visit; if treated with penicillin by 18th week, fetus will probably not be affected
- Herpes II: if active lesions are present at time of delivery, a cesarean will be performed to protect infant from exposure; if membranes rupture and active lesions are present, a cesarean should be performed within 4 hours

TORCH (Organisms That May Seriously Damage Embryo or Fetus)

T: toxoplasmosis (mother has flulike symptoms)

O: other (includes syphilis)

R: rubella (a titer is done at first prenatal visit—if less than 1:8, client should receive rubella vaccine after delivery and be instructed to avoid pregnancy for 2–3 months

C: cytomegalovirus (mother has mononucleosislike symptoms)

H: herpes II

10

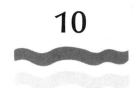

Nursing Care During the Intrapartal Period

The Client Undergoing Normal Labor and Delivery

Assessment

Processes of Labor (5 p's): Essential Factors That Influence the Process of Labor

- *Passage:* configuration (gynecoid most favorable) and diameters of pelvis (are the inlet, mid-pelvis, and outlet adequate?)
- *Powers:* strength, duration, and frequency of contractions
- *Passenger:* size, presentation, and position of fetus (problems include cephalopelvic disproportion, malposition)
- *Placenta:* site of insertion (fundal or low-lying)
- *Psychologic* state of client (*e.g.,* fearful, tense)

Stages of Labor

First Stage

The first stage begins with the onset of regular contractions and is complete when the cervix is completely dilated (dilation stage).

- Latent phase: cervix dilates to approximately 3–4 cm
- Active phase: cervix dilates from 3 or 4 cm to 8 cm; contractions are moderate to strong, lasting 30–45 seconds, occurring every 3–5 minutes; if membranes rupture, assess fluid for color and odor, and assess fetal heart rate (FHR) for deceleration (could indicate prolapsed cord)
- Transition phase: cervix dilates from 8 cm to 10 cm ("complete"); contractions are strong, lasting 45–60 seconds and occurring every 2–3 minutes; client may experience nausea and vomiting, be irritable, and find it more difficult to relax between contractions and to maintain control

Second Stage

The second stage begins when the cervix is fully dilated and ends with the delivery of the baby (expulsive stage). The client "pushes," the presenting part descends to the pelvic floor, and the baby is delivered.

- *Caution:* Client should not push until cervix is completely dilated or edema and lacerations of cervix will result (if client wants to push before cervix is completely dilated, panting will block urge)

Table 10-1. Definitions in Assessing Progress of Labor

Engagement: when the biparietal diameter of the head passes the pelvic inlet

Descent: progress of the presenting part through the pelvis

Effacement: thinning and shortening or obliteration of the cervix

Dilation: stretching of the external os from an opening a few millimeters in size to an opening large enough to allow for delivery of the infant

Station: relationship of the presenting part to an imaginary line drawn between the ischial spines

Contraction pattern
a) phases of contractions—increment (increase or rise), acme (peak), decrement (decline)
b) frequency—timed from the beginning of a contraction to the beginning of the next contraction
c) duration—timed from the beginning to the end of a contraction
d) Intensity—mild, moderate, or strong

Note: Effacement, dilation, station, bloody show, contraction pattern, vital signs and psychosocial response are monitored throughout labor to assess progress of labor and maternal and fetal well-being

---

Third Stage

The third stage extends from the birth of the baby until the delivery of the placenta (placental stage).

- *Caution:* do not knead uterus or push fundus downward to encourage placental separation (can result in incomplete separation of placenta and excessive bleeding)
- A gush of blood and extension of cord indicate placental separation
- Examine placenta to assess for intactness, retained placenta, or infarcts

Fourth Stage

The fourth stage is the first 2 hours after delivery when the mother makes her initial readjustment to the nonpregnant state.

- Critical time for mother in regard to homeostasis and hemorrhage in particular
- Important to begin family interaction (bonding) and breast-feeding

Monitoring Vital Signs

- Protocol varies from hospital to hospital

Maternal

- Assess blood pressure (BP), pulse (P), respiration (R) every 30–60 minutes unless otherwise indicated
- Check temperature every 4 hours unless otherwise indicated

Fetal

- Assess FHR every 15–30 minutes by fetoscope, or continuously by electronic means
- Electronic monitoring (external or internal) is used particularly for high-risk clients: external monitoring instruments and belts may limit mother's movement and positioning; internal monitoring with fetal scalp electrode (FSE) does not interfere with positioning—however, range of motion (ROM) exercises are necessary; FSE gives better reading

Fetal Response to Labor

FHR Decelerations

- Indicates hypoxia
- Early deceleration: transitory decrease below baseline rate, concurrent with uterine contractions; caused by head compression; a reassuring pattern, not ominous
- Late deceleration: transitory decrease below baseline rate, in contracting phase; caused by uteroplacental insufficiency; indicates significant fetal hypoxia
    Nursing measures: change maternal position and correct maternal hypotension, increase IV rate, discontinue oxytocin (Pitocin) if infusing, administer oxygen at 10–12 L/min per face mask

Table 10-2. Definitions of Fetal Heart Rate

Normal FHR: baseline rate between contractions, 120–160 beats/min

Baseline variability: normal irregularity of the cardiac rhythm caused by the autonomic nervous system (absence of baseline variability indicates CNS depression)

Tachycardia: FHR of over 160 beats/min, lasting longer than 10 minutes

Bradycardia: FHR below 120 beats/min, lasting longer than 10 minutes

---

- Variable deceleration: abrupt transitory decrease that is variable in duration, intensity, and timing relative to contractions; caused by cord compression; serious if rate falls below 70 beats/min
  Nursing measures: see late decelerations

Meconium Stained Amniotic Fluid

- Indicates fetal hypoxia has occurred at some time
- Dangers: degree of hypoxia experienced by fetus; aspiration of meconium at birth (requires careful suctioning)

Support During Labor

Relaxation and Breathing Techniques

- Help decrease tension and increase effectiveness of contractions
- Mother takes cleansing breath at beginning and end of each contraction, breathing in through nose and out through mouth
- Abdominal or chest breathing may be used during active phase
- 4:1 pattern (breath, breath, breath, breath, puff) may be used during transition (more difficult to concentrate on breathing techniques)
- Pushing during second stage consists of client holding her breath for no more than 5 seconds while being instructed to "push the baby out"
- Assist client to relax completely between contractions to conserve her energy and prevent exhaustion
- Assist father or significant other to become involved with relaxation, breathing, and comfort measures

Comfort Measures

- Keep client informed, give support and reassurance
- Position client comfortably with pillows; place cold cloth on forehead, provide quiet atmosphere, provide good hygiene
- Assess voiding needs every 1–2 hours

Analgesia

- Recognize and assess cultural implications of pain (some clients may experience what appears to be excessive pain; others may deny pain)
- Assess status and stage of labor:
  If analgesia is given before 3–4 cm dilation, labor process slows
  Do not administer if birth is expected in 2 hours
  For nullipara give before complete dilation
  For multipara give before 7 cm dilation
- After administration, assess for side-effects: respiratory depression, FHR decelerations and variability, nausea, vomiting
- Analgesia may slow labor or it may speed up labor as client relaxes

Anesthesia

Peripheral Nerve Block

- Pudendal: used for delivery and repair of lacerations and episiotomy; affects lower ⅔ of vagina and perineum; lasts 30 minutes; does not depress neonate's heart rate

Regional Blocks

- Common types: epidural, caudal, spinal
- Monitor vascular status and fetal response closely
- Side-effects: hypotension and fetal bradycardia; bearing-down reflex partially or completely eliminated

- *Nursing measures* in response to side-effects: change maternal position to side-lying, administer oxygen 10–12 L/min, discontinue oxytocin (Pitocin) if infusing, increase IV rate

Delivery

Vaginal

- Various positions now employed: lithotomy, side-lying, sitting
- Fathers in attendance need support, including information about care, assistance with coaching and with initiating attachment with newborn
- Siblings in attendance must have attended classes for siblings and have an adult with them
- As mother pushes, baby's head will crown; an episiotomy may be performed to facilitate delivery of head and prevent lacerations
- After delivery of head, physician will aspirate infant's mouth and nose and check for nuchal cord
- Body is then delivered, cord clamped and body placed head down (to facilitate drainage of mucus) and "skin to skin" on mother's chest
- Placenta separates and is expelled; IV oxytocin (Pitocin) is administered to help uterus contract and help prevent hemorrhage
- Maintaining clear airway and preventing heat loss are crucial for newborn

Cesarean

- Maternal indications: cephalopelvic disproportion (CPD) (most common), previous cesarean, pregnancy-induced hypertension (PIH), placenta previa, abruptio placentae, dystocia, pelvic tumors, gonorrhea, herpes II
- Fetal indications: fetal distress, prolapsed cord, hydrocephalus, breech and shoulder presentations
- Anchor indwelling urinary catheter and administer IV fluids as for any abdominal surgery
- Unless general anesthetic is employed, father may be permitted in OR
- Encourage early contact with infant for both parents
- Recovery period similar to that for any abdominal surgery
- Although information about cesarean section is included in childbirth education (CBE), an unplanned cesarean is a cruel blow to parents, and mother may feel a failure—support and reassure parents, especially mother

Immediate Care of the Newborn

Apgar Scoring

- Criteria: respiratory effort, heart rate, reflex, irritability (cry), color, and muscle tone
- Assess at 1 minute and 5 minutes after birth; give maximum of 2 points for each criterion; score of 7–10 indicates newborn is in good condition, 4–6 fair condition, and 0–3 poor condition

Other Procedures

- Perform physical examination checking number of vessels in cord (less than three may indicate presence of anomalies), and noting passage of meconium and urine
- Assess gestational age, weight, length, head and chest circumferences
- Implement identification procedures
- Administer silver nitrate or penicillin to eyes to prevent ophthalmia neonatorum, which results from gonorrhea or chlamydia organisms present in birth canal at delivery
- Administer vitamin K: routine in some institutions to increase coagulation (E. coli must be present in intestines for synthesis of vitamin K)

Facilitating Bonding

- Provide for and assist with early contact between newborn and both parents; give support, praise, and reassurance

- Assess eye-to-eye contact, touch, level of interest in infant
- Warning signs: passive or hostile reaction to newborn, disappointment over sex of infant, no eye contact with infant, nonsupportive interaction between parents

Maternal Physiological Assessments During Fourth Stage

- Assess fundus every 15 minutes for position and consistency (if soft, massage until firm)
- Assess amount of lochial flow, the perineum, BP and P, and check for full bladder, every 15 minutes

The High Risk Labor Client

Complications of Labor

Dystocia

Dystocia is prolonged, difficult birth due to deviation from normal in the interrelationship of any of the 5 p's (see processes of labor section).

Pelvic

Size or configuration of pelvis is abnormal or inadequate, contributing to CPD

Of Fetal Origin

Large fetus, fetal anomalies, malpresentation (breech, shoulder), malposition (posterior vs. anterior)

Uterine

Primary inertia: inefficient contractions persist from onset of labor

Secondary inertia: well-established efficient contractions become weak and inefficient or stop altogether

Medical Interventions

- Oxytocin (Pitocin) augmentation to stimulate uterus to contract (contraindicated for CPD)
- Artificial rupture of membranes may stimulate labor
- Episiotomy to allow for more room for delivery
- Forceps or vacuum extraction to assist forces of labor and delivery
- Cesarean delivery
- Forceps deliveries and hemorrhage more likely with dystocia

Nursing Measures

- Support and reassure client
- Provide comfort measures
- Assist with relaxation and breathing techniques

Prolapsed Cord

- Assess by noting significant decrease (20 beats/min or more) in FHR and by vaginal examination
- May occur with rupture of membranes, footling breech
- *Priority intervention:* prevent compression of cord between presenting part and bony pelvis by having client assume knee-chest or Trendelenberg position, and by vaginal support of presenting part with fingers to keep presenting part away from prolapsed cord
- Deliver promptly

Induction of Labor with Oxytocin

- Used when mother or fetus is in jeopardy if pregnancy continues

Administration

- Prostaglandin gel may be applied to cervix to soften
- Administered by infusion pump; dosage carefully regulated

Hazards

Tumultuous labor and tetanic contractions
Premature separation of placenta
Rupture of uterus
Laceration of cervix

Hemorrhage

Fetal hypoxia and injury

Nursing Measures
- Carefully monitor vital signs and FHR (watch for deceleration)
- Carefully monitor contractions for uterine tetany: sudden increase in frequency, duration, intensity of contractions, and decrease in relaxation between contractions—discontinue oxytocin

Episiotomy/Lacerations
- Episiotomy is performed to prevent tearing of perineum, but lacerations may occur anyway and extend episiotomy
- A 3° episiotomy or laceration extends into anal sphincter; a 4° episiotomy or laceration extends through anal sphincter and into rectal mucosa

Indications for Forceps Delivery
- Maternal: to shorten second stage for client with dystocia or for cardiac client
- Fetal: to shorten second stage when fetus is jeopardized
- *Nursing assessments:* closely monitor FHR; monitor mother for excessive bleeding after procedure; examine neonate for cerebral trauma or nerve damage

Premature Labor

Prevention

Good prenatal care

Occurs more frequently in adolescents and in clients with hypertension, cardiac disease, renal disease, anemia, multiple gestation, occult cervicitis, amnionitis

Management
- Administer ritodrine to relax uterus; watch for side-effects (pulmonary edema)
- If unable to stop labor and fetus is preterm, administer glucocorticoid (*e.g.*, betamethasone sodium—Celestone) to mother before delivery to accelerate fetal lung maturity and to prevent infant respiratory distress syndrome (IRDS)

Precipitate or Emergency Delivery
- As baby's head crowns, instruct client to pant-blow and to avoid urge to push
- Place hand on exposed fetal head and apply *gentle* pressure to prevent head from popping out (prevent subdural tears)
- Check for cord around neck
- Support head as body is delivered
- Keep head down to drain mucus
- Dry baby and keep at same level as mother's uterus to prevent gravity flow of baby's blood to or from placenta, which could result in hypovolemia or hypervolemia in newborn
- As soon as baby cries, place on mother's abdomen, cover and keep warm
- Wait for placenta to deliver—do not cut cord; wrap cord and placenta together
- Check firmness of uterus; prevent or manage boggy uterus by gentle massage, putting baby to breast, keeping bladder from filling, expelling any clots

Uterine Rupture

May occur in cases of dystocia, labor stress, or overstimulation with oxytocin

Client experiences intraabdominal hemorrhage, pain, and collapse; laparotomy or hysterectomy is performed

Inversion of Uterus

May be complete or partial; caused by traction applied to fundus or on cord

Client experiences profound shock; treat shock; uterus is replaced manually or surgically if necessary

11

Nursing Care During the Postpartal Period

The Normal Postpartum Client

Physiological Adaptation: Assessment and Interventions

Breasts

- Assess for engorgement: appears 2nd to 4th day, lasts 36–48 hours; nursing measures include providing snug supportive bra, analgesics
- Assess nipples of breast-feeding mother for irritation, cracks, or fissures
- To treat for suppressed lactation, provide snug bra and administer nonhormonal milk suppressant drug, *e.g.,* bromocriptine mesylate (Parlodel)

Fundus

- *Position:* fundus descends from umbilicus one finger breadth per day until 10th day when fundus is no longer palpable; a full bladder may displace fundus upward and to the right—employ nursing measures to empty bladder
- *Consistency:* fundus should be firmly contracted to prevent excess bleeding: if boggy, massage gently until firm—if fundus does not stay firm, examine for and remove clots; administration of an oxytoxic drug may be necessary
- Afterpains are common for 2–3 days in the multipara

Lochia

- Rubra (red): until 3rd day postpartum
- Serosa (pinkish): 4–10 days
- Alba (white): 10th day to 6th week
- Assess amount (important in regard to hemorrhage): gradually diminishes from large amount the first few hours to moderate amount 2nd and 3rd days, followed by scant amount; flow is excessive if pad is soaked through in 15 minutes
- *Interventions:* if fundus is relaxed, massage; if clots are present, expel by pushing downward on fundus

Episiotomy

- Assess for edema, inflammation, purulent discharge, bruising, intactness
- *Interventions:* apply ice first 12 hours; apply heat after first 12–24 hours; apply topical analgesics and anti-inflammatory preparations, perineal cleanse; teach Kegel exercises to strengthen and tighten perineal muscles

Hemorrhoids

- *Interventions:* teach about appropriate diet, fluids, timing; offer rubber ring and treatments as ordered by physician

Elimination

- Voiding: assess for bladder distention and stasis of urine (due to decreased bladder sensation), which could cause infection and interfere with contraction of uterus; institute nursing measures to encourage voiding if client unable; may need physician's order for catheterization
- Diuresis: reversal of fluids accumulated during pregnancy, occurring approximately 12 hours after delivery; adds to voiding problems
- Diaphoresis: profuse sweating may occur, especially at night (night sweats) for 2–3 days after delivery
- Bowel evacuation: most women do not have bowel movement for 2–3 days after delivery; laxative or stool softener may be ordered; suppositories and enemas are contraindicated for women with 3° or 4° episiotomies

Vital Signs

- Temperature may be elevated slightly first day or two
- Bradycardia is not unusual
- Blood pressure should remain at baseline

Activity and Exercise

- Vaginally delivered clients may be up *ad lib* and shower as soon as effects of anesthesia are gone
- Nonstrenuous exercises such as lifting head off pillow may begin immediately; more strenuous exercises need physician approval

Nutrition

- Ensure good nutrition for client during restorative period

Cesarean Birth: Assessment and Nursing Measures

- Monitor indwelling catheter and IV fluids
- Record intake and output (I and O); diet is advanced from clear liquid to full diet as bowel sounds are heard (varies from 2–3 days to several days)
- Postpartum assessment: *carefully* evaluate fundus
- Control pain—time administration of analgesics so mother will be fairly comfortable when she has contact with infant
- Promote attachment process, arrange pillows for comfort when mother holding infant
- Promote ambulation, turn, cough, deep breath
- Client may shower with physician's order

Lactation and Breast-feeding

Mother's Needs

Diet and Fluids

- Increase caloric intake, especially of protein, by 500 calories/day and supplement diet with vitamin and iron tablets
- Increase fluid intake to 2–3 quarts/day

Medications

- Consult physician
- Most medications are secreted in milk; should particularly avoid administering anticoagulants, antibiotics, and antimicrobials

Care of Breasts

- Clean with soap and water only once a day if at all
- Ensure client wears well-fitting, supportive bra
- Air-dry nipples after each feeding to prevent irritation

Family Planning

- Advise client to avoid birth control pills because estrogen interferes with production of prolactin, which is necessary for milk production

Putting Baby to Breast

- Put baby to breast soon after delivery and often, to stimulate production of milk; colostrum is beneficial—increased protein and immune bodies
- Ensure mother's comfort in order to decrease tension
- Ensure infant has portion of areola in mouth, to nurse efficiently
- Alternate beginning breast to equalize sucking and stimulation of milk production
- Awaken sleepy baby by unwrapping him or her or tapping on sole of feet, or assist with sucking motion by putting mother's thumb under baby's chin
- Baby is getting enough milk if he or she sleeps 2–4 hours between feedings or has 6 or more straw-colored voidings in 24 hours

Psychosocial Adaptation

Parental Attachment

- Promote attachment by providing for contact with infant and teaching infant care experientially
- Assess eye-to-eye contact, touch behaviors

Parental Tasks and Roles

Parents must:

Reconcile actual child with fantasy child

Accept child as a separate being with many needs

Learn to care for infant and learn his or her cues

Establish relationships within family group

Establish primary importance of adult relationship (set aside time for each other)

Siblings' Common Behaviors

2, 3, or 4-year-olds may regress to infantile behavior

Young child may act jealous and aggressive

Set aside special time for child

Divert aggressive behavior directed toward baby

Let older child participate in plans, help care for baby

Grandparents

Grandparents must work through unresolved differing opinions and conflicts with adult child

Grandparents can be helpful and supportive to parents and can have positive relationship with child

Educational Needs

Self-care

- Provide anticipatory guidance about lochial changes, activities, exercises, complications
- Tell client to expect return of menses within 3–4 months if she is not lactating
- Advise resuming intercourse if desired 6 weeks postpartum after medical check-up

Infant Care

Cord

Teach client to:

- Apply alcohol to cord stump each day until it drops off in 7–14 days
- Avoid tub bathing until stump drops off

Circumcision

Teach client to:

- Assess frequently for bleeding during first 12 hours
- Watch for first voiding

Safety

- Promote safety measures in home, including use of car seat

Signs of Illness

- Inform parents to contact physician if they notice change in infant's behavior (irritability, lethargy), fever, vomiting, diarrhea

Bottle Feeding

Teach parents to:

- Elevate infant's head to prevent eustachian tube filling with formula—could result in otitis media; do not prop bottles for same reason, and for promotion of attachment
- Ensure nipple is full of milk so infant does not ingest air
- Burp baby mid-feeding, at end of feeding, and as necessary
- Place infant in side-lying position on abdomen after feeding to prevent aspiration if he or she spits up formula

Family Planning

Inform couple of methods and advantages and disadvantages of each.

Less effective methods include natural, jelly, and foam. Natural methods include:

- Rhythm or calendar method: involves using formula to determine woman's fertile period based on time of menstrual period and recognizing signs of ovulation
- Basal body temperature (BBT) method: BBT drops 24–36 hours before ovulation, then rises 24–48 hours after ovulation
- Cervical mucus method: at time of ovulation woman has a feeling of wetness and mucus is slippery

More effective methods include:

- Diaphragm with spermicide: check for placement over os; leave in place at least 6 hours after intercourse; must be refitted after gain or loss of 10 pounds or more, abortion, or delivery of a baby
- Sponge: saturated with spermicide; may be left in place 2 days
- Condoms with spermicide: help prevent sexually transmitted diseases
- Birth control pills (BCP): contraindicated if client has diabetes (interfere with carbohydrate metabolism—women with vascular problems run increased risk for thrombus), hypertension, stroke, thromboembolic disease, or is over 40 years of age
- Surgical methods: bilateral tubal ligation and vasectomy are most popular methods, particularly among couples over 35 years of age

The High Risk Postpartum Client

Assessing the High Risk Mother

Physical Factors

Hemorrhage (monitor for conditions that predispose to hemorrhage)

Infection

Abnormal vital signs

Traumatic labor or delivery: prolonged labor, malposition of fetus, large fetus, instrument delivery

Multiple pregnancy

Psychosocial Factors

Preexisting major health problem, including mental illness or alcoholism

Poverty (parents may not have been able to afford prenatal care)

Insufficient support system

Family disruption or dissolution

Poor coping skills

Complications of the Postpartal Period

Hemorrhage

Assessment

Loss of 500 mL or more of blood indicates hemorrhage

Early postpartum hemorrhage (first 24 hours) is usually due to uterine atony or lacerations

Late postpartum hemorrhage (from 24 hours–28th day) is usually caused by subinvolution, retained placental tissue, or infection

Interventions

- Quickly assess, diagnose and treat cause, administer oxygen
- For uterine atony, massage fundus and administer oxytoxic agent
- For lacerations, repair

Infection

Episiotomy Wound Infection

- Assess for discharge, inflammation
- Have culture of discharge taken and administer appropriate antibiotic; institute supportive health measures

Endometritis

- Assess for foul-smelling lochia, abdominal discomfort, back ache
- Provide care as for episiotomy wound infection and administer oxytoxic agent

Mastitis (Unilateral)

- Develops after flow of milk is established (3–4 weeks); causative organism is usually *Staphylococcus aureus*
- Assess for chills, fever, localized tenderness, redness, and warmth
- Administer antibiotics, apply heat to breast, provide supportive health measures; nursing may or may not be discontinued on affected side—if discontinued, breast must be pumped to maintain milk supply

Urinary Tract Infection

- Assess voiding pattern for frequency, residual urine, dysuria
- Administer antibiotics and provide supportive health measures

Thrombophlebitis

- Assess for edema, warmth, leg pain
- Apply hot, moist packs; provide elastic stockings; administer anticoagulant if necessary (heparin is not excreted in breast milk)

Psychosocial Problems

Postpartum Psychosis

Etiology: drastic change in body chemistry and sleep deprivation may precipitate manic depression or other psychiatric disorders

Most common condition involves severe depression (different from "baby blues"); lasts from 6 months to 1 year

Crisis Caused by Delivering High Risk Infant (Defective or Premature), Abortion, Ectopic Pregnancy, or Fetal Loss

Parents will experience denial, blame, guilt, grief

Interventions

- If baby lives, provide for early parent–child interaction, include siblings, encourage parents to talk about crisis and support each other
- In case of fetal loss, let parents see and hold infant, give parents memento (picture, crib tag) as concrete evidence child existed

12

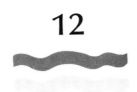

Nursing Care of the Neonate and Family

The Normal Newborn

Physiological Changes

Establishment of Respiration

Establishment of respiration within 1 minute after birth is vital to subsequent central nervous system (CNS) functioning. The change is caused by a combination of cold, gravity, light and noise, with changes in partial pressure of oxygen in arterial blood (PaO_2) and partial pressure of carbon dioxide in arterial blood ($PaCO_2$).

Transformation of Fetal Circulation to Newborn Circulation

Independent circulation is initiated by the infant's first breath, which causes changes in pulmonary blood flow and results in changes in pressure. Changes in pressure in the right and left atrium cause a functional closing of the foramen ovale. Increased PO_2 causes the ductus arteriosus to constrict, but permanent closure is not accomplished immediately. The umbilical vein and ductus venosus close immediately when the cord is clamped and cut.

Thermoregulation

Thermoregulation is vital to systemic adaptation. Cold stress increases the infant's need for oxygen.

Physical Assessment

General

- Assess posture, symmetry of head, and presence of flexed extremities

Skin

- Acrocyanosis, erythematous flush present first few days
- Milia, lanugo gradually disappear
- Mongolian spots, telangiectatic nevi (stork bites), erythema toxicum are normal variations
- Jaundice may be physiologic or hemolytic; note degree of jaundice present

Head

Assess for:

- Caput succedaneum—normal variation
- Cephalhematoma—possible problem

- Bulging or depressed fontanelles—indicate intracranial pressure or dehydration

Eyes

Assess for:

- Discharge—could indicate infection
- Transient strabismus—may be present 3–4 months

Mouth

Assess for:

- Epstein's pearls—normal variation
- Intact palate

Abdomen

- Assess for distention—possible problem

Genitalia

Assess for:

- Pseudomenorrhea in girls—normal variation
- Undescended testicles and phimosis in boys—possible problems

Reflexes and Activity

Assess for:

- Normal reflexes—Moro's embrace, tonic-neck (fencing position), grasping, sucking, rooting, swallowing and gagging, sneezing and coughing, stepping, hand to mouth, Babinski (plantar)
- Lethargy or jitteriness—may indicate infection or hypoglycemia

Vital Signs

Assess for normal values, including:

- Temperature: 97.6°–98.6°
- Respirations: 30 breaths/min–60 breaths/min
- Pulse: 110 beats/min–160 beats/min

Measurement

- Weight: average 7–7.5 pounds (loss of 5%–10% birth weight is normal, regained in 1–2 weeks)
- Length: average 19–21 inches
- Head and chest circumferences average: 13–14 inches

Laboratory Tests

Hematocrit
Blood glucose level (Dextrostix)
Phenylketonuria (PKU)
T_4
Bilirubin level

Nutritional Needs

- Provide 120 calories/kg a day for newborn; formula: 20 calories/ounce; premie formula: 24 calories/ounce
- Offer water at first feeding to rule out tracheal-esophageal fistula
- Ensure early feedings to prevent hypoglycemia
- Expect infant to spit up some mucus first few days; may also spit up some milk due to immature cardiac sphincter
- Follow infant's schedule: will demand feeding every 2–5 hours—infant is getting enough formula if he or she sleeps 3–5 hours between feedings
- Instruct parents not to offer solids for at least 4–6 months, due to digestive immaturity of newborn

Complications That May Affect the Newborn

Respiratory Problems

- Excess mucus: position on side for drainage, elevate foot of crib, suction oropharynx
- Gagging and choking: suction

- Cyanosis, bradycardia, prolonged periods of apnea: ensure prone position, provide warmth, gavage, or IV fluids

Jaundice

Physiologic Hyperbilirubinemia

Physiologic hyperbilirubinemia refers to a progressive increase in serum levels of unconjugated bilirubin due to immature liver functioning or bruising at the time of delivery.

- Occurs when infant is 2–4 days old (a day or two later in premature infant); peaks at 3–6 days of age and disappears at 7–10 days of age (the later days for premature infant)
- Bilirubin concentration does not exceed 12 mg/dL in term infants and 15 mg/dL in premature infants—levels at which damage to brain (kernicterus) may occur, however, are unpredictable, especially in immature infants
- Assess degree of jaundice by blanching skin cephalocaudally (newborn jaundice develops cephalocaudally)—jaundice visible at 4–6 mg/dL of total bilirubin (higher level applies to black infants)

Interventions

For the well, term infant, treatment is probably not necessary. The condition can be prevented by providing adequate fluids early to encourage passage of meconium and to prevent hypoglycemia, which can cause an increase in bilirubin level.

Phototherapy involves the use of fluorescent lights to cause photo-oxidation of bilirubin. It may be started at levels of 10–14 mg/mL for the term infant and lower levels for the more immature infant.

Procedure

- Remove clothing to expose skin
- Cover eyes to prevent injury to conjunctiva or retina
- Cover genitalia
- Monitor temperature
- Evaluate fluid loss (loose greenish stools are common)
- Discontinue light, remove eye covering and hold infant to feed
- Provide parent–infant interaction and appropriate education for parents

Pathologic Hyperbilirubinemia

Pathologic hyperbilirubinemia may develop during the first 24 hours of an infant's life. Isoimmune hemolytic disease is based on antigen-antibody response.

Rh Incompatibility

Usually does not occur with first pregnancy

Can be detected prenatally by rising serum antibody titers

Isoimmunization occurs when an Rh− woman receives Rh+ blood by transfusion or from an Rh+ fetus when placenta separates—will not affect mother, but with next Rh+ fetus, antibodies will pass through placenta resulting in hemolysis of the fetus' RBCs

Diagnosis: bloodtype and Rh determined at first prenatal visit; after delivery, baby's Rh is determined and Coombs' test determines whether mother is already sensitized

Interventions

- IM injections of Rho (Du) immune globin (Rhogam) prenatally at 28–30 weeks of gestation or by 32 weeks of gestation
- If mother is Rh−, baby is Rh+, and Coombs' test result is negative, mother will be given Rhogam within 72 hours after delivery
- Assess infant for jaundice; monitor bilirubin levels; infant may require phototherapy
- Occasionally, exchange transfusion performed if bilirubin level is rising rapidly or reaches 20 mg/100 mL in term infant or 15 mg/100 mL in preterm infant, depending on maturity
- All Rh− women should receive Rhogam after an abortion

ABO Incompatibility

Occurs in first-born child; cannot be predicted; occurs when mother has O blood type and baby has A, B, or AB blood type

Mother's O blood has A and B antibodies that cross placenta and attack baby's RBCs

Infant's jaundice is usually mild and of short duration

Interventions
- Assess infant for jaundice
- Monitor bilirubin levels
- Carry out phototherapy if ordered

Feeding Problems

- Small babies (5½ to 6½ pounds) may need smaller, softer nipple or, if breast-feeding, may be slow to nurse at first
- For allergies to cow's milk, give goat's milk or soy formula
- Infant with respiratory problem or premature infant may require gavage (aspirate for residual formula in stomach before procedure—if more than 1 mL, check with physician before continuing)

Infection

- All newborn infants have increased susceptibility to infection; handwashing is vitally important
- Assess for lethargy, tachypnea, tachycardia, skin rash, temperature instability
- Diagnosis: cultures done from ears, nose, cord, urine, spinal fluid
- Interventions: administer antibiotics, provide supportive therapy and nursing care (oxygen, fluids, warmth)

Congenital Anomalies (See Chapters 13–16)

Nervous System
Spina bifida
Meningocele
Myelomeningocele
Hydrocephaly
Anencephaly
Down's Syndrome
Peripheral nerve injuries
CNS damage

Cardiovascular System
Transposition of great vessels
Tetralogy of Fallot
Patent ductus

Gastrointestinal System
Cleft lip and palate
Tracheoesophageal fistula
Pyloric stenosis
Biliary tract abnormalities
Imperforate anus
Omphalocele
Phenylketonuria

Genitourinary System
Extrophy of bladder
Bilateral renal agenesis
Polycystic kidneys
Hypospadias
Phimosis
Hydrocele
Undescended testicles

Musculoskeletal System
Fractures
Polydactyly
Congenital club foot
Congenital dislocation of hips

Care of the High Risk Infant

The Preterm Infant (Born Between Conception to 37 Weeks Gestation)

Characteristics include thin skin, plentiful lanugo, minimal sole creases, minimal or no ear cartilage; all systems immature

Infant Respiratory Distress Syndrome (IRDS)

Due to deficient surfactant

Assessment
- Usually develops within 2–6 hours after birth
- Initially revealed by expiratory grunting with nasal flaring, tachypnea (more than 60 respirations/min)
- Retractions, hypotension, shock, respiratory acidosis, decreased muscle tone, drop in temperature follow

Interventions
- Administer oxygen
- Apply continuous positive airway pressure
- Provide umbilical arterial catheter for blood gases

Complications

Intracranial hemorrhage

Pneumothorax

Necrotizing enterocolitis

Bronchial pulmonary dysplasia

Retrolental fibroplasia

Cold Stress

Temperature below 98°F—results in increased need for oxygen

Imposes metabolic and physiologic problems on *all infants*, especially preterm, hypoxic infants

Vicious cycle resulting in hypoglycemia, metabolic and respiratory acidosis, hyperbilirubinemia, kernicterus

Post-term Infant (Born 43rd Week of Gestation or Later)

Characteristics usually include large size, but otherwise infants are normal with advanced development and bone age. The *wasted-appearing infant* is the exception; characteristics include:

Large appearing head

Decreased subcutaneous fat

Desquamating skin

Absent vernix

Hazards include placental insufficiency resulting in perinatal asphyxia; heat loss, CNS trauma, infection

Small-for-Gestational-Age (SGA) Infant

Weight is below 10th percentile for given gestational week

Indicates slowed intrauterine growth

Characteristics include reduced body dimensions and subcutaneous fat

Loose dry skin

Decreased muscle mass over buttocks and cheeks

Sparse scalp hair

Wide sutures

Alert, wide-eyed appearance due to hypoxia

Hazards include perinatal asphyxia, heat loss, hypoglycemia, infection (neonatal mortality 8 times higher than appropriate-for-gestational-age AGA infants)

Appropriate-for-Gestational-Age (AGA) Infant

Weight falls between 10th and 90th percentiles for age

Large-for-Gestational-Age (LGA) Infant

Weight is above 90th percentile for age

Indicates increased intrauterine growth

Characteristics include weight over 400 g (8 pounds, 13 ounces)

Hazards include birth trauma (CPD) and increased incidence of cesarean birth, hypoglycemia

Effects of Maternal Problems on the Newborn

Diabetes

Infants of gestational diabetics and insulin-dependent diabetics *without* vascular disease are likely to be LGA—CPD or CS likely

Infants of insulin-dependent diabetics *with* vascular disease are likely to be SGA

Monitor infants for hypoglycemia (most likely to occur within 3 hours after birth), hypocalcemia, RDS, hyperbilirubinemia

Drug Dependence

Signs usually appear within several hours of birth, caused by withdrawal rather than narcosis

May be depressed initially; may be jittery and hyperactive, have shrill persistent cry, yawn or sneeze frequently; tendon reflexes increased

Administer phenobarbital, perhaps paregoric

Most drug-dependent infants recover by 10 days of age

If not treated, may develop fever, vomiting, diarrhea, dehydration, apnea, convulsions, and die

Cesarean Birth

Increased likelihood of respiratory problems due to excess mucus (not having gone through labor process)

Maternal chronic health problems and problems present when emergency CS is done could result in problems for newborn

Infections

Gonorrhea, chlamydia (see Chapter 10)

Moniliasis: *Candida albicans* organism present at time of birth can cause thrush in newborn; treat with nystatin liquid

Herpes II: transplacental transmission is rare; cultures are done on infant if mother has active lesions; without treatment, most infants will die from CNS damage

Bibliography for Unit III
Care of the Client During Childbearing

Bobak IM, Jensen MD: Essentials of Maternity Nursing: The Nurse and the Childbearing Family, 2nd ed. St Louis, CV Mosby, 1987

Jensen MD, Bobak IM: Maternity and Gynecologic Care: The Nurse and the Family, 3rd ed. St Louis, CV Mosby, 1985

Ladewig PA, London ML, Olds SB: Essentials of Maternal-Newborn Nursing. Menlo Park, CA, Addison-Wesley, 1986

Neeson JD, May KA: Comprehensive Maternity Nursing. Philadelphia, JB Lippincott, 1986

Olds SB, London ML, Ladewig PA: Maternal-Newborn Nursing: A Family-centered Approach, 3rd ed. Menlo Park, CA, Addison-Wesley, 1988

Pillitteri A: Maternal-Newborn Nursing: Care of the Growing Family, 3rd ed. Boston, Little, Brown & Co, 1985

Reeder SR, Martin LL: Maternity Nursing: Family, Newborn, and Women's Health Care, 16th ed. Philadelphia, JB Lippincott, 1987

IV

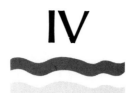

Care of the Child

13

Nursing Care of the Infant

Growth and Development

Developmental Assessment

- For developmental milestones that serve as standards of reference, see Table 13-1
- Assess parent–child interaction—optimal times are when child is age 2 weeks, 2 months, 4 months, 6 months, 9 months, 12 months, and every year thereafter

Health Promotion

Routine Health Assessment

Health History

- 60% of medical conditions affecting infants can be diagnosed by health history
- Assess prenatal, postnatal, neonatal history; obtain obstetrical records, apgar scores
- Review child's health history including immunizations (see Table 13-2), illnesses, hospitalizations
- Perform or review family assessment

Health Screening

- Measure height, weight, occipital–frontal head circumference, and plot on growth charts at each visit
- Record vital signs and blood pressure (BP), hemoglobin, hematocrit; perform vision and hearing screening

Nutrition: Recommendations for Parents

- From birth to age 6 months, breast-feeding is preferred method: supplement with iron, vitamin D, and fluoride; if using formula with iron, no supplements except fluoride (depending on fluoride content of local water); if using evaporated milk formula, supplement with vitamin C and iron
- After age 6 months, introduce iron-fortified cereals and continue until age 18 months; continue breast-feeding or using formula until age 1 year; begin feeding vitamin D whole milk if intake of solids approximates 200 g daily—provide vitamin C with whole milk
- Introduce solids at age 5 or 6 months: begin with rice cereals, introduce one new solid at a time for no more than one or two new foods in the same week, to assess for allergy
- Introduce textured foods between ages 8–12 months
- Avoid using bottle as pacifier, may cause dental caries

Family Relationships

Bonding

- Note consistency of parenting
- Assess mother–child interaction

Table 13-1. Growth and Development: Infant through Preschool Age

Age	Gross Motor Skills	Fine Motor Skills	Language	Cognitive	Social Adaptive
Infant					
1–3 months	Raises head 45° at 2 months Raises head 90° at 3 months	Hands are open Follows past midline Holds objects	Coos	Deliberate actions replace reflexes	Smiles responsively Alert Responsive
3–6 months	Rolls over Increased strength Sits with supports	Reaches for and grasps objects	Responds to noise Localizes sounds at 5 months	Recognizes familiar faces Pursues activity for result	Reciprocity between parent and child
6–9 months	Sits alone Crawls backwards Crawls forward at 9 months	Transfers Rakes small objects	Says "mama," "dada" nonspecifically Locates sound	Aware of object permanence Stranger anxiety	Explores environment
9–12 months	Pulls to stand Cruises	Bangs blocks together Neat-pincer grasp	Says "mama," "dada" specifically Vocalizes 5 words at 12 months	Curious	Increased attachment to parents

	Motor	Fine Motor/Adaptive	Language	Cognitive	Social
Toddler 12–24 months	Walks at 12–15 months Stoops and recovers at 15 months Walks well at 18 months	Controls and releases object Stacks blocks at 18 months Uses cup	Combines 1–2 words at 12 months Combines 2–3 words at 24 months Points to named body part	Aware of shapes and object permanence	Increased autonomy Negativism Security objects
2–4 years	Jumps, broad jumps, stands on one foot Pedals tricycle at 3 years	Draws a circle at 2 years Draws a cross at 3 years Stacks 7–8 blocks	Combines 2–3 words Says first and last name	Infers cause-effect Imaginative play Egocentric	Increased independence Temper tantrums begin to diminish Tolerates separation
4–5 years	Climbs jungle gym Catches ball Rides bike with training wheels	Draws square at 4 years Draws man with 3 parts Draws triangle at 5 years	Recognizes 3 colors Speaks in 4–5 word sentences Understands concepts *long* and *short*	Classifies objects according to similarity	Increased independence in daily activities Sexual curiosity Attachment to parent of same sex School

Table 13-2. Recommendations for Active Immunization of Normal Infants and Children

Recommended Age	Vaccine
2 months	DTP-1, OPV-1
4 months	DTP-2, OPV-2
6 months	DTP-3, OPV-3 (optional)
15 months	MMR
18 months	DTP-4, OPV-3
18–60 months	Haemophilus influenza type B (Hib)
4–6 years	DTP-5, OPV-4
14–16 years	Td (reduced dose of diphtheria, repeat every 10 years

DTP = Diptheria, Tetanus, Pertussis
MMR = Measles, Mumps, Rubella
OPV = Trivalent form of polio virus
The Redbook: Report of the Committee on Infectious Diseases, American Academy of Pediatrics, 1986

Separation Anxiety

Teach parents to:

Anticipate child's fears
Allow transitional objects (blanket, toys)
Have alternative caretakers (friends, family, and babysitter) visit often while parents home
Spend time with child and sitter before leaving

The Hospitalized Infant

Separation

- Allow child to bring transitional objects to hospital
- Promote primary care to establish trust
- Try to maintain routines similar to those at home
- Play hide-and-seek, peek-a-boo to help child learn about object permanence and to allay separation anxiety
- Encourage parents to room in at hospital
- Be alert to signs of stranger anxiety
- Help parents with separation
- Support child–staff attachments

Loss of Control

Recognize that:

- Child may regress to earlier stage of successful coping
- Hospitalized child is unable to control environment

Fear of Pain and Injury

- Perform tasks as quickly as possible, because infants will cry and thrash about during most procedures
- Maintain parent–child contact

Health Problems of the Infant

Myelomeningocele

Myelomeningocele is a cystic defect anywhere on the spine. It involves a hernial protrusion of a saclike cyst containing meninges, spinal fluid, and a portion of the spinal column with nerves. Eighty percent occur in the lumbar or lumbosacral area. Treatment consists of closure. Complications include hydrocephalus (results in 75% of cases), meningitis, and spinal cord dysfunction.

Assessment

Health Status

- Dysfunction related to level of injury on spine
- Musculoskeletal deformities, hip dislocation, joint contractures, foot deformities, scoliosis
- Pressure decubiti
- Bowel and bladder dysfunction; urinary tract infection, rectal prolapse
- Impaired cognitive or perceptual abilities
- Seizure activity

Diagnostic Factors

Sac illumination

Radiography to detect bony defects

Computed tomography (CT) scan to detect hydrocephalus

Urinalysis, culture and sensitivity, blood urea nitrogen (BUN) measurement, creatinine clearance level measurement

Prenatal: amniocentesis reveals increased concentration of α-feto protein

Nursing Plans and Interventions

Nursing Measures

Decrease infection of sac:

- Inspect frequently
- Position client prone with knees flexed
- Place pad between knees and small roll under ankles to maintain neutral foot position
- Change pads frequently

Prevent trauma:

- Observe for signs of hydrocephalus, such as increasing occipital–frontal circumference, bulging fontanelles, irritability, high-pitched cry and feeding difficulties
- Observe for signs of meningeal irritation, such as fever, nuchal rigidity, and irritability
- Observe for signs of urinary tract infection, such as fever, foul-smelling urine, or irritability

Prevent skin breakdown:

- Changing position frequently
- Gently massage skin
- Clean area
- Avoid pressure points
- Apply lotion with diaper change

Prevent hip and lower extremity deformity:

- Assist with passive range of motion (ROM) exercises
- Take care to avoid fractures
- Maintain hips in moderate abduction

Cleanse area with sterile solution and use sterile dressings

Nutrition Therapy

- Provide or encourage parents to provide high-calorie foods and whole milk to promote growth and development

Client/Family Teaching

Teach parents aspects of child's care, encourage questions, encourage involvement in care, allow supervised practice, and teach signs of complications

Refer family to support groups (*e.g.,* Spina Bifida Association) and to social work and financial assistance agencies

Teach family how to promote normal growth and development, refer family to agencies with physical and occupational therapists, discuss age-appropriate activities, suggest adaptive devices

Evaluation

Treatment and client teaching are successful if:

- Infection has decreased or disappeared
- Child shows increased flexibility without deformities
- Child has clean and intact skin without decubiti
- Family demonstrates skills, provides care, and communicates understanding of child's care
- Family promotes normal growth and development
- Family follows up agency referrals and keeps medical reevaluation appointments

Hydrocephalus

Hydrocephalus results from an imbalance in production and absorption of cerebral spinal fluid (CSF). Impaired absorption of CSF in the subarachnoid space is called *communicating*. Obstructed flow of CSF in the ventricle is called *noncommunication*. Treatment is the ventricular peritoneal (VP) shunt, which is threaded subcutaneously against the cranium down the chest to the abdominal wall. A catheter drains CSF into the peritoneal cavity with a unidirectional flow valve.

Assessment

Health Status

- Increased occipital–frontal circumference
- Bulging fontanelles
- Irritability, high-pitched cry, poor feeding
- Seizures

Diagnostic Factors

Change in head circumference
CT scan
Percussion reveals "cracked-pot" sound (Macewen sign)

Nursing Plans and Interventions

Nursing Measures

- To care for child with postoperative VP shunt, keep pressure off valve and keep child flat
- Assess for signs of shunt obstruction, such as pupil dilation, irritability, poor feeding, vomiting, decreased responsiveness, or seizures

Client/Family Teaching

Teach signs of complications and signs of increased intracranial pressure
Refer to community agencies for support, financial assistance, physical or occupational therapy
Assess parents' understanding of surgery
Promote normal growth and development

Evaluation

Treatment and client teaching are successful if:

- Child shows no signs of increased intracranial pressure after surgery
- Parents are aware of complications and signs of shunt malfunction
- Family promotes normal growth and development and follows up agency referrals if applicable

Cleft Lip and Cleft Palate

Cleft lip and cleft palate are the most common facial defects. They result from failure of fusion of the primary or secondary palates during gestation. Transmission is multifactorial. Treatment is repair first of cleft lip and later of the cleft palate, between ages 6 months to 5 years.

Assessment

Health Status

- Visual and manual examination of lip and palate reveals cleft
- Assessment may reveal impaired sucking capabilities
- Other birth defects may be present

Diagnostic Factors

Digital examination to assess degree and depth of cleft (may also be bifid uvula)

Nursing Plans and Interventions

Nursing Measures

- Teach parents optimal feeding technique for adequate fluid and caloric intake: hold baby upright during feeding; burp frequently; use compressible bottles with soft nipples and enlarged slit; if child vomits, suction thoroughly
- Postoperatively, restrain child's arms; enforce prone position; feed with clear liquids; do not use tube, syringe, or fork; suction

carefully, clean suture site with sterile water; prevent trauma to suture site
- Offer support with feeding to parents, allow expression of feelings, maintain follow-up care

Evaluation

Treatment and client teaching are successful if:

- Child maintains adequate fluid and caloric intake
- Parents understand feeding techniques and feel supported by professional
- Postoperatively, suture site remains free of trauma and infection
- Parents seek follow-up care after discharge

Congenital Hip Dysplasia

Congenital hip dysplasia is imperfect hip development affecting the femoral head and acetabulum. The condition is more common among females than among males, and affects the left hip more frequently than the right. Treatment involves reducing the dislocation by maintaining the hip in abduction while the acetabulum develops. This goal is accomplished by splinting with pillow or commercial splints in the case of partial dislocation, by closed reduction with no surgical incision in the case of complete dislocation (hip spica cast is applied) or by open reduction. Treatment before 2 months of age increases the rate of success.

Assessment

Health Status

- Difference in shape of lower extremity, such as uneven gluteal folds, prominent trochanter, uneven appearance of thighs; affected limb is shorter (Allis's sign)
- Abduction may be painful or impossible
- Ortolani's sign: click is felt when flexed legs are abducted
- Trendelenberg's sign: pelvic dropping occurs if child's weight is supported on affected leg
- Child walks late with uneven or limp, waddling gait

Diagnostic Factors

History and Ortolani's sign
X-rays in older infants and children

Nursing Plans and Interventions

Nursing Measures

Encourage normal growth and development:

- Wean from bottle
- Offer finger foods
- Promote use of upper extremities for grasping and holding
- Vary the environment
- Provide affection

Provide cast care:

- Check neurovascular signs: pulse, color, temperature, movement, sensation and presence of swelling
- Turn frequently
- Prevent soiling of cast
- Maintain clean, intact skin
- Petal cast
- Use cool blow dryer to relieve itching
- Check for small items under cast

Work with physical therapist to help client resume exercise and walking.

Client/Family Teaching

Teach parents about splint and cast care and about how to apply splint when changing diaper

Evaluation

Treatment and client teaching are successful if:

- Growth and development are promoted
- Cast care is maintained without signs of infection

- Parents learn splint and cast care and are ready for child's discharge

Strabismus

Strabismus is neuromuscular incoordination affecting the alignment of the eyes. The eyes see two different images, but in the case of strabismus the brain suppresses images from the weaker eye. If uncorrected the problem may result in amblyopia. Treatment involves several options, including eye muscle exercises, corrective lenses, patching the unaffected eye, and surgery if other options do not correct the problem. Strabismus must be corrected before the child is 6 years old.

Assessment

Health Status

- Parents report seeing child's eye turn in (normal in infants under 4 months old)
- Corneal light reflex test reveals reflection of light falls on two different places on each eye
- Esotropia: eyes turn in towards nose
- Exotropia: eyes deviate outwards
- Hypertropia: eyes are at different levels

Diagnostic Factors

Cover/uncover test: blank card held over child's eye while child looks with uncovered eye at examiner's nose—when card is removed there should be no movement of eye that had been covered

Corneal light reflex test

Nursing Plans and Interventions

Nursing Measures

- Detect early and refer to ophthalmologist to prevent blindness

Client/Family Teaching

Teach parents and family importance of treatment

Emphasize child's positive qualities, allow child to express feelings

Offer support and follow-up to family

Evaluation

Treatment and client teaching are successful if:

- Child's strabismus is detected and treated early
- Family understands importance of treatment and follow-up
- Child's growth and development is not impaired, positive self-image is maintained

Congenital Heart Disease

Congenital heart disease includes acyanotic and cyanotic heart disease. Acyanotic heart disease occurs when there is no mixing of desaturated blood. Cyanotic heart disease occurs when desaturated blood enters systemic circulation, and may involve right-to-left shunting of blood due to increased pulmonary resistance. Treatment involves closed heart surgery, which is merely palliative, or open heart surgery to correct defects.

Assessment

Health Status

- Growth retardation
- Decreased exercise tolerance
- Dyspnea
- Tachycardia
- Cyanosis
- Tissue hypoxia

Diagnostic Factors

Electrocardiogram (ECG)
Chest x-ray
Cardiac catheterization
Angiography
Complete blood count

Nursing Plans and Interventions

Nursing Measures

- Prevent injury by observing for signs of increased distress or cardiac disease, such as poor weight gain, feeding or exercise intolerance, and respiratory infections
- Place child in knee-chest position to increase comfort and decrease work load of heart
- Keep child warm
- Prevent activity intolerance by feeding slowly, allowing rest, encouraging quiet games
- Caution parents about high altitude

Drug Therapy

Digitalis (Lanoxin)

Increases force of contraction, decreases heart rate, slows conduction of impulses through AV node, and indirectly enhances diuresis by improving renal perfusion

Give at regular 12-hour intervals

Give 1 hour before or 2 hours after meals, do not mix with other foods

Administer missed dose if less than 4 hours have elapsed

If child vomits, do not give second dose

Assess for signs of toxicity: vomiting, diarrhea, anorexia, nausea, bradycardia, arrhythmias, fatigue, muscle weakness, headaches, drowsiness, blurred vision

Furosemide (Lasix)

Eliminates excess water and sodium

Observe for signs of dehydration

Assess for side-effects: nausea, vomiting, diarrhea, hypokalemia, digitalis toxicity

Encourage foods high in potassium

Monitor chloride level and acid-base balance

Nutrition Therapy

- Encourage well-balanced diet with high-potassium and iron-rich foods
- Administer small frequent meals and provide frequent rest periods
- Discourage high-sodium foods

Client/Family Teaching

Increase family's understanding of child's condition

Encourage family members to take active role in child's care

Prepare family for home care

Teach cardiopulmonary resuscitation (CPR)

Refer to agencies for financial and developmental support

Evaluation

Treatment and client teaching are successful if:

- Child remains free of infection
- Signs of complications are detected early
- Child consumes adequate amounts of calories for growth
- Child engages in age-appropriate activities
- Family and child demonstrate understanding of illness, tests, medications, and therapy
- Family learns CPR and becomes involved with support groups

Tracheoesophageal Fistula

Tracheoesophageal fistula results from failure of the esophagus to develop a continuous passage, resulting in a patent fistula between two structures. There are five types. In type C, the most common type, the proximal esophageal segment terminates in a blind pouch. The distal segment is connected to the trachea. Treatment is immediate, and involves preventing aspiration and placing a drainage tube. Surgical repair includes fistula ligations, possible esophagostomy, ostomy, and placing a gastrostomy tube, all with the goal of eventually creating a new passage.

Assessment

Health Status

- Excessive salivation at birth
- Choking, coughing, or sneezing at birth or shortly after
- Cyanosis from laryngospasms

Diagnostic Factors

Failure to pass nasogastric (NG) tube into stomach

Fluoroscopic studies and bronchoscopy to determine extent of defect

Nursing Plans and Interventions

Goals

Preoperative

- Detect and prevent aspiration
- Maintain client in head-up position with frequent suctioning
- Monitor intake and output (I and O) and urine specific gravity
- Maintain intravenous fluid

Postoperative

- Care for surgical site
- Monitor chest tubes
- Provide respiratory support

Nursing Measures

- Assess for signs of respiratory difficulty such as increased respirations, fever, cyanosis, use of accessory muscles
- Care for gastrostomy tube, and teach parents to feed child with tube and clean tube
- Monitor I and O
- Provide meticulous skin care around cervical esophagostomy site

Client/Family Teaching

Teach parents to encourage child to suck, using pacifier

Support parents and encourage them to hold, cuddle, and comfort child during disruption of feeding periods

Teach parents to care for gastrostomy tube (demonstrate)

Evaluation

Treatment and client teaching are successful if:

- Infant does not experience aspiration or respiratory problems
- Parents become involved in care, learn gastrostomy tube care, hold and comfort child during feeding
- Infant remains well hydrated before and after surgery
- Parents encourage normal growth and development
- Skin integrity is maintained around esophagostomy site

Acute Respiratory Infections

Acute respiratory infections involve infection of the upper respiratory tract. Most causes are viral. Croup is caused by swelling of the larynx. There are three kinds of croup, acute spasmodic croup, laryngotracheobronchitis (LTB), and bacterial croup (acute epiglottitis). Treatment consists of maintaining a patent airway by maintaining a high humidity environment, providing oxygen and inhalation therapy, and possibly intubating and administering IV fluids.

Assessment

Health Status

- Barking cough
- Hoarseness
- Cyanosis pallor
- Stridor or labored breathing
- Fever
- Sore throat
- Restlessness
- Nasal flaring
- Decreased or absent breath sounds

Diagnostic Factors

Blood cultures, blood gas measurement, complete blood count, chest x-ray, sinus x-ray

Thoracentesis or venipuncture, lumbar puncture

Throat and sputum cultures

Nursing Plans and Interventions

Nursing Measures

- Prevent spread of infection by isolating client, teaching good handwashing, discouraging sharing utensils at home
- Control fever by ensuring cool mist environment, monitoring temperature, providing cool liquids as tolerated, providing light clothing
- Assess respiratory status closely by observing respirations, listening to lungs, monitoring heart rate, observing color, watching for behavior changes such as restlessness or decreased responsiveness; do not observe throat if epiglottitis is suspected
- Prevent dehydration by monitoring I and O, testing urine specific gravity, monitoring weight daily, encouraging liquids when acute phase ends
- Maintain patent airway by positioning to promote drainage, suctioning as needed, using croup tent, reducing anxiety, preventing aspiration

Nutrition Therapy

- Provide high-calorie foods as tolerated
- Conserve child's energy by promoting rest, decreasing anxiety, discouraging excessive coughing

Client/Family Teaching

Reduce parents' and child's anxiety by explaining procedures, allowing child to keep transitional objects, allowing parents to room in, and providing for comfort

Teach administration of and side-effects of medications: antibiotics or antihistamines

Teach parents how to make necessary environmental changes at home, such as reducing allergens, handwashing, avoiding smoke, avoiding pets, having children use own utensils

Teach signs of respiratory distress and measures to take if reinfection occurs

Evaluation

Client treatment and teaching are successful if:

- Parents understand and communicate signs of respiratory distress
- Child rests and becomes free of infection without signs of increasing respiratory distress
- Child is well hydrated and takes nourishment
- Parents and child are ready for discharge
- Household members are free of infection

Pyloric Stenosis

In pyloric stenosis, the circular muscle of the pylorus becomes enlarged and obstructs the pyloric outlet. Treatment involves surgery (pyloromyotomy).

Assessment

Health Status

- Regurgitation or vomiting in second or third week of life, projectile vomiting shortly after feeding; emesis contains gastric secretions and undigested formula
- Infant remains hungry
- Decreased weight gain, dehydration
- Distended upper abdomen
- Palpable tumor in epigastric area

Diagnostic Factors

Observation of emesis patterns

Palpation of tumor in epigastric region

Contrast studies to locate obstruction

Radiographs show delayed gastric emptying, narrowed pylorus

Nursing Plans and Interventions

Goals

- Preoperatively, observe for signs of pyloric stenosis
- Strictly monitor I and O
- Monitor urine specific gravity
- Rehydrate infant

Nursing Measures

- Monitor I and O
- Assess operative site for signs of infection and drainage
- Prevent infection

Nutrition Therapy

- Monitor feeding regimens as feeding is increased
- Position on right side or in Fowler's position to promote gastric emptying

Client/Family Teaching

Encourage parents to hold and cuddle infant; reassure parents

Teach care of ostomy site

Evaluation

Treatment and client teaching are successful if:

- Child is diagnosed and treated immediately
- Child remains well hydrated
- Parents cuddle, hold, and interact closely with infant
- Parents learn ostomy care

Diarrhea and Dehydration

Diarrhea and dehydration result in an increase in the number of stools, a decrease in the consistency of stools, and voluminous losses of fluid and electrolytes. Treatment involves rehydration, administering antimicrobial medications, and treating fungal infections with protective ointments.

Assessment

Health Status

- Sudden increase in number, reduction in consistency, increased fluid content, or change in color (green) of stool
- Diarrhea with vomiting, reduced fluid intake
- High specific gravity of urine, dry mucous membranes, lack of tears, sunken fontanelle
- Increased irritability, decreased responsiveness

Diagnostic Factors

Age of child may indicate cause: peak incidence of *E. coli* is 1–3 months of age; of shigellosis, 2–4 years; of salmonella, birth to 2 years

History regarding exposure

CBC, serum electrolyte measurement, BUN level

Stool cultures, pH, and test for presence of sugar in urine (Clinitest)

Bulky stools (malabsorption)

Breath hydrogen test (carbohydrate malabsorption)

Watery stools with pus and mucous abdominal cramps (*Shigella*)

Nursing Plans and Interventions

Nursing Measures

- Prevent spread of infection by isolating client, washing hands carefully, using gown and glove, assessing child's home environment
- Maintain fluid and electrolyte balance by rehydrating with appropriate fluids (npo initially); monitoring I and O, urine specific gravity, daily weight, vital signs, and neurologic status every 4 hours or more
- Prevent injury by changing position every 2 hours, observing pressure areas, vital

signs and neurologic status, assessing for behavior changes and decreased responsiveness
- Prevent skin breakdown by changing diapers often, keeping baby meticulously clean, washing and drying thoroughly, applying protective ointments, exposing reddened area to heat lamp and air drying, using cloth diapers, providing for comfort
- Protect mucous membranes by providing mouth care and applying ointments during dehydration phase

Nutrition Therapy

- Maintain IV fluids
- Begin offering rehydration fluids such as orally administered rehydration solutions (Pedialyte), fruit juices, soft drinks (decaffeinated); delay milk intake 24–36 hours
- Gradually reintroduce foods
- Monitor I and O
- Observe consistency and frequency of stools
- Weigh daily

Client/Family Teaching

Teach family about:

Dietary planning, preparation, and food storage

Good handwashing, care and disposal of waste, good hygiene

Evaluation

Treatment and client teaching are successful if:

- Skin remains free of breakdown
- Child is rehydrated and alert
- Stools decrease in consistency and frequency
- Child's nutritional status improves
- Family understands proper care of food and proper handwashing and waste elimination
- Family feels supported and less anxious
- Family members are prepared for discharge and understand signs of complications

Iron Deficiency Anemia

Iron deficiency anemia results from an inadequate supply, intake, or absorption of iron, resulting in smaller red blood cells and decreased hemoglobin synthesis. Treatment involves supplementation of diet with iron products.

Assessment

Health Status

- Pallor, fatigue, irritability
- History of iron-deficient diet
- Underweight and poor muscle development
- Short attention span
- Spoon finger nails
- Increased susceptibility to infection

Diagnostic Factors

RBC normal or slightly elevated

Hemoglobin below normal for child's age

Hematocrit below normal for child's age

Decrease in size and concentration of red blood cells

Low reticulocyte count

Reduced serum iron concentration and elevated total iron binding capacity

Stool culture for occult blood

Nursing Plans and Interventions

Nursing Measures

- Prevent iron deficiency anemia by promoting optimal nutrition with iron-rich foods; supplementing iron through food sources; discouraging use of whole milk before age 1 year; supplementing diet with iron cereals at age 4–6 months for full-term baby, 2 months for premature baby (limit amount of milk to no more than 1 L daily)
- Promote optimal development by teaching age-appropriate skills

Client/Family Teaching

Teach family proper administration of iron products: give as directed, give in combination with ascorbic acid, give divided doses between meals, do not give with milk, tea or antacids, prevent contact with teeth, rinse mouth after administration

Teach family to seek routine medical examinations (hemoglobin levels should be checked every 6 months)

Assess family's understanding of diet and medication

Evaluation

Treatment and client teaching are successful if:

- Parents communicate understanding of diet modification
- Parents can explain proper administration of iron preparation
- Parents keep follow-up appointments
- Parents understand and are able to assess for signs of reoccurrence
- Child is alert and active and performs age-appropriate tasks
- Parents keep medication out of reach and only give as prescribed

Intussusception

Intussusception is telescoping or invagination of one portion of the intestine into another. Treatment involves hydrostatic reduction with a barium enema if detected within 24 hours. If this procedure not successful, surgery is performed.

Assessment

Health Status

- Severe paroxysmal pain
- Vomiting, eventually bile-stained
- Weakness
- Currant-jelly-like stools
- Distension of abdomen, mass in upper right quadrant

Diagnostic Factors

History of onset of pain
Barium enema may reveal obstruction

Nursing Plans and Interventions

Nursing Measures

- Document pain, vomiting, stools
- Preoperatively, monitor for signs of obstruction
- Prepare parents by using drawings to explain procedure
- Keep child well hydrated
- Assess for signs of recurrence
- Decrease anxiety

Evaluation

Treatment and client teaching are successful if:

- Intussusception is detected early and treated
- Parents understand child's problem and treatment
- Parents' anxiety is decreased
- Parents recognize signs of recurrence

Hirschsprung's Disease (Congenital Aganglionic Megacolon)

Hirschsprung's disease is the absence of autonomic parasympathetic ganglion cells of the myenteric and submucous plexuses, with a lack of peristalsis within the affected segment of the colon. Treatment involves surgical intervention (colostomy). Later a "pull-through" procedure is performed, involving removing the aganglionic colon with reanastomosis of the normal colon.

Assessment

Health Status

- Constipation or obstruction
- Infants may have vomiting and abdominal distension

- Emesis may be bile stained
- Failure to thrive
- With older children, fecal mass in lower left quadrant may be palpable

Diagnostic Factors

Rectal biopsy
For neonates, anorectal manometry
History of onset and stool pattern
Barium enema

Nursing Plans and Interventions

Nursing Measures

- Assess for signs of obstruction

Client/Family Teaching

Teach family to:

Care for ostomy and stoma
Maintain I and O records, monitor urine specific gravity, record ostomy drainage
Maintain IV fluids

Evaluation

Treatment and client teaching are successful if:

- Parents understand treatment
- Parents understand care of stoma and know who to contact with questions
- Child remains well hydrated
- Normal growth and development is promoted
- Parents praise child's accomplishments to build self-esteem
- Parents seek home care follow-up if needed

Allergies

Allergies result from a hypersensitive immune system response. IgE causes immediate hypersensitivity. T lymphocytes cause delayed hypersensitivity. The allergic response may be local or generalized. Treatment involves desensitization.

Assessment

Health Status

- Skin: rashes, eczema, urticaria, lesions, pruritis, hives, wheals, erythema with vesicles and crusting
- Mucous membranes: red and edematous eyes and upper respiratory tract, increased mucoid discharge, conjunctivitis, sneezing, dark circles under eyes, sinus headache
- Systemic allergic reactions: GI tract—abdominal cramping, nausea, vomiting, diarrhea, colic; respiratory tract—bronchospasm, asthma; vascular system—migraine headaches
- Anaphylaxis: systemic response with sneezing, urticaria, weakness, restlessness, laryngal spasms, edema, GI symptoms, eventually circulatory collapse

Diagnostic Factors

History from family
Skin test; scratch, prick, injection
Radioallergosorbent test (RAST)—in vitro blood testing
Food diary
Urine tests

Nursing Plans and Interventions

Nursing Measures

- Assist child and family to adjust to long-term illness: teach family to allow child increased independence, praise positive behavior, allow expression of feelings, *not* allow child to manipulate parents
- Assist child to adapt to change in body image by allowing expression of feelings, minimizing appearance changes caused by medication, encouraging sports like swimming, providing support for child and family
- Decrease anxiety and stress by eliminating allergens in environment, reducing internal and external stress, teaching relaxation

techniques, helping parents become aware of stress factors and effects on child

Client/Family Teaching

Refer family to social services for financial assistance

Teach parents about medication side-effects, signs of complications, and actions to take in emergency situations

Evaluation

Treatment and client teaching are successful if:

- Allergies are detected and both family and child are aware of them
- Family decreases allergens in child's environment
- Parents understand effects of stress on child
- Parents learn to handle stress more effectively
- Family follows up on referral to social service agencies
- Child maintains a positive self-image

Child Abuse

Child abuse or neglect may be physical, sexual, or emotional.

Assessment

Health Status

- Bruises on eyes, mouth, lips, torso, buttocks, genital areas, burns, fractures, face, skull, long bones; lacerations or abrasions on mouth, lip, gums, eyes, genitals
- Presenting behavior: flat affect, fear of parents, inappropriate responses, extreme aggressiveness or withdrawal
- In the case of sexual abuse, laceration of labia, vagina, or perineum; injury, pain or itching, hematomas in genital area; vaginal or penile discharge; dysuria; sexually transmitted disease; pregnancy; unexplained vaginal or rectal bleeding
- Reported behavior changes; fear of home, reluctance to take showers or sudden reluctance to participate in sports, sleep disturbance, fear of being alone, poor peer relations, change of performance in school, somatic complaints
- In the case of emotional abuse, change in behavior at school, poor peer relations, withdrawal, fear of home, sleep disturbances

Diagnostic Factors

History and clinical findings

Documentation of child's appearance and of interactions with peers, parents, or other adults

Development assessment

History of substance abuse, poor medical care

Nursing Plans and Interventions

Nursing Measures

- Assess for high-risk situations, such as children living with parents who are isolated, single, have low self-esteem, many unmet needs, history of substance abuse, lack of knowledge of normal growth and development, multiple stressors in life, lack patience, or are impulsive
- Assist parents to cope effectively by discussing parents' self-concept and ways to cope with stressors, and referring to appropriate community services
- Increase parents' knowledge of normal growth and development by discussing child's needs, providing anticipatory guidance, listening to parents discuss ways to promote development
- Make sure child is not in danger of additional trauma
- Elevate head if injured
- Apply emergency treatment if needed, maintain patent airway
- Stop bleeding

- Assess extent of injury
- Determine state of consciousness
- Evaluate pain
- Assess for any other injuries
- Assess home environment
- Document all physical and behavioral findings concerning child and parents
- Allow trust to develop between child and health care worker and between parents and health care worker
- Suggest counseling if child's interactions with peers warrants
- Refer family to child protective agency if necessary (always inform family)

Client/Family Teaching

Refer family to community resources such as welfare, mental health center, emergency shelter, Women, Infants, and Children Program (WIC), family counseling center, religious group

Evaluation

Treatment is successful if:

- Child abuse is detected early
- All findings are documented
- Counseling of parents begins immediately and referrals to outside agencies are made if necessary
- Child's behavior is assessed and counseling is recommended as needed
- Child is placed in foster care with loving, consistent caregivers, if warranted
- Parents can explain normal growth and development and how to cope with stress
- Child is not in danger of abuse reoccurring

Sudden Infant Death Syndrome

Sudden infant death syndrome (SIDS) refers to the sudden unexpected death of a healthy infant. Peak incidence is at ages 2–4 months. Death usually occurs during sleep. Treatment includes resuscitation and apnea monitoring for siblings and for infants who have experienced "near miss" SIDS.

Assessment

Health Status

- Apnea lasting 20 seconds or more
- Higher incidence among siblings
- Infant under 1 year of age
- May be neurological

Diagnostic Factors

History or monitoring reveals apnea

Nursing Plans and Interventions

Nursing Measures

- Support and assist parents to cope with grief by offering counseling
- Assess family's support systems
- Refer to local Foundation of Sudden Infant Death (provide number for contact person)

Client/Family Teaching

Teach use of apnea monitor in the case of "near miss" SIDS and for siblings

Evaluation

Client teaching is successful if:

- Family successfully completes grief process
- Family follows up referrals to appropriate agencies, support groups, or counseling
- Parents do not feel guilt over child's death
- Contact person maintains contact with family to offer support

Phenylketonuria

Phenylketonuria is an inborn error of metabolism. The body is unable to metabolize phenylalanine. Abnormal byproducts of phenylalanine accumulate in the bloodstream, or are stored in CSF or body tissue, and are excreted in urine and sweat. Treatment is minimizing intake of phenylalanine.

Assessment

Health Status

- If untreated, moderate to severe mental retardation due to degeneration of brain and defective myelination of nerves
- Eczema or seborrhea
- Mousy odor to urine or sweat
- May develop seizures or hyperactivity
- Characteristically, blond hair, blue eyes, and fair skin

Diagnostic Factors

Phenylketonuria screening within 24–48 hours of ingestion
Test infants at 14–28 days of age

Nursing Plans and Interventions

Nursing Measures

- Encourage child to have as much control as possible while staying within limitations
- Be supportive of family and child
- Assist family and child to understand need for strict diet and followup

Nutrition Therapy

- Minimize phenylalanine in diet
- Low phenylalanine formula (Lofenalac)
- Low-phenylalanine foods, meal planning based on exchange list
- Teach preschoolers to become involved in meal planning
- Child maintains diet until 7–9 years of age; family needs support, child needs confidence

Client/Family Teaching

Teach parents about:

Diet
Signs of complications, such as metabolic acidosis, skin rashes, and height or weight changes

Evaluation

Treatment and client teaching are successful if:

- Child maintains strict diet
- Child and family are supported in adhering to diet
- Parents understand diet and importance of follow-up
- Family receives genetic counseling if necessary
- Child has adequate weight gain and attains normal developmental milestones
- Family promotes normal growth and development
- Child participates in meal planning

Failure to Thrive

Infants or children whose weight, height, or height for weight falls below the fifth percentile for their age are described as experiencing failure to thrive. Organic failure to thrive has physical causes. Nonorganic failure to thrive is usually caused by psychosocial factors.

Assessment

Health Status

Nonorganic Failure to Thrive

- Infant or child is below fifth percentile in weight but shows weight gain with adequate nurturing
- May demonstrate developmental retardation that improves with appropriate stimulation
- No evidence of physical cause or congenital abnormality that caused developmental or growth failure
- May appear withdrawn, irritable, apathetic
- May demonstrate poor personal hygiene, poor parent–child interaction, oral-defensive behavior with solids

Organic Failure to Thrive

- Height, weight, or height for weight is below fifth percentile with physical cause or congenital malformation

Diagnostic Factors

History and physical examination

Plotting of height, weight, height for weight, and head circumference on growth charts

3-day diet history

Developmental testing (Denver Developmental Screening Tool)

Skin fold measurements

Home environment assessment

Nursing Plans and Interventions

Nursing Measures

- Assess mother–child interaction (if mother is primary caregiver)
- Identify high-risk parents such as those with low self-esteem or history of maternal deprivation, or those experiencing isolation, single parenthood, multiple family crises
- Create trusting atmosphere with parents
- Set up structured meal plan (three meals daily plus two snacks)
- Suggest increasing child's caloric intake with whole milk, eliminating juices, pop, and water from diet, and including high-calorie foods
- Ask patients to keep diet record for child
- Limit time of each meal to 30 minutes
- Give parents suggestions for creating more nurturing environment such as providing age-appropriate toys, holding child during feeding, maintaining eye-to-eye contact with child and ensuring calm mealtime
- Assess parents' anxiety level and stressors, particularly mother's if she is child's primary caregiver
- Suggest counseling if needed, recommend social worker
- Arrange for public health nurse to visit family to encourage and support parents and monitor child's weight gain and development
- Follow family closely, assessing child's weight and development
- Child may need hospitalization for teaching and observation

Evaluation

Treatment and client teaching are successful if:

- Mother's or primary caregiver's anxiety decreases
- Child's interaction with mother (or primary caregiver) improves
- Child gains weight in more nurturing environment
- Home environment is more nurturing; age-appropriate developmental activities are provided
- Family maintains consistent contact with public health nurse
- Mother or primary caregiver receives appropriate counseling to cope with stress

14

Nursing Care of the Toddler and Preschooler

Growth and Development

- For developmental milestones that serve as standards of reference, see table 13-1
- Assess growth and development at 18 months and then once a year until age 5

Health Promotion

- Maintain immunization schedule (see table 13-2)

Nutrition: Recommendations for Parents

- Provide on daily basis 2–3 glasses whole milk (avoid skim milk until 2 years of age); 2 servings meat, poultry, or fish; 4 servings fruit or vegetables; 4 servings bread, pasta, or potatoes

Dental Health

- Promote oral hygiene
- Teach tooth brushing
- Advise parents to schedule dental visit before child is 3
- Advise parents to avoid fluoridated toothpaste until child is 3 (child may swallow toothpaste with fluoride)

Family Relationships

Discipline

Teach parents to:

Set clear, consistent limits (child tries to control environment but wants limits)

Reason with child, praise desirable behavior, express disapproval or ignore bad behavior

Follow discipline with understanding

Take pride in child's accomplishments

Toilet Training

Physical signs of readiness include:

Voluntary anal control and urethral sphincter control

Ability to stay dry for 2 hours (wakes from nap dry)

Regular bowel movements

Ability to sit, walk, squat, remove clothing

Mental signs of readiness include:

Ability to recognize urge to go

Ability to communicate (verbally or nonverbally) wetness or urge to go

Cognitive signs of readiness include:

Ability to imitate and follow directions

Psychological signs of readiness include:

Willingness to please parents

Ability to sit on toilet for 5–10 minutes

Curiosity in wanting to be changed

Sibling Rivalry

Teach parents to:

Expect firstborn child to display most pronounced rivalry

Expect children under age 2 to experience particular difficulty

Prepare child 1 or 2 months in advance

Understand child's fears of abandonment and separation anxiety

Allow time for each child

Allow siblings to become involved in care of new baby

The Hospitalized Toddler and Preschooler

Separation

- Encourage parents to room in
- Help parents with separation
- Have parents leave while child is awake
- Allow use of transitional objects (blanket, toys, pictures)

Loss of Control

- Recognize that child is unable to control environment (allow as much control as possible over times of treatment, etc.)
- Toddlers may view illness or hospitalization as punishment (provide reassurance)
- Try to maintain routines similar to home routines
- Choose words carefully, because toddlers often use "magical thinking"
- Use doll play to enable child to act out feelings

Fear of Pain and Injury

- Recognize that toddlers have poorly developed body image
- Recognize that preschoolers may view illness as punishment, have fears of mutilation and castration, and are vulnerable to threats of bodily injury
- Anticipate aggressive or dependent reaction
- Explain procedures by use of drawing or dolls
- Allow child to play with equipment
- Perform procedures quickly

Health Problems of the Toddler and Preschooler

Tonsillitis and Tonsillectomy

Tonsillitis is infection of the tonsils and pharynx; it can be viral or bacterial in origin. Treatment may require tonsillectomy and adenoidectomy. The condition is initially treated with antibiotics.

Assessment

Health Status: Nonbacterial Tonsillitis

- Low-grade fever, loss of appetite, mild headache
- Sore throat, hoarse voice, productive cough

Health Status: Bacterial Tonsillitis

- Most common cause group A β-hemolytic *Streptococcus*
- Fever 38–40°C
- Muscle aches, headache, and vomiting, lasting 18–24 hours
- Skin rash, peritonsillar abscess, sinusitis, otitis media

Diagnostic Factors

Throat culture to determine causative agent

Nursing Plans and Interventions

Goals: Preoperative

- Use doll play, involve parent in care
- Reassure child, explain throat will be sore
- Assess clotting and bleeding studies
- Check mouth for loose teeth

Nursing Measures: Postoperative

- Observe for bleeding
- Maintain client in prone position with head slightly lower than chest
- Perform frequent throat and nasal checks
- Monitor vital signs and blood pressure frequently
- Assess for signs of hemorrhage: increased pulse rate, restlessness, low blood pressure
- Monitor hydration using ice chips, clear liquids
- Monitor intake and output (I and O) records and urine specific gravity
- Comfort child, use ice packs, use mouth sprays (no utensils in mouth), do not allow child to gargle
- Administer medications such as ampicillin (observe for side-effects such as diarrhea), administer acetaminophen rather than aspirin (aspirin prolongs bleeding time)

Nutrition Therapy

- Clear liquids and ice chips as tolerated
- Soft diet after 7–10 days (gradual change)

Client/Family Teaching

Alert family to signs of complications, such as increased bleeding, altered levels of consciousness

Inform family that child may return to school 1–2 weeks postoperatively

Evaluation

Treatment and client teaching are successful if:

- Client shows no signs of further infection
- Client is as comfortable as possible
- Client shows no signs of alteration in vital signs
- Parents are prepared to care for child at home
- Child was well prepared before and after surgery with teaching and play therapy

Otitis Media

Otitis media is inflammation of the middle ear caused by bacteria, blockage of the eustachian tubes, or allergies. The condition may be chronic or acute, and is treated with antibiotics for 10 days; if this treatment is not successful and the condition recurs, insertion of myringotomy tubes may be indicated.

Assessment

Health Status

- Increased irritability
- Loss of appetite
- Upper respiratory infection
- Tugging at ear
- May be febrile
- Enlarged lymph nodes (postauricular or cervical)
- May be drainage from ears if tympanic membrane has perforated

Diagnostic Factors

Otoscopic examination reveals loss of landmarks, bulging of tympanic membrane, increased redness, or no movement of tympanic membrane with use of pneumatic bulb

Tympanometry reveals decreased tympanic membrane compliance (tympanometry also measures middle ear pressure)

Nursing Plans and Interventions

Nursing Measures

- Administer ampicillin for 10 days as ordered
- Assess for infection
- Comfort child with analgesics (*e.g.,* acetaminophen, warm cloths to ear)

- Stress to parents importance of child's ears being rechecked 10 days after treatment
- Assess for hearing loss by noting any delays in language development

Nutrition Therapy

- Lactose-free diet to counteract diarrhea (side-effect of amoxicillin)

Client/Family Teaching

Teach parents to:

Prevent ear infection by feeding child upright, encouraging gentle nose blowing, discouraging use of bottle while child lying in bed, eliminating allergens such as smoke at home

In the case of myringotomy tube insertion, teach parents that:

Tubes allow drainage of fluid and ventilation of middle ear

Tubes remain approximately 6 months before ear spontaneously rejects them

Bath, shampoo, and lake water should be kept out of ears

Ear plugs should be worn in the water

Diving, jumping, and submerging in the water should be avoided

Evaluation

Treatment and client teaching are successful if:

- Infection is detected early and treated
- Parents understand importance of administering antibiotic for prescribed time, enforcing lactose-free diet, and following up after 10 days
- Child is comforted by acetaminophen and warm cloth to ear
- Parents understand and prevent further ear infections
- Parents are alert to signs of further complications, such as hearing loss, recurrent otitis, or meningitis

Cystic Fibrosis

Cystic fibrosis is generalized dysfunction of the exocrine glands. It is inherited as an autosomal recessive tract, and causes defects of multiple organs, including the respiratory and digestive tract, pancreas, and sweat glands. Treatment includes administering pancreatic enzymes with each meal and with snacks, aggressive pulmonary care, and measures to improve nutrition.

Assessment

Health Status

- In the case of meconium ileus, intestinal obstruction, vomiting, and failure to pass stools
- Foul-smelling, bulky, fatty stools
- Voracious appetite but failure to thrive, abdominal distension, and thin extremities
- Rectal prolapse
- Respiratory complications, such as wheezing, dry nonproductive cough, pulmonary infections, barrel-shaped chest, clubbing of nails, nasal polyps, and episodes of bronchitis and pneumonia
- In girls, increased viscosity and dehydration of cervical mucus, possible cervical polyps

Diagnostic Factors

Sweat test: two tests recommended, results of 40–60 mEq/L highly suggestive of disease

Duodenal enzyme activity measurement

Fat absorption test

Radiography

Nursing Plans and Interventions

Nursing Measures

Encourage normal growth and development:

- Incorporate primary caregivers into care
- Encourage parents to room in
- Establish trust
- Provide tactile sensory stimulation
- Be alert to signs of separation anxiety

- Allow child to ventilate feelings
- Maintain routine similar to home routine
- Encourage child to keep transitional objects
- Play hide-and-seek
- Reassure child

Drug Therapy

Pancreatic enzymes (teach parents to mix with pureed fruit, clean child's face and lips afterward, and administer with all meals and snacks)

Nutrition Therapy

- High-calorie, high-protein diet, additional fat soluble vitamins (A, D, E, K), medium chain triglycerides (MCT) oil, supplementary iron, diet supplements, and pancreatic enzymes with meals and snacks as prescribed
- Extra fluids and salt in heat and exercise

Client/Family Teaching

Assess family's understanding of disease
Teach parents and child about disease
Recommend genetic counseling
Teach family to assess for signs of complications such as dehydration
Teach family about pulmonary therapy: percussion and postural drainage, breathing exercises, and sports that promote lung expansion, such as swimming
Support family emotionally by referring to support groups in community, creating trust, using doll play, supporting siblings, and promoting normal growth and development

Evaluation

Treatment and client teaching are successful if:

- Family understands illness and recognizes signs of complications
- Parents are prepared for discharge
- Family follows up referrals to appropriate agencies for financial and emotional support
- Child is encouraged to participate in normal growth and developmental tasks
- Child maintains high-calorie diet

Ingestion of Poisonous Substances

The most frequently ingested poisons include plants, cleaning supplies, cosmetics, hydrocarbons, alcohol, analgesics, vitamins, topical preparations, and sedative hypnotics. Treatment includes emergency measures, maintenance of respiratory function, reduction of effects of shock, gastric decontamination, gastric lavage if indicated, use of activated charcoal, administration of cathartics and administration of antidotes in the case of certain poisons.

Assessment

Health Status

- Gastrointestinal system complications, such as abdominal pain, vomiting, diarrhea, or anorexia
- Respiratory system complications, including depressed respirations, labored respirations, cyanosis, and signs of shock
- Central nervous system complications, such as convulsions, overstimulation, loss of consciousness, dizziness, stupor, lethargy, and coma

Diagnostic Factors

History (parents called poison control center)
Laboratory evaluation
Chest x-ray

Nursing Plans and Interventions

Nursing Measures

- Maintain respiratory function
- Reduce effects of shock by elevating head and legs to heart level, providing warmth and rest and circulatory support as needed
- Decrease parents' anxiety by not placing blame, explaining procedures, and comforting

Client/Family Teaching

Delay teaching how to child-proof home until child is stable

Prevent recurrence by assessing support systems, assessing stress factors in family, visiting home if possible, administering questionnaire about poisons, offering suggestions such as use of child-resistant closures and poison stickers, providing information about poison control center

Evaluation

Treatment and client teaching are successful if:

- Child is treated immediately
- Parents and child are comforted during acute phase
- Parents' and child's anxiety is decreased
- Family understands how to child-proof home
- Home assessment has been made
- Parents understand they should contact poison control center with questions or in case of further complications

Celiac Disease

Celiac disease is a common malabsorption disorder in children, involving intolerance for gluten. The defect is believed to be an inborn error of metabolism or of immunologic response. Treatment involves a gluten-restricted diet with supplemental vitamins.

Assessment

Health Status

- Steatorrhea
- General malnutrition
- Abdominal distension
- Secondary vitamin deficiency

Diagnostic Factors

Stool analysis for fecal fat excretion

Hematologic studies for hypoproteinemia; anemia; hypothrombinemia; serum iron, folic acid, vitamin B12, and immunoglobulin levels

Roentgenographic studies for bone age

Bowel studies

Sweat test and pancreatic function studies

Small bowel biopsy (three biopsies recommended)

Nursing Plans and Interventions

Nursing Measures

- Recommend genetic counseling
- Comfort parents and child
- Stress long-range complications if child does not adhere to diet
- Allow family and child to express feelings, concerns

Nutrition Therapy

- Life-long gluten-free diet even when asymptomatic (make diet interesting and involve child in planning)

Client/Family Teaching

Educate family on how to anticipate crisis and avoid exposure to infections (vomiting and diarrhea are warning signs)

Refer family to counseling as needed, to cope with chronic illness

Evaluation

Treatment and client teaching are successful if:

- Family and child understand need for life-long dietary modifications
- Family is able to anticipate signs of complications
- Family follows up referrals to appropriate community resources for support
- Child maintains normal growth and development
- Child becomes involved in diet planning
- Family and child feel supported
- Family pursues long-term follow-up care

Appendicitis

Appendicitis is inflammation of the vermiform appendix. It is an acute condition usually caused by obstruction. Treatment includes an appendectomy.

Assessment

Health Status

- Colicky abdominal pain, initially generalized then descending to lower right quadrant (McBurney's point)
- Rigid abdomen with decreased bowel sounds
- Rebound tenderness
- Vomiting following onset of pain
- Anorexia
- Low-grade fever

Diagnostic Factors

History and examination
Increased white blood cell count
Abdominal x-ray

Nursing Plans and Interventions

Nursing Measures

- Assess behavior changes of younger child, if child unable to identify pain
- Prepare child for surgery; nasogastric (NG) tube may be placed to suction
- Assess hydration status carefully
- Decrease anxiety by giving age-appropriate explanations to child
- Comfort parents
- Postoperatively, assess surgical site and vital signs frequently
- In the case of ruptured appendix, place client in semi-Fowler's position on right side, with frequent dressing changes, wound and skin precautions and sterile dressing changes
- Prevent injury by ensuring complete bedrest, avoiding application of heat to abdomen, applying cold packs, assessing bowel activity, preventing abdominal distension

Evaluation

Treatment is successful if:

- Child is diagnosed early and treated
- Family's anxiety is decreased and child understands surgery
- Child is prepared for surgery
- No signs of infection are evident postoperatively
- Child remains well hydrated
- Child recovers and resumes normal growth and development activities
- Family and child feel supported

Nephrosis

Nephrosis is glomerular injury with massive proteinuria, hypoalbuminemia, hyperlipidemia, and edema.

Assessment

Health Status

- Edema (periorbital or on scrotum or abdomen)
- Weight gain
- Pallor, fatigue, anorexia
- Decreased urine volume, high urine specific gravity
- Increased susceptibility to infection

Diagnostic Factors

History
Proteinuria
Increased blood cholesterol level, low serum sodium level, decreased serum protein level
Renal biopsy

Nursing Plans and Interventions

Nursing Measures

- Increase comfort by allowing child to rest, recommending age-appropriate diversionary activity
- Prevent fluid volume deficit by monitoring I and O, urine specific gravity and albumin, abdominal girth, daily weight; restricting

fluid during short-term occurrence of massive edema
- Maintain skin care with frequent position change, special care in perineal area, and protection of scrotum if edematous (use scrotal supports)
- Protect from infection using careful handwashing (teach family members also), monitoring temperature and signs of infection

Drug Therapy

Teach family about medication therapy (corticosteroids): monitor levels, administer according to regular schedule; side-effects include weight gain in trunk and face due to water and sodium retention, GI irritation, bleeding ulcers, increased susceptibility to infection, mood swings; drug must be tapered off during illness

Nutrition Therapy

- Initial small, frequent feedings
- Increased protein during edema phase
- Restricted salt (in renal failure discontinue high-protein diet)

Client/Family Teaching

Prepare family for discharge by teaching signs of relapse, how to protect child from infection

Discuss body image and how to promote child's self-esteem

Listen to and comfort family and child

Evaluation

Treatment and client teaching are successful if:

- Child is free of infection
- Child does not have any skin breakdown
- Family understands medication and side-effects
- Parents demonstrate knowledge of disease process and signs of relapse
- Family promotes normal growth and development and enhances child's self-esteem
- Family keeps medical follow-up appointments

Hemophilia

Hemophilia refers to a group of bleeding disorders involving deficiency of one of the factors necessary for coagulation of blood. It is transmitted as an X-linked recessive disorder. The most common types are classic hemophilia (hemophilia A or Factor VIII deficiency) and Christman disease (hemophilia B or Factor IX deficiency).

Assessment

Health Status

- Excessive bleeding
- Hematomas from minor bumps, immunizations
- Bleeding gums
- Hemarthrosis (bleeding into a joint cavity)
- Long-term contractures, crippling
- May have blood in urine

Diagnostic Factors

History of accident with **prolonged bleeding time**

Blood coagulation studies to determine missing factor

Prothrombin time, partial thromboplastin time, thromboblastin generation test, prothrombin consumption test

Nursing Plans and Interventions

Nursing Measures

- Prevent injury by assessing for pain, positioning client to support affected joint, providing diversionary activities, administering aspirin-free medications
- Support child and family by encouraging normal growth and development, enhancing self-esteem, listening, establishing trust, referring to public health nurse in community for assistance, suggesting genetic

counseling, fostering child's independence, referring to outside support groups for financial and emotional support (*e.g.*, National Hemophilia Foundation)

Client/Family Teaching

Instruct child to avoid contact sports (suggest activities such as swimming and bike riding)

Teach good health practices

Instruct family on illness and administration of antihemophilic factor concentrates

Teach child and family importance of child wearing med-alert tag at all times

Teach child and family signs of complications, such as internal or external bleeding

Teach emergency measures, such as applying pressure for 10–15 minutes, immobilizing joint, applying cold packs, elevating joint above heart level, maintaining range of motion (ROM) exercises

Evaluation

Treatment and client teaching are successful if:

- Child and family understand disease process
- Family and child can identify signs of complications and emergency measures to take
- Child does not sustain further injury
- Child feels supported by hospital, schools, and community
- Child's independence is promoted with age-appropriate activities

Accidents

The major type of accidents affecting both boys and girls 1–4 years old is motor vehicle accidents, followed by burns, drownings, ingestion of poison, suffocation, and falls.

Client/Family Teaching

Teach parents safe behavior practices:

Infancy

Use crib sides and bumper pads
Do not use pillows or extra blankets
Use infant car seats correctly
Do not leave child on high places
Test bath water (should be lukewarm)
Protect from sun
Child-proof home
Select safe toys without movable parts
Use plastic bottles
Cover electrical outlets
Protect stairways with gates
Do not leave child unattended while eating
Cut food into small pieces, no peanuts or popcorn

Early Childhood

Child-proof home
Lock up poisonous substances
Do not leave child unattended in tub
Teach danger of fire and hot stove
Prevent falls (use siderails on crib or bed)

3–5 Years of Age

Teach bicycle safety and riding in streets
Teach medication safety
Fence pools, observe children in water
Teach Halloween safety (check candy)
Do not let children run with objects in mouth
Encourage safe play with peers and street safety
Know whereabouts of child at all times

15

Nursing Care of the School-age Child

Growth and Development

Psychosocial

According to Erikson, child struggles between industry and inferiority

Assumes more responsibility and learns new skills

Needs support and praise from family and peers

Develops moral judgment, sees rules as less absolute, moves from judging an act as right or wrong to taking into consideration different points of view

Develops sense of accomplishment in relating to others, in academic achievement, and in mastering new physical skills

Cognitive

According to Piaget, child develops understanding of concrete operations

Learns to see things from different viewpoints

Understands concept of conservation (understands relation of two or more dimensions, *e.g.*, volume of short fat glass of water = volume of tall thin glass of water)

Develops classification ability (can group and sort objects based on attributes and dissimilarities)

Develops combination skills (learns alphabet and how to arrange words in many ways)

Physical

Grows 1–2 inches per year

Gains 3–5 pounds per year

Vision reaches 20/20 by age 9–11

Permanent teeth appear

Moves more gracefully than preschooler

Motor Skills

6 years: uses scissors, climbs, hops, skips, jumps

7 years: swims, rides bicycle, eye-hand coordination not fully developed

8 years: movements more graceful

9 years: fully developed eye-hand coordination, hands ready for crafts, works to perfect skills

10 years: develops greater stamina, strength, coordination

11 years: clumsy, fidgety

Play

6 years: rough and tumble, table games

7 years: more careful, collecting, some sex play

8 years: likes competition, needs supervised play, likes to read and watch TV

9 years: loves crafts and table games

10 years: noisy, likes reading, enjoys "messing around"

11 years: likes popular music, team games, humor, comic and joke books

Social Interactions and Fears

6 years: life centers around school and friends, is unpredictable, forgets manners; fears loud noises, parental death, the supernatural; wants night light, is superstitious

7 years: very talkative, likes to help, more polite than 6-year-old; complains about parents; fears trying new activity, dark, ghosts, spies

8 years: very busy, silly, giggles a lot, easy to get along with, has fewer fears, worries less

9 years: very sociable, peer-oriented, begins hero worship, has fewer but more realistic fears

10 years: very competitive, same sex groups, has "best friend"; fears wild animals, fires, dark

11 years: very sociable, loves conversations, rebellious with parents, argues about everything, fears being alone and being disliked, worries about money and parents' health

Health Promotion

Sleep and Rest

- Amount needed depends on child's age, health status, and amount of activity: usually 9–12 hours per night, decreasing in amount as child grows older

Nutrition

- Needs less calories than toddler because not growing as fast
- Needs approximately 2400–2800 calories depending on exercise, state of health, height, and weight
- Needs basic four food groups
- Has more independence and some money, so eats more junk food than preschooler

Exercise

- Most children are very active with jumping, climbing, and bike riding
- Encourage child to exercise every day if not particularly active

Dental Health

- Teach child to brush teeth well at least two times per day
- Encourage parents to schedule dental visit every 6 months for check-up and to watch for teeth crowding and malocclusion problems

Sexuality

- Develops interest in opposite sex
- Wants information about conception, pregnancy, birth, menstruation, wet dreams
- Engages in mild sex play
- Is interested in changes occurring in body (breast buds, erections)
- Needs factual information from parents

Family Relationships

- Is more interested in friends than family
- Is more cooperative
- Still relies on family for some emotional support

The Hospitalized School-aged Child

Children ages 2½ years and older should be prepared for hospitalization with explanations about why they are there and what might happen, and about their physical surroundings.

Separation

- Is better able to handle separation from family, friends, and activities
- Is better able to cope with strange people and environment
- May try to act brave, not to complain of pain, not to cry

Loss of Control

- Is not able to make decisions as he or she does at home
- Feels dependent, may be on bedrest or have to use bed pan
- Is not as involved in family activities as preschooler

Fear of Pain and Injury
- Wants to know what procedures are for, if they will hurt, and if they have long-term consequences
- Needs to know what to expect

Administration of Medications
- Most drugs are administered intravenously:

$$\text{Drops/min} = \frac{\text{Volume infused} \times \text{drops/ml}}{\text{Total infusion time (min)}}$$

Adaptation of Procedures for Children
- Consider developmental level of child and family
- Explain procedures repeatedly, if necessary
- Use puppets or dolls to foster understanding
- Restrain child during procedure if necessary to prevent injury
- Provide emotional support to family
- Allow family to be with child before and after procedure

Preparation for Diagnostic Tests
- Use developmental level of child and family to determine teaching plan
- Speak in language that child and family understand
- Explain what will occur before, during, or after diagnostic test
- Explain to child and family what they should do during procedure

Health Problems of the School-age Child

Accidents

Accidents are the chief cause of death in children 5–14 years of age. Motor vehicle accidents are the leading cause of accidental death, followed by bicycle and water accidents.

Nursing Plans and Interventions

Goals
- Client will learn to wear seat belts always

Client/Family Teaching

Teach child and family to:

Cross at corners
Not ride in open trucks
Practice water safety
Practice bicycle safety
Understand traffic signals

Evaluation

Client teaching is successful if:
- Parents and child are able to repeat safety rules
- All family members use seat belts

Helminthic Infections

Pinworms are the most common parasitic infection in children; they are transmitted by the fecal-oral route or by contact with contaminated articles.

Assessment

Health Status
- Rectal itch
- In girls, vaginal itch, frequency, urgency

Diagnostic Factors

Observation of eggs collected on scotch tape from anus

Nursing Plans and Interventions

Nursing Measures
- Have parent use cellophane tape at night on rectum
- Have parent bring tape to office/clinic in morning to be examined for eggs

Drug Therapy

Administer mebendazole (Vermox) to affected child and entire family

Client/Family Teaching

Teach client and family that:

Bed linens and underwear of affected child should be washed in hot water daily

Good handwashing prevents spread to other family members

Evaluation

Treatment and client teaching are successful if:

- Pinworms are gone when checked by scotch tape method
- Family uses good handwashing techniques

Mental Retardation

Mental retardation is characterized by subaverage general intelligence and deficits in adaptive behavior. Mental retardation may be caused by genetic or environmental factors in the prenatal period; by birth injury or prematurity in the neonatal or perinatal period; by infections such as meningitis in the postnatal period; by degenerative disease such as Tay-Sachs, by head injury or asphyxia, by brain tumors, or by neglect or malnutrition.

Assessment

Developmental Factors

- Developmental delays
- IQ score less than 70

Nursing Plans and Interventions

Nursing Measures

- Encourage child to be as independent as abilities allow
- Encourage child to be in school or alternative and to progress as far as possible
- Support family in their decisions about independence and school

Client/Family Teaching

Teach family to:

Encourage child to be as independent as abilities allow

Encourage child to be in school or alternative and to progress as far as possible

Evaluation

Client teaching is successful if:

- Child is allowed to be as independent as possible
- Child is in school or program for stimulation

Acute Lymphocytic Leukemia

Leukemia is the most common malignancy of childhood. It accounts for about 33% of all childhood cancers. Normal bone marrow cells are replaced with immature blast cells, resulting in anemia, infection, and bleeding. Treatment is chemotherapy, radiation, or bone marrow transplantation.

Assessment

Health Status

- Fatigue
- Bruising
- Petechiae
- Fever
- Anorexia
- Weight loss
- Hepatosplenomegaly
- Lymphadenopathy

Nursing Plans and Interventions

Nursing Measures

- Assess skin for petechiae and bruises
- Use soft toothbrush to prevent bleeding

- Encourage good mouth care
- Observe for side-effects of oncovin (Vincristine), such as alopecia, jaw pain, constipation, neurotoxicity
- Watch for side-effects of cyclophosphamide (Cytoxan), such as hemorrhagic cystitis, mouth ulcers, nausea, and vomiting
- Watch for side-effects of radiation (dependent on site radiated)
- Immunizations are not given to an immunosuppressed child
- Offer psychosocial support about grieving

Drug Therapy

Chemotherapy with specified protocols

Cyclophosphamide (Cytoxan), vincaleukoblastine (Vincristine), methotrexate, prednisone

Nutrition Therapy

- Offer nutritious and attractive meals
- High-fiber diet for child receiving oncovin to prevent constipation
- Force fluids because of increasing amounts of uric acid due to breakdown of cells

Client/Family Teaching

Teach family:

About use of nonaspirin products

About the disease

About medications

To treat child as normally as possible

Evaluation

Treatment and client teaching are successful if:

- Child has normal uric acid level
- Child has regular bowel movements
- Child has no mouth ulcers
- Family is able to express fears and feelings

Brain Tumor

Brain tumors are the most common type of solid neoplasm and are most commonly seen in the 6- to 10-year-old age group. Brain tumors are either *infratentorial*, in the cerebellum, brain stem, optic chiasm and fourth ventricle, or *supratentorial*, in the cerebrum and optic nerve. Meduloblastomas are the most common type. Treatment is usually craniotomy followed by chemotherapy or radiation therapy.

Assessment

Health Status

- Depends on age of child and location of tumor
- Headache upon awakening
- Nausea and vomiting
- Seizures
- Change in school performance
- Diplopia and visual field defects
- Ataxia and clumsiness

Nursing Plans and Interventions

Preoperative Nursing Measures

- Assess neurological system for changes
- Encourage eating again after vomiting
- Supply cool cloth and pain medicine for headache
- Protect from hazards in environment
- Raise head 30–45° to decrease intracranial pressure
- Support child and family through diagnostic tests and surgery
- Support child and family during grieving

Preoperative Client/Family Teaching

Teach about diagnostic procedures and surgery

Postoperative Nursing Measures

- Monitor vital signs frequently until stable
- Assess neurological system for changes
- Have client turn, cough, and deep breathe to prevent respiratory infection
- Assess breath sounds to identify rales or rhonchi (because of immobility)

- Offer pain medication as needed for headache
- Observe head dressing for drainage
- Monitor IV fluids
- Provide good mouth care to prevent oral infection
- Support family
- Encourage family members to discuss feelings

Evaluation

Treatment and client teaching are successful if:

- No changes in neurological system result
- No physical injuries result
- Headaches are helped by cool cloths and pain medication
- Child does not lose weight from vomiting
- Child and family are able to repeat teaching verbally

Acute Glomerulonephritis

Acute glomerulonephritis (AGN) follows a group A β-hemolytic *streptococcal* infection that occurred 10 to 14 days prior to the onset of symptoms. AGN is thought to be an antigen-antibody response to the invading streptococcus, and involves inflammation and obstruction in the glomeruli. Medical treatment is supportive and includes fluids, hypertensive medications, and a restricted sodium diet. Recovery is spontaneous without further complications in most cases.

Assessment

Health Status

- Mild periorbital edema in morning, due to fluid retention
- Decreased amount of brown, cloudy urine
- Increased specific gravity due to fluid retention
- Lethargy due to increasing blood urea nitrogen (BUN) level
- Pallor due to blood loss in urine
- Increased BUN and creatinine levels
- Hypertension and decreased pulse rate

Nursing Plans and Interventions

Nursing Measures

- Monitor vital signs for increasing blood pressure
- Measure weight and I and O because of edema
- Provide appropriate diversional activities
- May be on bedrest because of severe edema
- Encourage a no-added-salt diet if symptoms are mild

Client/Family Teaching

Teach family and child about diagnosis and expected outcomes

Evaluation

Treatment and client teaching are successful if:

- Vital signs are stable
- No weight gain occurs
- Appropriate diversional activities are provided
- Family and child are able to discuss diagnosis and expected outcomes

Asthma

Asthma is the most common chronic illness in children. It affects about 5% to 10% of all children. The most common inhaled allergens that cause asthma are pollens, house dust, molds, and cat and dog danders. Foods that may cause asthma are wheat, chocolate, cow's milk, and citrus fruits. Other factors that aggravate asthma are respiratory infections, weather changes, stress, and air pollutants.

Medical treatment is an oral theophylline preparation that may be taken daily or only when symptoms appear. If hospitalized, hydrocortisone and aminophylline will be administered, in addition to an antibiotic if an infection is present. The child will also be given humidified oxygen.

Assessment

Health Status

- Wheezing
- Dry cough may be paroxysmal
- Use of accessary respiration muscles
- Theophylline blood level may be low if child has not received any recently

Nursing Plans and Interventions

Nursing Measures

- Assess vital signs for changes
- Assess breath sounds for increasing wheezing
- Encourage fluid intake
- Observe for side-effects of aminophylline (headache, jitteriness, nausea, vomiting, arrhythmias)
- Measure I and O
- Monitor amount of oxygen being administered
- Provide emotional support to child and parents

Evaluation

Treatment is successful if:

- Vital signs are stable
- Breath sounds are clear
- Child is well hydrated
- No side-effects from theophylline result
- I and O is normal
- Emotional support is provided to child and family
- Theophylline blood level is therapeutic

Cystic Fibrosis

Cystic fibrosis is the most common inherited disease in children. It is inherited as an autosomal recessive trait, meaning the child inherits the defective genes from both parents. It affects the exocrine glands, mucus is thick and tenacious, sticking to the walls of the pancreatic and bile ducts and bronchi, eventually causing obstructions. Obstructions cause fibrosis and eventually chronic lung disease. The heart develops right ventricular hypertrophy in adaptation to pulmonary hypertension. Medical treatment includes prescribing pancreatic enzymes with meals and snacks, water soluble vitamins, and a high-caloric, moderate fat, high-protein diet. The character of stools helps determine how much of the pancreatic enzymes the client should take. If the child has to be admitted to the hospital for severe respiratory infection he or she will receive IV antibiotics such as tobramycin sulfate (Nebcin), as well as frequent aerosol treatments to help cough up the mucus.

Assessment

Health Status

- History of frequent respiratory infections
- Barrel-shaped chest
- Clubbed toes and fingers
- Productive cough
- Small stature
- Thinness
- Possible rales and rhonchi

Nursing Plans and Interventions

Nursing Measures

- Maintain open airway
- Encourage productive coughing
- Supervise administration of aerosols and bronchodilator treatments
- Weigh daily
- Assess character of feces
- Assess for side-effects of antibiotics if applicable (tobramycin and gentamicin: hearing loss, nephrotoxicity; nafcillin: rash, anaphylactic reaction)

Drug Therapy

Pancreatic enzymes with meals and snacks
Antibiotics (tobramycin, gentamicin, nafcillin)

Nutrition Therapy

- High-calorie, moderate-fat, and high-protein diet with snacks

Client/Family Teaching

Teach family how to prevent respiratory infection by getting enough rest, eating well, avoiding others with respiratory infection

Encourage family to treat child as normally as possible

Collaborate with respiratory therapy professionals to teach family about chest physiotherapy

Evaluation

Treatment and client teaching are successful if:

- Breath sounds are clearer
- Coughing is productive
- Child follows prescribed diet
- Child does not lose weight
- Pancreatic enzymes are taken with meals and snacks
- Vitamins are taken as ordered
- Family is able to repeat how to prevent respiratory infections
- Family understands importance of treating child as normally as possible

Inguinal Hernia

Inguinal hernia is due to a defect in the closure of the processus vaginalis during the 8th month of gestation. It precedes the testicle through the inguinal canal into the scrotum. The proximal portion of the processus vaginalis normally closes and the distal portion envelops the testicle in the scrotum. When the proximal portion fails to close, abdominal fluid or an abdominal structure can be forced into it, creating a bulge or hernia. The problem occurs in boys more often than in girls. The hernia appears as the intestine pushes through this defect. Treatment is surgical reduction.

Assessment

Health Status

- Painless inguinal swelling
- Swelling more prominent during straining or crying

Nursing Plans and Interventions

- Provide preoperative teaching to reduce child's and parents' anxiety
- Postoperatively allow child to be as active as desired
- Child may have collodion rather than dressing over incision
- Mild pain medication as needed for several days

Evaluation

Treatment is successful if:

- Child's and parents' anxiety are reduced
- Child is active
- Need for pain medication decreases

Appendicitis

Appendicitis is inflammation of the appendix. It affects boys more often than girls. Treatment is surgical removal.

Assessment

Health Status

- Abdominal pain, usually periumbilical first, then localizing to right lower quadrant (McBurney's point)
- Nausea and vomiting
- Low-grade fever
- Possible elevated white blood cell count
- Walks bent over

Nursing Plans and Interventions

Nursing Measures

Preoperative Care

- Keep client as comfortable as possible by administering pain medication
- Maintain npo
- Offer no enemas or laxatives
- Do not apply heat to abdomen (prevent rupture of appendix)
- Offer support to child and family

Postoperative Care

- Keep as comfortable as possible by administering pain medication as needed
- Offer clear liquids when bowel sounds are heard
- Maintain IV fluids as ordered
- Check abdominal dressing for drainage (change as ordered)
- Encourage child to be up as much as possible
- Monitor I and O while fluids are infusing
- Offer support to child and family

Client/Family Teaching

Inform parents of what is occurring and what to expect

Evaluation

Treatment is successful if:

- Child is free of pain
- I and O are maintained
- Bowel sounds are present a few hours after surgery
- Abdominal dressing is free or nearly free from drainage
- Parents are able to repeat what will occur

Acute Rheumatic Fever

Acute rheumatic fever (ARF) is a systemic inflammatory disease caused by a preceding group A β-hemolytic *Streptococcus* infection. It is most commonly seen in children 5–15 years old. It usually resolves in 3 weeks. Diagnosis is based on the use of Jones' criteria (Table 15-1). The presence of two major criteria or one major and two minor criteria suggests the child may have ARF. Carditis occurs in 50% of children with ARF. Mitral and aortic valves are the most susceptible to damage from vegetation. Aspirin and steroids are frequently used.

Assessment

Health Status

- Vital signs
- I and O
- Hydration
- Breath sounds
- Heart murmur
- Tachycardia
- Signs of aspirin toxicity tinnitus

Table 15-1. Jones' Criteria

Major	Minor
Carditis	Fever
Chorea	Arthralgia
Arthritis	Previous streptococcal infection
Erythema marginatum	Positive C reactive protein
Subcutaneous nodules	Elevated sedimentation rate
	Previous history of ARF
	Prolonged PR interval

Nursing Plans and Interventions

Nursing Measures

- Provide rest periods
- Explain medications (penicillin, aspirin, prednisone) to child and family
- Provide appropriate diversional activities
- Provide support to child and family
- Encourage child to keep up with school work

Client/Family Teaching

Teach child and family about disease

Teach child and family about penicillin prophylaxis (receive IM monthly or orally daily, also before dental procedures or after intrusive procedures)

Evaluation

Treatment and client teaching are successful if:

- Vital signs are stable
- I and O is maintained
- Breath sounds are clear
- Heart sounds are normal
- Resting heart rate is normal
- No signs of aspirin toxicity are present
- Rest periods are provided
- Child and family can repeat information about medication
- Child is provided with activities, including homework
- Child and family can explain penicillin prophylaxis program

Sickle Cell Anemia

Sickle cell disease is an autosomal recessive hereditary disorder found predominately in blacks. A person may have the trait or the disease. A child inherits the defective genes from both parents. Those with the trait usually do not have symptoms of the disease but those with the disease always have symptoms. When deoxygenation occurs, the sickle hemoglobin molecule increases blood viscosity, which results in stasis of cells and causes further deoxygenation. A crisis may result. Treatment is supportive, including fluids, pain medications, and the application of heat to painful areas.

Assessment

- Crisis caused by infection, vigorous exercise, or emotional stress

Health Status

- Joint pain
- Nausea and vomiting
- Fever
- Irritability

Nursing Plans and Intervention

Nursing Measures

- Offer pain medication as needed
- Encourage fluid intake to prevent dehydration
- Record I and O
- Organize care to provide rest periods to decrease oxygen needs
- Apply dry heat to painful area(s) as needed
- Provide emotional support
- Monitor IV flow rate
- Encourage well-balanced meals

Client/Family Teaching

Teach client and family to:

Keep away from others with infections

Learn to deal with stressful situations

Avoid places of low-oxygen tension, *e.g.,* mountains, unpressurized airplanes

Take penicillin daily if prescribed

Maintain high fluid intake

Maintain nutritious diet

Evaluation

Treatment and client teaching are successful if:

- Need for pain medication decreases as crisis subsides
- Fluid intake increases greatly

Diabetes Mellitus

Diabetes mellitus is a disease of metabolism involving a deficiency of the hormone insulin. It is the most common metabolic disease in the United States. Type I occurs in children and is treated with insulin and diet. The onset of diabetes mellitus in children is quite rapid. Children of all ages can develop it. The pancreas does not produce enough insulin, so carbohydrates are used for energy and glucose accumulates in the blood stream. Short-acting and intermediate-acting insulins are administered twice daily. The American Dietary Association (ADA) exchange diet is commonly used and provides three meals and two or three snacks per day. The ADA diet substitutes one food for another within the same list. A bedtime snack is included to prevent late night hypoglycemia.

Assessment

Health Status

- Polyuria
- Polydipsia
- Polyphagia
- Weight loss
- Fatigue
- Lethargy
- Nausea and vomiting
- Abdominal pain

Nursing Plans and Interventions

Nursing Measures

- Assess glucose levels with reagent strip (Dextrostix) or glucometer
- Provide emotional support to child and family

Client/Family Teaching

Begin teaching about diabetes when diagnosed. Teach child and family about:

Dietary requirements
How to plan menus
How to administer insulin
Signs of hypoglycemia (insulin reaction)—regular insulin peaks in 2–3 hours, NPH insulin peaks in 8–10 hours—shakiness, irritability, headache, sweating
Signs of hyperglycemia (insulin shock)—weakness, thirst, nausea and vomiting, abdominal pain
Importance of notifying physician when ill
Need for exercise program
Need for insulin when child is sick

Evaluation

Treatment and client teaching are successful if:

- Child and family plan diet, administer insulin, and plan exercise
- Child and family can state signs of hypoglycemia and hyperglycemia
- Child and family can explain what to do when child is ill

Burns

Burns are the second most common cause of accidental death in children from birth to age 15 years. In partial thickness burns, part of the dermis and epidermis are destroyed. These burns are also called first-degree and second-degree burns. They usually heal in 2–10 days. Full thickness burns are also called third-degree burns. The dermis layer is destroyed down to the subcutaneous fat. Burns can be caused by chemical, thermal, or electric substances. Most result from thermal exposure (fire or hot water). First aid treatment for burns is applying cool water to the burn site and notifying a physician. If the child is on fire, wrap the child in a blanket or available clothing and call an ambulance. Treatment for partial thickness burns involves cleansing and debriding the wound, then covering with an antimicrobial cream and dressing. For full thickness burns, establish and maintain an airway and establish IV infusion for fluids. Cleanse the burns in a whirlpool, debride, then cover with antimicrobial cream and dressing. Skin grafting may be needed.

Assessment

Health Status

- Extent of burn
- Depth of burn
- Vital signs
- Breath sounds for rales and rhonchi
- Nose and nasal hair for signs of smoke inhalation
- Gastrointestinal bleeding
- Weight

Nursing Plans and Interventions

Nursing Measures

- Maintain protective isolation to prevent wound infection
- Administer pain medications as needed
- Provide age-appropriate distraction
- Keep child from picking and scratching wound
- Monitor side-effects if antibiotics ordered for wound infection
- Measure I and O because of fluid shifts and diuresis
- Promote self-help skills
- Offer support to child and family

Nutrition Therapy

- High-calorie, high-carbohydrate, high-protein diet

Evaluation

Treatment is successful if:

- Vital signs become more stable as burns heal
- Need for pain medication decreases as burns heal
- Child becomes more independent as burns heal
- Child and family adjust to burn scars

Fractures

Fractures have many causes, from birth injury and child abuse to motor vehicle accidents. Childrens' bones are more easily injured because they are still developing and becoming harder. Serious injury may occur if the epiphysis is damaged while the child is still growing. A *simple or closed* fracture involves no break in the skin. In an *open or compound* fracture, the bone protrudes through the skin. In a *complicated* fracture, bone fragments cause damage to other organs. In a *comminuted* fracture, fragments of bone lie in surrounding tissue.

Assessment

Health Status

- Swelling
- Pain
- Tenderness
- Decreased use of affected part

Nursing Plans and Interventions

Traction is used to immobilize the fracture site to promote healing. Pressure traction is a type of skin traction.

Nursing Measures (Traction)

- Perform neurovascular assessment of involved extremity
- Assess movement distal to fracture
- Assess for swelling
- Assess traction ropes for fraying
- Maintain hip flexion to prevent nerve damage
- Make sure weights hang free
- Have child pull self up in bed, or help him or her
- Do not lift weights to reduce pull on fracture site

A cast (plaster or synthetic) is used to immobilize the area around the fracture site to aid healing.

Nursing Measures (Cast)

- Perform neurovascular assessment of involved extremity
- Assess movement of extremity distal to cast
- Turn a wet cast using palms of hands
- Petal cast edges when cast is dry

Client/Family Teaching

Teach client and family:

That plaster cast produces heat as it sets

To use cool hair dryer to blow down cast if it becomes too hot

To insert no foreign objects in cast

To assess cast for foul odor

Evaluation

Treatment and client teaching are successful if child has no complications from traction or cast

16

Nursing Care of the Adolescent

Growth and Development

Psychosocial

According to Erikson, adolescent tries to establish own identity while coping with role diffusion
Sees self as an individual
Belongs to a crowd
Relies on peers for support, praise, reassurance
Reassesses values and beliefs
Gains independence from parents

Cognitive

According to Piaget, adolescent develops understanding of formal operations
Is capable of scientific reasoning and formal logic
Sees self and world more realistically
Can think abstractly

Physical

Both sexes undergo growth spurt
Girls grow 2–8 inches and gain 15–55 pounds between ages 10–14
Boys grow 4–14 inches and gain 15–65 pounds between ages 12–16

Females develop secondary sex characteristics:

Increase in pelvic diameter
Breast development
Change in vaginal secretions
Axillary and pubic hair growth
Menarche: average age is 12.5 years

Males develop secondary sex characteristics:

Increase in size of genitalia
Breast swelling
Pubic, axillary, chest, and facial hair growth
Changes in voice
Increase in shoulder breadth
Nocturnal emissions, spermatogenesis

Health Promotion

Sleep and Rest

- Needs more sleep than when younger, due to growth spurts
- Stays out later so may want to sleep later

Nutrition

- Girls need about 2100 calories per day
- Boys need about 3000 calories per day
- Protein and calorie needs high because of growth spurt
- Adolescents frequently do not eat enough fruits and vegetables
- Adolescents eat snacks that are easily accessible but not necessarily nutritious
- **Girls may be iron deficient at menarche**

Leisure Activities
- Talking on phone
- Competitive sports
- Movies
- Video games
- Daydreaming
- Parties
- Hobbies

Dental Health
- Regular dental visits are still important
- Adolescence is frequently the time for wearing braces so teeth and gum care becomes more important

Sexuality
- Needs information about how pregnancy occurs
- Needs to know about venereal disease
- Forms social relations with peers and may explore sexuality

Family Relationships
- Relationships may be strained as adolescent tries to become more independent
- Adolescents may be moody; need more understanding from parents
- Adolescents do not share feelings or activities with family members as readily as younger children

The Hospitalized Adolescent

Separation
- Finds it difficult to be separated from peer group

Loss of Control
- Has well-developed coping mechanisms to deal with stress
- Fears loss of control due to illness or hospitalization

Fear of Pain and Injury
- Reacts to pain with self-control
- Is very concerned about body image

Health Problems of the Adolescent

Accidents

Adolescents are risk takers and act impulsively. Motor vehicle accidents are the leading cause of death in adolescence, followed by drownings, falls, and firearms.

Client/Family Teaching

Teach motor vehicle safety:

Do not drink and drive

Do not ride with driver who has been drinking

Always wear seat belt

Evaluation

Client teaching is successful if client:
- Can repeat teaching about motor vehicle safety
- Always wears seat belt

Obesity

Obesity develops in response to a particular life stressor or develops as a result of bad eating habits. It may also have a genetic or endocrine basis. It is considered a form of malnutrition.

Assessment

Health Status
- Height and weight
- Duration of obesity
- Eating patterns
- Adolescent's self-perception
- Family's attitude toward adolescent
- Recent stressors for adolescent
- Recent stressors for family
- Family's problem-solving skills

Nursing Plans and Interventions

Nursing Measures
- Set goals with adolescent and family for realistic weight loss

- Encourage adolescent to increase physical activity if necessary
- Help adolescent adjust eating patterns to decrease calorie intake
- Use adolescent's strengths to improve self-concept
- Provide positive reinforcement
- May use behavior modification program to change eating habits and improve self-esteem

Evaluation

Treatment is successful if client:

- Loses weight according to goals set
- Develops healthy ways to handle stress
- Increases physical activity if necessary

Bone Tumors

The following discussion pertains to osteogenic sarcoma, the most frequently occurring bone tumor in children. The tumor arises from the bone-forming mesenchyme tissue. More than 50% are located near the knee. Peak age is 15–19 years. Tumors may be related to adolescent growth spurt. Metastasis to the lung is common. Treatment usually is amputation and chemotherapy.

Assessment

Health Status

- Pain
- May have swelling at site
- Limited movement of joint

Nursing Plans and Interventions

Nursing Measures

- Provide preoperative teaching for probable limb amputation
- Support adolescent and parents during grieving
- Introduce adolescent to another adolescent who has had same diagnosis and treatment
- Provide support during chemotherapy

Client/Family Teaching

Teach adolescent and parent about disease and treatment (limb prosthesis a possibility)

Evaluation

Treatment and client teaching are successful if:

Adolescent and parents are able to grieve

Adolescent and parents can repeat teaching about disease and treatment

Scoliosis

Scoliosis is lateral curvature of the spine with some rotation of the vertebrae; it can occur at any age. Types of scoliosis include *functional* (due to posture or leg length discrepancy), and *structural*. Two subtypes of structural scoliosis include *paralytic*, which may be caused by muscular disorders such as myelomeningocele, and *idiopathic*, which includes approximately 70% of the cases, usually occurs after age 10, and affects girls more often than boys. Treatment depends on the severity of the curve. Bracing may be used to correct curvature until growth stops. The brace is worn 23 hours a day. If the curve is severe, spinal fusion with rod placement is performed.

Assessment

Health Status

- Hem length discrepancy
- One shoulder higher than other
- One hip more prominent than other
- Girls wear bra and shorts during screening

Client/Family Teaching

Teach client to:

Wear undershirt under brace

Shower and wash hair during hour out of brace

Inspect skin daily for redness and breakdown

Avoid using lotions, creams, or powders under brace

Wear loose-fitting clothes outside of brace

Wear low-heel shoes

Avoid contact sports and vigorous gymnastics

Continue in physical education class (usually possible)

Wear brace until growth stops or other treatment is planned

Offer emotional support to client and family, and talk to adolescent's peers about scoliosis and treatment if possible.

Evaluation

Client teaching is successful if adolescent complies with treatment plan

Convulsive Disorder/Epilepsy

Seizures are not a specific disease but an indication of a brain dysfunction. There are many different causes of seizures. Epilepsy is a chronic, recurring seizure disorder. Seizure is a disorder in brain function caused by the erratic discharge of electrical impulses in the brain. An international classification system divides seizures into two categories: generalized and partial seizures. Seizures are treated with anticonvulsant medications. Anticonvulsant medication blood levels are measured periodically.

Assessment

Health Status

- May have aura before seizure
- Witness observes tonic-clonic episodes
- Eye-rolling
- Daydreaming or short periods of inattentiveness
- Repetitive movements
- Lapses in consciousness

Nursing Plans and Interventions

Nursing Measures

During seizure:

- Help client to floor
- Place pillow under head
- Protect from harm
- Time seizure activity
- Note activity during seizure
- Suction as needed

After seizure, client may sleep, and later awaken with a headache and no memory of seizure activity; provide emotional support to adolescent and family.

Medical Treatment

For Generalized Seizures

Phenytoin (Dilantin) (side-effects: gingival hyperplasia, rash)

Phenobarbital (side-effects: drowsiness, hyperactivity)

For Partial Seizures

Ethosuximide (Zarontin) (side-effects: nausea, vertigo)

Client/Family Teaching

Teach client and family:

Not to put object in adolescent's mouth during seizure

With good seizure control, activities are not limited

To avoid alcohol

To consult physician before client takes other medication

About medication, including side-effects

Evaluation

Treatment and client teaching are successful if adolescent and family understand epilepsy and treatment

Venereal Disease

Venereal disease is sexually transmitted disease (disease transmitted primarily through sexual contact). Conditions may involve the genital, rectal, or oral areas, and may be caused by bacterial, viral, or fungal organisms. There is a high incidence among 15–25 year olds, possibly because they experience more sexual freedom than other age groups. Common diseases include gonorrhea, which is caused by *Neisseria gonorrhoeae*, and chlamydia, which is caused by *Chlamydia trachomatis*. Medical treatment is high doses of penicillin for gonorrhea and tetracycline for chlamydia. Partners are also treated. (See also chapter 8).

Assessment

(See Chapter 8)

Client/Family Teaching

Client teaching is primarily aimed at prevention. Teach client to:

Clean perineal area daily
Urinate after intercourse
Wipe front to back (girls)
Avoid bubble baths, douches, and hygiene sprays (girls)
Use condoms
Avoid sex with infected partner

Evaluation

Treatment and client teaching are successful if adolescent can repeat instructions for prevention, and is free of infection

Drug Abuse

Drug abuse is higher among adolescents than in the general population. The most common drug used is marijuana; many marijuana users experiment with other drugs, such as hallucinogens and cocaine.

Assessment

Health Status

- More likely to occur in adolescent with poor self-esteem and poor school performance
- Slurred speech
- Decreased attention span
- Nasal irritation

Nursing Plans and Interventions

Nursing Measures

- Be nonjudgmental when eliciting information
- Interview adolescent alone
- Discuss adolescent's behavior with parents
- Refer to drug rehabilitation program if necessary
- Provide emotional support to family

Evaluation

Treatment and client teaching are successful if adolescent is knowledgeable about drugs and does not abuse drugs

Suicide

Suicide attempts are on the rise. Adolescents at risk should be identified and helped, in order to prevent a suicide attempt.

Assessment

Health Status

- Family history of suicide
- Peer suicide
- Substance abuse
- Recent loss
- Depression

Nursing Plans and Interventions

Nursing Measures

- Refer to psychologist or psychiatrist
- Encourage adolescent to follow up with counseling
- Remove articles at home that can be used in another attempt (*e.g.*, firearms, medicines)

Client/Family Teaching

Teach client and family:

Side-effects of antidepressive medication if applicable
About need for frequent follow-up

Evaluation

Treatment and client teaching are successful if no suicide attempt occurs

Acne

Acne is the most common skin condition of adolescence; its degree of severity varies. Acne involves the sebaceous glands and hair follicles. During adolescence, more androgen is produced, and more sebum is secreted, which blocks the sebaceous follicles. This blocking can produce either open or closed comedones.

Assessment

Health Status

Assess:

- Extent of lesions
- Distribution of lesions
- Scarring
- Progress, if client in treatment

Nursing Plans and Interventions

Client Teaching

Teach client to:

Cleanse face with mild soap once or twice daily

Not pick at face

Eat nutritious foods

Not rub or scrub face hard

Not use greasy products on affected areas

Keep scheduled appointments with physician or nurse practitioner

Learn to deal positively with stress because stress may worsen problem

Provide support to adolescent.

Evaluation

Treatment and client teaching are successful if adolescent has positive self-image, and little or no scarring results

Bibliography for Unit IV
Care of the Child

Bindler RM: Home care for a child with a cardiac defect. Issue Comp Pediatr Nurs 3(7):48–60, 1979

Biro, Thompson: Screening young children for communication disorders. Matern Child Nurs J 9: 410, 1984

Capute, Shapiro, Palmer, Ross, Wachtel: Normal gross motor development: The influences of race, sex, and socioeconomic status. Dev Med Child Neurol 27:635–643, 1985

Castigna, Petrini: Selecting a developmental screening tool. Pediatr Nurs (11) (1), 1985

DeBenhem B et al: Initial assessment and management of chronic diarrhea in toddlers. Pediatr Nurs 11:281–285, 1985

Denehy: What do school-age children know about their bodies? Pediatr Nurs 10:290–298, 1984

Ellund: Teenage thinking: Implications for care. Pediatr Nurs 10:383–387, 1986

Gaddy PS, Wood A: The leukemias. In Fachtman D, Foley GU (eds): Nursing Care of Children with Cancer. Boston, Little, Brown & Co, 1982

Jackson DL: Digoxin therapy at home: Keeping the child safe. MCN 4:105–109, 1979

McGrath B: Fluids, electrolytes and replacement therapy in pediatric nursing. MCN 5:58–62, 1980

Mott S, Fazekas N, James S: Nursing Care of Children and Families. Menlo Park, CA, Addison-Wesley, 1985

Petrillo M, Songer S: Emotional Care of Hospitalized Children. Philadelphia, JB Lippincott, 1980

Rice: Nutritional problems of developmentally disabled children. Pediatr Nurs 7:15–18, 1981

Rushton CH: Preparing children and families for cardiac surgery: Nursing interventions. Issue Comp Pediatr Nurs 6:235–248, 1983

Scipien G et al: Comprehensive Pediatric Nursing. New York, McGraw-Hill, 1986

Sper J, Sachs B: Selecting the appropriate family assessment tool. Pediatr Nurs 11:349–356, 1985

Whaley L, Wong D: Nursing Care of Infants and Children. St Louis, CV Mosby, 1983

Winnelstein: Overfeeding in infancy: The early introduction of solid foods. Pediatr Nurs 10:205–210, 1984

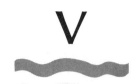

Care of the Client with a Mental Health Problem

17

General Psychiatric Nursing Treatment Modalities

Basic Assumptions of Nursing as a Practice Profession

- Goals of nursing practice are based on helping human individuals achieve maximum health
- Goals can be met in many settings, but are most effectively met within the framework of the nursing process
- Individuals and their problems or needs are best viewed holistically: their biological, psychological, and sociological aspects considered together
- Nurses encounter individuals of all ages and in all health settings who are functioning at less than optimal psychological wellness
- Psychiatric nursing focuses on psychological problems as the primary dysfunctional pattern encountered with clients

Foundations of Psychiatric Nursing

- Humans interact holistically with the environment throughout life
- Mentally healthy people cope effectively with the environment
- Mental illness implies behavior that is a dysfunctional interaction with the environment
- Psychiatric nurse practitioners identify therapeutic communication as the critical intervention for dysfunctional behavior
- Therapeutic communication occurs within the context of a therapeutic nurse/client relationship
- This relationship should be a warm, trusting relationship between nurse and client for the purpose of helping client (the client must trust the nurse and the nurse must accept the client)

Therapeutic Communication as Process

- Therapeutic communication is an ongoing, dynamic, ever-changing series of events, and can occur on three levels: intrapersonal (within self), interpersonal (within dyads and small groups), and public (in speech and mass media)
- Influences that affect both nurse and client include perception, values, and culture

Principles the Nurse Can Use to Enhance Therapeutic Communication

- See chapter 4 for details
- Facilitation: helps initiate, build, and maintain trusting relationships
- Facilitative intimacy: has therapeutic goals; is specifically focused on client's problem; encourages self-disclosure with the purpose of understanding circumstances and moving toward resolution; encourages sharing of feelings; all messages (verbal and nonverbal) are recognized and open to discussion
- Encouragement of interpersonal relationships
- Feedback
- Confrontation: results from examination of discrepancy between what person says and what person does; requires careful attention to nonverbal messages
- Empathy
- Respect: demonstrates that nurse values client's integrity
- Genuineness: ability to be real or honest; timing important; used when client is ready
- Immediacy: response to the here and now

Phases of the Therapeutic Relationship

Orientation Phase

Assessment begins

Nurse/client contract is made

Working Phase

Nurse and client identify and explore patterns of dysfunctional behavior and establish goals for their resolution

Barriers that may arise include excessive dependence, hostility, self-destructive behavior, manipulation, withdrawal, detachment

Termination Phase

Termination is first discussed when contract is made (in orientation)

Goal is to achieve positive separation

Mental Status Interview (To Evaluate Psychological Functioning)

The usefulness of the mental status interview is universally recognized by mental health practitioners; it evaluates present level of psychological function in five basic assessment areas:

- Appearance, attitude, and behavior
- Affect (mood and emotional reactions)
- Thought processes and content
- Intellectual function
- Judgment and insight

See Table 17-1 for summary assessment.

Psychotropic Medications

Pharmacologic agents affect mood and behavior and are an important part of a total treatment plan. Dosage ranges vary widely and are adjusted according to control of target symptoms vs. appearance of primary side-effects, which include:

- Extrapyramidal symptoms (EPS)
- Anticholinergic effects
- Sedative effects

Nurses must be client advocates in order to combat noncompliance. Noncompliance with drug therapy is the primary reason for hospital readmission of psychiatric clients. Reasons for noncompliance include:

- Reliance on medication may be a blow to person's self-image (wants to see self as autonomous, capable individual)
- May be embarrassed to be judged "out of control"
- May view medication regimen as attempt by others to gain control
- May fear being poisoned
- May fear addiction
- May be unwilling to accept troublesome side-effects, such as decreased libido, impaired sexual function, weight gain

Table 17-1. Summary Mental Status Assessment of an Adult

A. Appearance, Attitude, and Behavior
   1. Attitude toward interview and interviewer
   2. Dress and physical appearance
   3. Posture, gait, motor activity, types of movement
   4. Facial expression
B. Affect (Mood and Emotional Reactions)
   1. Objective observations of interviewer and subjective report of client
   2. Predominant emotion/attitude
   3. Reaction of client (expressed by client or perceived by interviewer) to topics discussed
   4. Physiological indicators
C. Thought Processes and Content
   1. Both verbal and nonverbal expression is measured
   2. Form, sequence, quantity, choice of language
   3. Psychomotor activity accompanying speech
   4. Content (organized around one of four modes)
      a. Selective attention
      b. Overdetermined attitudes (includes prejudices and biases)
      c. Preoccupations or exaggerated concerns
      d. Distortion or denial of reality
D. Intellectual Function
   1. Sensorium
      a. Time, place, person, self
      b. Recent/remote memory
      c. Retention and recall
   2. Intellectual capacity
      a. General information
      b. Calculation
      c. Abstraction and comprehension of current events, proverbs
E. Judgment and Insight
   1. Past responsibilities and interpersonal relationships
   2. Changes that have occurred in present
   3. Plans for future
   4. Awareness of emotional nature of illness

- May be unwilling to give up secondary gains from sick role

Antipsychotic/Neuroleptic Agents

Action

Principal action is to counteract effects of psychosis (particularly of schizophrenia):

- Formal thought disorders
- Blunted affect
- Bizarre behavior
- Social withdrawal
- Hallucinations
- Belligerence
- Paranoid thinking
- Confusion

Antipsychotic/neuroleptic agents prevent the neurotransmitter dopamine from crossing the neuron membrane and inhibit the transmission of neural impulses.

Administration

Oral

- Absorbed rapidly within 30–60 min from gastrointestinal (GI) tract
- Absorption rate decreases with presence of food in stomach and with concurrent administration of anticholinergic agents, antiparkinson drugs, antacids

Intramuscular (IM)

- Produces calming effects within 10 minutes
- Use Z-tract to avoid subcutaneous tissue irritation
- Do not mix with other injectables
- Short-acting injectables used mainly to help client gain control and to avoid potential violent behavior
- Long-acting injectables use an oil base for 2–4 week absorption (use combats problem of noncompliance): category includes haloperidol (Haldol), fluphenazine decanoate (Prolixin Decanoate)

Metabolism
- Metabolites accumulate in fatty tissue and may remain in body for weeks or months
- Dosage is carefully monitored to decrease cumulative effect
- Drugs may cross placental barrier, but do not cause congenital malformations
- Watch for jaundice, EPS, and anticholinergic side-effects in infant if taken in third trimester or at birth
- Unclear which drugs may be excreted in breast milk (Haldol has been found); consider risks and benefits for lactating woman

Drug Classes, Generic and Trade Names, and Dosage Ranges
- See Table 17-2

Side-effects and Nursing Implications
- See Table 17-3

Antidepressant Agents

Action
- Work specifically to correct abnormal state of depression (do not influence or improve the mood of an emotionally stable individual)
- Principal action of tricyclics and tetracyclics is to block reuptake of norepinephrine, serotonin, or both
- Increase neurotransmitters within synapses, and delay metabolism

Table 17-2. Examples of Antipsychotic/Neuroleptic Drugs

Class	Generic Name	Trade Name	Dosage (mg/day)
Phenothiazine	Chlorpromazine	Thorazine	L: 400–1500 M: 200–1000
	Triflupromazine	Vesprin	L: 60–400 M: 20–200
	Thioridazine	Mellaril	L: 400–800 M: 25–800
	Mesoridazine	Serentil	L: 20–600 M: 10–400
	Trifluoperazine	Stelazine	L: 20–100 M: 10–40
	Fluphenazine hydrochloride	Prolixin	L: 20–80 M: 5–40
	Fluphenazine decanoate	Prolixin Decanoate	L: 12.5–25 M: up to 100
Butyrophenones	Haloperidol	Haldol	L: 20–100 M: 5–40
Thioxanthenes	Thiothixene	Navane	L: 20–100 M: 5–40
	Chlorprothixene	Taractan	— M: 10–100
Dihydroindolones	Molindone	Moban	L: 50–400 M: 25–100
Dibenzoxazepines	Loxapine	Loxitane	L: 50–250 M: 25–100

L = loading dose   M = maintenance dose

Table 17-3. Side-effects and Nursing Implications for Antipsychotic/Neuroleptic Drugs

Side-effects	Nursing Implications*
Most Common *Extrapyramidal Reactions (reversible)* Parkinsonism Akathisia (continuous restless pacing beyond conscious control) Dyskinesia (defect in voluntary movement) Dystonias (impaired tonicity of muscle tissue): acute dystonic reaction occurs with initial dose and is characterized by severe muscle contractions of tongue, face, and extraocular muscles *Anticholingeric Symptoms* Blurred vision, dry mouth and lips, constipation, urinary retention, delayed micturition, diaphoresis Sedation Photosensitivity Postural hypotension Weight gain **Others** Agranulocytosis Dermatitis Decreased libido Inhibition of ejaculation Menstrual irregularities *Tardive Dyskinesia (generally irreversible)* May occur after 2 years of high doses; some physicians order drug holidays to avoid; prime symptoms are excessive blinking and fine vermiform movements of tongue	Review concurrent medications for CNS depressants, narcotic analgesics and anesthetics (neuroleptics potentiate their action) Caution client regarding sedative action Supervise ambulation and smoking in early drug therapy Monitor BP q 4 hr until stable during 1st 48 hr of therapy Take BP lying and standing Offer fluids frequently, gum or sugarless mints for dry mouth Watch for and monitor bladder for distension especially in immobile and elderly clients Provide fluids and roughage for constipation Weigh clients regularly Carefully monitor client with history of seizures (seizure threshold is lowered) If indicated, rule out pregnancy before therapy (may give false pregnancy results) Supervise client carefully to be certain medicine is taken Administer oral concentrates with 40 oz of orange or apple juice and follow with 8 oz of water Complete liver function tests, ophthalmoscopic exams, CBC, and ECG studies, and periodically review Instruct clients to protect themselves from ultraviolet rays Encourage client to take drugs regularly and as prescribed Instruct clients to report fever, sore throat, or general malaise (r/o agranulocytosis) Instruct clients to move slowly from sitting to standing and to avoid hot baths and showers to prevent effects of hypotension

* Applicable to all antipsychotic/neuroleptic drugs.

Administration and Metabolism

- Absorbed completely from GI tract
- Maximum therapeutic effects occur within 1–3 weeks
- Antidepressants are long-acting drugs with half-lives ranging from 8–80 hours or longer
- Metabolized in liver
- Excreted through urinary system

Dosage

- Begins at lower end of range
- Often administered in divided doses
- Increased as tolerance to side-effects develops
- Should be continued for several months and discontinued gradually
- Forms include tablets, capsules, solutions (doxepin) and IM injectables
- Combination products (perphenazine-amitriptyline hydrochloride [Triavil and Etrafon]) should not be initial choice to treat symptoms of depression

Drug Classes, Generic and Trade Names, and Dosage Ranges

- See Table 17-4

Side-effects and Nursing Implications

- See Table 17-5

Antimania Agent: Lithium Carbonate

Action

- Treatment of choice for clients with bipolar affective disorder
- Used prophylactically to prevent future episodes
- Used on an experimental basis to treat al-

Table 17-4. Examples of Antidepressant Drugs

Class	Generic Name	Trade Name	Dosage (mg/day)
Trycyclic	Amitriptyline hydrochloride	Elavil	U: 75–200 E: 50–300
	Desipramine hydrochloride	Norpramin Pertofrane	U: 100–200 E: 25–300
	Doxepin hydrochloride	Adapin Sinequan	U: 75–150 E: 25–300
	Imipramine hydrochloride	Tofranil	U: 100–200 E: 30–300
	Nortriptyline hydrochloride	Aventyl	U: 75–100 E: 20–150
	Amoxapine	Asendin	U: 150–300 E: 75–600
Tetracyclic	Maprotiline hydrochloride	Ludiomil	U: 75–150 E: 50–300
	Trazodone	Desyrel	U: 150–400 E: 50–600
Monoamine Oxidase Inhibitors	Isocarboxazid	Marplan	I: 30 M: 10–20
	Phenelzine sulfate	Nardil	I: 45–90 tid M: 15 qod

U = usual dose   E = extreme dose   I = initial dose   M = maintenance dose

coholism, personality disorders, mood disorders associated with premenstrual tension, and anorexia nervosa
- Exact mechanism of action is unknown, but it is known to travel across cell membranes in a manner similar to that of sodium

Administration and Metabolism

- Absorbed completely through GI tract when given orally
- Peak plasma levels are reached 1–2 hours
- Excreted by kidneys (half of single dose is excreted within 24 hours)
- Competes with sodium for absorption
- Elderly persons and persons with sodium imbalances risk toxic reaction at lower doses than other persons
- Drug is contraindicated for clients with heart failure, kidney disorders, or hypertension

Table 17-5. Side-effects and Nursing Implications for Antidepressant Drugs

Side-effects	Nursing Implications
Tricyclics and Tetracyclics	**Tricyclics and Tetracyclics**
Most Common	Assess for suicidal potential routinely
Orthostatic hypotension	Measure BP lying and standing
Tachycardia	Teach precautions for orthostatic hypotension
Blurred vision	Caution against driving or use of heavy machinery
Constipation	Give with food
Mydrioses	Caution to avoid over-the-counter medicines without checking with physician
MI, CHF	Withhold if systolic pressure falls more than 20 mm Hg or if pulse rate rises suddenly
Disturbed concentration	Encourage oral hygiene to prevent dry mucous membranes
Insomnia, nightmares	May alter certain diagnostic tests
Dizziness, atoxia	
Nausea and vomiting	
Bone marrow depression	
Diaphoresis	**MAO Inhibitors**
Other	Assess for suicidal potential routinely
Agranulocytosis	Do not give at HS (causes insomnia)
Cholestatic jaundice	Caution not to take *any* other drug without consulting physician
Leukocytosis, leukopenia	Must be on low-tyramine diet
MAO Inhibitors	Be alert to cues for both hypotension and hypertension
Most Common	
Orthostatic hypotension	
Dizziness	
Edema	
Urinary retention	
Delayed ejaculation	
Constipation, dry mouth	
Hypertensive crisis	
Other	
Confusion, transition from retarded to agitated depression	

Dosage

- Based on achieving and maintaining therapeutic serum level
- Range is 0.6 to 1.2 mEq/L (in acute stage, may be 0.8 to 1.5 mEq/L)
- Level of drug in blood measured 8–12 hours after last dose (typically in morning before first daily dose would normally be given)
- During acute stage, level of drug in blood measured every 2 to 3 days
- During maintenance stage, level of drug in blood measured weekly until stable, and then measured monthly
- Dosage in acute phase is 600 mg tid to load; 300 mg tid or bid to maintain
- Laboratory tests to establish baseline data before starting lithium treatment include T_3, T_4, blood urea nitrogen (BUN) level, creatinine clearance level, and ECG

Side-effects and Nursing Implications

- See Table 17-6

Antianxiety Agents (Sedatives and Hypnotics)

Action

- Principal action is to produce state of calmness or relaxation (sedatives) or to induce sleep (hypnotics)
- Alleviate specific anxiety or sleep problems but do *not* alter factors creating problems
- Use is symptom-specific, noncurative; helps decrease distress so that client may cope with underlying causes of problems
- Almost all produce psychologic and physiologic dependency
- Classified as barbiturates or nonbarbiturates
- Have no antipsychotic potential but are extremely effective in combatting neurotic reactions
- Major action is depression of central nervous system (CNS)
- Interfere with rapid eye movement (REM) sleep, so client awakens feeling unrested despite extended sleep

Administration and Metabolism

Nonbarbiturate Benzodiazepines

- Absorption rate varies
- Diazepam (Valium) is absorbed rapidly, is fat soluble and is widely distributed throughout body fat
- Chlorazepate dipotassium (Tranxene), prazepam (Verstran), and oxazepam (Serax) form active metabolites
- Temazepam (Restoril), triazolam (Halcion), and lorazepam (Ativan) have shortest (3–20 hour) half-life and do not produce active metabolites
- Chlordiazepoxide (Librium) is absorbed more slowly (1–2 days), and its metabolites have cumulative effect

Barbiturates

- With oral administration, absorbed rapidly
- Rate of absorption increases when food is in stomach
- Absorbed through colon (may be administered rectally)
- Rapidly cross placental barrier; contraindicated for pregnant clients
- Tolerance develops within 7–14 days and dependency within 1 month
- Cumulative effect creates morning "hangover"

Barbiturates vs. Nonbarbiturates (Benzodiazepines)

- Use of barbiturates as sedatives not recommended due to advantages of benzodiazepine; used only when nonbarbiturates are ineffective in lowering anxiety
- Benzodiazepines cause less drowsiness and less dermatitis, have fewer disinhibiting effects, and are less addictive
- Barbiturates appear helpful for depression

Table 17-6. Side-effects and Nursing Implications for Lithium

Side-effects	Nursing Implications
Cardiovascular Arrhythmias, hypotension, peripheral circulatory collapse, and reversible changes of T waves on ECG readings	Teach client to expect minor side-effects* Encourage staying on routine schedule Encourage drinking 2–3 qt of water Monitor baseline laboratory values Monitor serum lithium levels closely
CNS Seizures, blackouts, slurred speech, dizziness, vertigo, urinary and fecal incontinence, restlessness, confusion, stupor, and coma	Be alert for toxicity if sodium or water depletion occurs Encourage exercise and diet to prevent weight gain
Dermatologic Drying and thinning of hair, alopecia, chronic folliculitis, psoriasis, pruritus	Give medicine with meals Recommend ID medicine card to be carried at all times Encourage client to avoid food and drinks containing high levels of caffeine
Endocrine Goiter, hypothyroidism	
GI Anorexia, nausea, vomiting, diarrhea*	
GU Albinuria, oliguria, polyuria,* glycosuria	
Neurologic Fine resting tremor of hands,* ataxia, hyperactive deep tendon reflexes	
Other Anticholingeric symptoms, increased thirst, fatigue, lethargy	

* Initial side effects usually subside after 2–3 weeks when maintenance dose is established

occurring with early morning awakening and as anesthetics (alone or in combination with other drugs)

Drug Classes, Generic and Trade Names, and Dosage Ranges

- See Table 17-7

Side-effects and Nursing Implications

- See Table 17-8

Antiparkinsonian and Antihistamine Agents

- Used to control EPS associated with antipsychotic drugs
- Should always be kept (in injectable form) as emergency antidote on units where antipsychotic medicines are given
- Antiparkinsonian agents include trihexyphenidyl hydrochloride (Artane), benz-

Table 17-7. Examples of Antianxiety Drugs (Sedatives and Hypnotics)

Class	Generic Name	Trade Name	Dosage (mg/day)
Benzodiazepines	Chlordiazepoxide hydrochloride	Librium	I: 10–100 (tid) M: reduced to most effective dose
	Clorazepate dipotasium	Tranxene	I: 15 M: 15–30
	Diazepam	Valium	I: 2–10 bid or qid
	Temazepam	Restoril	I: 15–30 M: 15–30
	Lorazepam	Ativan	I: 2–10 M: 2–10
	Flurazepam	Dalmane	I: 15–30 M: 15–30 Elderly 15
	Alprazolam	Xanax	I: 0.75–4 M: 0.75–4
Propanediol Carbamates	Meprobamate	Miltown Equanil	I: 200–1200 M: 200–1200
Other nonbarbiturates	Chloral hydrate	Noctec Somnos	I, M (hypnotic) 500–1000 I, M (sedative) 250 tid
	Ethchlorvynol	Placidyl	I, M 500–1000
	Methyprylon	Noludar	I, M (hypnotic) 200–400 I, M (sedative) 50–100
Barbiturates	Secobarbital	Seconal	I, M 100–200
	Pentobarbital	Nembutal	I, M 100–200
	Butabarbital	Butisol	I, M (hypnotic) 45–100 I, M (sedative) 15–60
	Amobarbital	Amytal	I, M (hypnotic) 65–200 I, M (sedative) 50–300 Anticonvulsant 65–500
	Phenobarbital	Luminal	I, M 15–100

I = initial dose   M = maintenance dose

Table 17-8. Side-effects and Nursing Implications for Antianxiety Drugs

Side-effects	Nursing Implications
Benzodiazepines	*Benzodiazepines*
Most Common	Give orally when possible
Drowsiness, headache, vertigo, dizziness, mental confusion, slurred speech, lethargy	Evaluate for tolerance, dependency
	Withdrawal may not develop until 7–10 days because of long half-life
Other	Caution client that drowsiness, lightheadedness, and dizziness may occur
Mild hypotension	
Anticholinergic symptoms	*Propanediol*
Hematologic problems	Assess for tolerance, dependence, and withdrawal
Weight gain	Assess suicide potential
Propanediol	*Other Nonbarbiturates*
Most Common	Watch for dependency
Hangover effect	Noctec has very unpleasant taste—don't break capsule
Dermatologic reactions	
Other Nonbarbiturates	*Barbiturates*
Most Common	Tolerance develops within 7–14 days
GI irritation	Assess suicide potential
Nausea and vomiting	Check for cues of dependency
Flatulence	
Barbiturates	
Most Common	
Hangover effect	
Slurred speech	
Drowsiness	

tropine mesylate (Cogentin), biperiden hydrochloride (Akineton), carbidopa (Sinemet)
- Antihistamines include diphenhydramine hydrochloride (Benadryl), Phenoxene

Electroconvulsive Therapy

Electroconvulsive therapy (ECT) is indicated primarily in treatment of major depression with melancholia, when accompanied by:

- Unresponsiveness to chemotherapy
- Severe suicidal risk
- Acute psychomotor retardation
- Anorexia

ECT has evolved into a routine, benign treatment since its introduction in 1938; improvements include:

- Short-acting IV barbiturate e.g., methohexital sodium (Brevital) is used as anesthetic before treatment
- IV succinylcholine is used to provide muscle relaxation and to reduce effects of convulsion
- Client feels no sensation and has only barely perceptible convulsion

- During paralysis and following treatment respiration is supported artificially
- Consciousness returns in a few minutes

Nursing Measures
- Similar to those for surgical procedure
- Enforce npo order after midnight the night before treatment
- Have client void in morning before treatment
- Check for dentures and hairpins and provide pajamas or loose-fitting clothes
- Record vital signs (VS)
- Following treatment, observe for respiratory distress until client fully oriented, alert, and able to get out of bed
- Observe and assist client in case of confusion for 1–2 hours following treatment
- Provide accurate and reassuring information about procedure to client

Psychosocial Therapies

Milieu Therapy

- Implies using total environment as therapeutic agent
- Provides safe, protective setting for client
- Provides relationships that help client learn more effective and socially acceptable means of coping
- Activities, rules, regulations are structured and explained to client
- Clients should not have to cope with staff tensions or staff needs for approval
- Clients are treated with respect
- Right to privacy is ensured

Group Therapy

- Provides for multiple situations within group for client to develop greater insight into own and others' behavior
- Allows staff to utilize time economically
- Provides climate for client to try out new patterns of behavior
- Can be used as setting to teach about medications, developmental tasks, activities of daily living (ADL)

Family Therapy

- Primary goal is to clarify and improve family communication and relationship patterns
- Family as a whole becomes client or system
- Successful therapy implies that every member's behavior is changed
- Identifies and protects potential scapegoats in family

Activity Therapy

- Task-oriented recreational and occupational activities are used to assess and develop social skills
- Well suited to clients who "act out"
- Provides nonthreatening environment with few formal demands; allows client to vent feelings on inanimate objects rather than to people

Behavior Therapy

- Based on learning or cognitive theory
- Focuses on overt maladaptive behaviors or symptoms rather than on underlying dynamics
- Desensitization effective for phobias
- Reciprocal inhibition therapy reduces anxiety by pairing anxiety-provoking stimulus with another stimulus associated with an opposite feeling strong enough to suppress the anxiety (meditation, yoga, biofeedback)

Crisis Intervention

- Short-term therapy with limited goal of assisting client to cope with stressful situation
- Client must define problem in initial stages
- Main function is to return client to precrisis level of coping
- Used for developmental crises, including independence from parents, new parenthood, divorce, retirement

- Used for situational crises, including natural disasters, rape, trauma, sudden unexpected loss

Suicide Intervention

- Suicide is culmination of self-destructive tendencies resulting from anger turned inward
- *Suicidal ideation* is thoughts about committing suicide or about how to commit suicide
- *Suicidal gesture* is action that is physically self-destructive like a suicide attempt, but is not lethal (may or may not be manipulative behavior)
- *Suicide attempt* is self-destructive behavior that is potentially lethal
- *Suicide precautions* are specific actions taken by nursing staff to protect a client and to ensure close observation

Assessment: Clients at Risk

Risk factors and warning signs include:

- Male sex over age 65 (highest rate in U.S.); men commit suicide more often than women
- Client has made a specific plan
- History of suicide attempts that have become increasingly painful, violent, or lethal
- Adolescence (high-risk group)
- Client is divorced, widowed, separated, or living alone without family
- Client gives away personal possessions, settles accounts, makes will, ties up "loose ends" in personal affairs
- Early stages of treatment with antidepressant medications when mood and activity level elevate
- Sudden mood or activity level change

Nursing Plans and Interventions

Goals

Client will:

- Be free of self-inflicted harm
- Express feelings verbally and nonverbally
- Direct anger and hostility outward in a safe manner
- Increase feelings of self-worth
- Communicate with others and participate in activities
- Maintain adequate nutrition, hydration, and elimination
- Maintain adequate rest, sleep, and activity patterns

Nursing Measures

- Provide safe environment by determining necessary level of precautions (assess daily)
- Provide one-to-one supervision at all times (including toileting and sleeping) if necessary
- Restrict client at risk to locked unit
- Permit client to use nothing that may cause harm
- Explain precautions to client
- Locate client's room near nursing station (avoid rooms at ends of hallways, near elevators, etc.)
- Lock windows of client's room
- Be aware of relationships client forms with other clients, family, or visitors
- Be alert for manipulative behavior
- Search visitors if necessary
- Monitor rumination or excessive talk about suicide
- Help relieve feelings of depression
- Convey that you believe client is a worthwhile human being
- Encourage ventilation of feelings
- Do not joke about death or belittle client's wishes or feelings
- Provide opportunities for success and give positive feedback even for small accomplishments
- Help client increase communication with others
- Help client develop insight and increase ability to express feelings
- Encourage and support expressions of anger (role playing may help)
- Provide opportunity to contact chaplain or other clergy if appropriate

18

Nursing Care of the Client with an Organic Mental Disorder

Delirium

Delirium is characterized by the reduced ability to maintain attention to external stimuli and to shift attention to new external stimuli. Delirium is disorganized thinking. Its causes vary widely:

- Infectious disease associated with elevated temperature: Streptococcal septicemia
- Metabolic disease: uremia, porphyria, hypoglycemia
- Medical/surgical conditions: Congestive heart failure (CHF), thyrotoxicosis, cardiac surgery
- Neurologic conditions: cerebral trauma, subdural hematoma
- Drug intoxication/withdrawal
- Environmental disruptions: elderly persons may become confused when hospitalized or relocated, or experience "sundowning" in evening from sensory deprivation

Assessment

Health Status

- Rambling, irrelevant, or incoherent speech
- Lowered level of consciousness
- Disorientation to time, place, person
- Perceptual disturbances causing misinterpretations of environment: illusions, hallucinations
- Disturbed sleep–wake cycle (dreams and nightmares common)
- Abrupt shift in psychomotor activity (behavior may range from restlessness and hyperactivity to sluggishness and stupor)

Developmental Assessment

Especially common in children and persons over age 60

Diagnostic Factors

Differentiated from other organic mental syndromes by rapid onset, short duration, and fluctuation in symptoms

Begins abruptly

Lasts 1 week to 1 month

Symptoms worsen during night or in dark

Lucid periods generally occur in morning

Psychosocial/Cultural Assessment

Client is easily distracted and has difficulty focusing attention

Goal-directed behavior is reduced

Emotional disturbances are common and result in rapid and unpredictable behavior

Disturbances include:

- Anxiety
- Fear
- Depression
- Irritability
- Anger
- Euphoria
- Apathy

Nursing Plans and Interventions

Goals

- Safety: client will be free from harm
- Orientation: client will be aware of environment and in touch with reality
- Functioning: client will be able to function at appropriate level of independence

Nursing Measures

- Protect severely agitated clients by providing constant staff presence
- Do not respond to delusional material without reinforcing reality
- Maintain tolerant, calm, unflustered manner
- Focus on areas of competent functioning and do only what client cannot do for self
- Use appropriate restraints (physical and chemical) if necessary
- Ensure adequate sensory perception day and night
- Maintain familiar surroundings and provide personal contact if needed
- Communicate face to face with simple, direct, descriptive statements
- Explain what you are doing
- Provide new information slowly and in small doses

Drug Therapy

Should be used cautiously: side-effects of sedatives/hypnotics often are contributing factor in delirium in persons over age 60

Carefully evaluate medicine client currently taking

Avoid barbiturates

Nonbarbiturate, antianxiety medication may help with emotional disturbances

Haloperidol (Haldol) 1–2 mg IM most often used for severe agitation and hallucinations

Evaluation

Treatment is successful if:

- Client returns to premorbid personality
- No residual organic brain symptoms are present
- Underlying cause of delirium (infections, postoperative factors, neurological factors, intoxicants, metabolic disorders) is under control
- Client's mental and physical energy is restored
- Client resumes preillness activities and responsibilities
- Client is oriented with adaptive reality testing (aware of environment, positive sensorium)

Dementias Arising in the Senium and Presenium

Primary degenerative dementia of the Alzheimer type is characterized by an insidious onset and a progressive and deteriorating course. Senile onset or senium refers to onset after age 65; presenile onset or presenium occurs at age 65 and before. Intellectual abilities (memory, judgement, and abstract thinking) are lost.

Assessment

Health Status

- Memory impairment is predominant early symptom
- Mild impairment: forgetfulness in daily life (need to have statements repeated)
- Severe impairment: forgets names of close relatives, own occupation, schooling, birthday, or even own name
- Short-term memory deficit is common

- Long-term memory may be intact
- Impaired judgement and impaired impulse control common (result in coarse language, inappropriate jokes, neglect of appearance and hygiene, general disregard for conventional social conduct)
- Thinking becomes very concrete
- Client cannot cope with novel situations, especially if pressed for time
- Client avoids situations and tasks that require complex processing
- Client has difficulty finding similarities and differences in situations

Developmental Assessment

Found predominately in elderly, however diagnosis may be made at any time after IQ is fairly stable (age 3 or 4)

Psychosocial/Cultural Assessment
- Personality change almost always present
- Alterations or accentuations of premorbid traits common *e.g.,* active person becomes apathetic and withdrawn, neat and meticulous person becomes unconcerned about personal behavior; or compulsive, impulsive, or paranoid person's traits are accentuated
- Client's range of social involvement narrows
- Client is especially vulnerable to psychosocial stresses (bereavement, retirement, change in residence)
- Diagnosis is confirmed when social or occupational functioning is compromised
- In severe cases client becomes oblivious to surroundings and requires constant care

Goals for Institutionalized Clients
- Client will avoid injury
- Client will not injure others or destroy property
- Client will establish or maintain adequate nutrition, hydration, elimination
- Client will establish or maintain balance of rest, sleep, and activity
- Client will increase or maximize contact with reality
- Client will demonstrate decreased agitation and restlessness (Schultz and Dark, 1986)

Nursing Measures
- Assess own response to regressive behavior of client
- Keep client mentally active within parameters of his or her limitations
- Promote independent functioning, responsibility for self, and self-determination
- Frequently orient client to time, place, person, using clocks, calendars, and visual aids
- Establish well-known, set routine for client to follow
- Reinforce client's sense of identity by frequently addressing him or her by name; avoid belittling and cute nicknames
- Give all directions in clear, distinct, step-by-step fashion
- Avoid confrontation of inappropriate behavior and probing for feelings
- Do not make false promises
- Encourage maintaining activities of daily living (ADL)
- Reassure client that he or she is safe
- Monitor environment for excess stimulation and decrease if necessary (may mean restricting visitors)
- Convey warmth and concern; touch client if appropriate
- Involve and support family in treatment plan

Evaluation

Evaluation of the care of a client with an organic mental disorder is highly individual, depending on the organic impairment and specific symptoms. Treatment is successful if

- Client's maximal level of functioning and independence is preserved
- Client's basic physical, emotional, intellectual, social, and spiritual needs are met
- Family is sustained and supported in interactions with client
- Secondary complications are prevented

- Interactions with client and caregivers are positive experiences that enhance the personal and professional growth of caregivers

Alcohol-induced Organic Mental Disorders

Alcohol intoxication is maladaptive behavioral change due to recent ingestion of alcohol.

Alcohol idiosyncratic intoxication is sometimes called *pathological intoxication* and is distinguished by a marked behavioral change, usually aggressiveness, after ingesting a quantity of alcohol insufficient to cause intoxication in most people. Amnesia usually follows the period of intoxication, which is brief, lasting only a few hours. The person's behavior is unlike his or her usual behavior when not drinking (for instance, a shy, well-mannered person becomes belligerent and assaultive after one weak drink).

Uncomplicated alcohol withdrawal is characterized by physiological and psychological symptoms that follow within several hours of cessation or reduction in alcohol intake by a person who has been drinking for several days or longer.

Alcohol withdrawal delirium has also been called *delirium tremens*.

Alcohol hallucinosis is an organic hallucinosis involving the development of vivid and persistent hallucinations by a person who has alcohol dependence.

Alcohol amnestic disorder due to thiamine deficiency is also called *Korsakoff's Syndrome*.

Dementia may be associated with alcohol when all other causes of dementia have been ruled out (the etiologic role of alcohol in dementia associated with prolonged heavy drinking is controversial).

Assessment

Health Status

Intoxication
- Slurred speech, incoordination, unsteady gait, nystagmus, flushed face
- Aggressiveness, impaired judgment, impaired attention, irritability, euphoria, emotional lability

Withdrawal
- Coarse tremors of hands, tongue, eyelids
- Nausea and vomiting
- Malaise or weakness
- Dry mouth, puffy, blotched complexion, mild peripheral edema
- Gastritis
- Headache, insomnia
- Tachycardia, sweating, elevated blood pressure
- Depressed mood, irritability, anxiety, transient hallucinations

Delirium Tremens (Most Severe Form of Withdrawal)
- Increased autonomic nervous system activity
- Insomnia or daytime drowsiness
- Increased or decreased psychomotor activity
- Vivid visual hallucinations, illusions, misinterpretations
- Clouding of consciousness
- Inability to shift, focus, and sustain attention to environmental stimuli
- Frequent agitation
- Major complication is motor seizures (rum fits)

Alcoholic Hallucinosis
- Occurs 48 hours after drinking has stopped
- Vivid, often threatening auditory hallucinations occur but consciousness remains clear
- Auditory hallucinations are usually voices but may be hissing or buzzing sounds
- Behavioral responses are fear and anxiety

Alcoholic Amnestic Disorder
- Heavy prolonged drinking accompanied by poor nutritional intake
- Short and long-term memory deficit
- Neuropathy, unsteady gait, myopathy may be present

Alcoholic Dementia

- Associated with prolonged, chronic alcoholic dependence
- Loss of intellectual ability severe enough to interfere with social or occupational functioning
- Memory impaired, abstract thinking and judgement compromised
- May lead to permanent brain damage

Developmental Assessment

Drinking patterns vary by age and sex for both males and females

Prevalence is highest and abstention lowest in 21–34 year age range

At all ages, 2 to 5 times more males than females are heavy drinkers

Abstainers outnumber drinkers among persons over age 65 of both sexes

Most alcohol consumed by a small percent of people: 10% of drinkers consume 50% of the total amount of alcohol consumed

Diagnostic Factors

Ethyl alcohol or ethanol (ETOH) is a CNS depressant; effects of ETOH are related to blood levels and concentration of alcohol in brain

Blood alcohol levels (BAL) are reported in mg of alcohol per mL of blood (mg%); most people become intoxicated when BAL = 0.10% to 0.20%

Degree of intoxication can also be measured by breathalyzers

Recent research in Canada is concentrating on measuring alcohol levels in urine and saliva by using litmus paper dipsticks

Alcohol concentration in blood depends on:

Rate of absorption (in stomach, mouth, small intestine)

Rate of transportation to CNS

Rate of redistribution to parts of body

Metabolism (liver metabolizes 1 ounce per hour)

Whether any alcohol has been eliminated

Presence of fatty foods in stomach (slow absorption)

Body size (light weight people reach greater blood alcohol concentrations more easily than heavy people)

Psychosocial/Cultural Assessment

- 35% to 64% of drivers in fatal accidents in U.S. have been drinking
- Between 45% to 60% of all fatal crashes involving teenage drivers are alcohol related
- Alcoholics are 10 times more likely to die in fires than nonalcoholics
- Half of all fire deaths are alcohol related
- Alcoholics' risk of suicide is 30 times greater than that of nonalcoholics
- 15% to 65% of persons who attempt suicide are alcoholics
- 80% of those who succeed are alcoholics
- Health professionals live and work in an environment conducive to developing substance abuse problems (15%–20% of all health professionals succumb to substance abuse)

Nursing Plans and Interventions

Goals

- Short-term goals include assuring client's physical safety, reality orientation, maintenance of homeostasis
- Intermediate goals address nutrition, defusing hostile or aggressive behavior, and achieving balance of rest, sleep, and activity
- Long-term goals include abstinence, optimal physical health, and agreement to participate in substance abuse program

Nursing Measures

Short-term Measures

- Intoxication requires no specific nursing intervention because no proven methods to speed up metabolism exist

- Restrain client experiencing pathologic intoxication, if necessary
- Assess client in alcohol coma for other injuries and complications: subdural hematoma, pneumonia, meningitis, hepatic failure, GI bleeding (gastric lavage unnecessary due to rapid absorption of alcohol in stomach)
- Monitor vital signs every 2 hours for client in alcohol withdrawal (vital signs increase prior to hallucinations and convulsions)
- Give liquid or foods high in glucose if vital signs remain elevated (8 ounces Kool-Aid with 1 or 2 tablespoons Karo Syrup)
- Encourage client in withdrawal to tolerate tremors and feelings of inner shakiness
- Reduce environmental stimuli and stay with client experiencing hallucinations
- Acknowledge that hallucinations are real to client but that nurse does not have same experience
- Let client know that experiences are the result of alcohol withdrawal and that they will abate

Intermediate Measures
- Be nonjudgmental and objective
- Be aware of wanting to rescue client
- Avoid using offensive terminology such as "drunk" or "boozer" when discussing condition
- Maintain hope but be aware that relapses and failures are common
- Structure interview questions to elicit specific, factual information about problem (client may be vague, defensive, and unreliable in providing information)
- Interview significant other for more reliable history
- Recognize and understand client's defensive maneuvers (*e.g.*, projection, rationalization, intellectualization, minimization, diversion, anger)

Long-term Measures
- Disulfiram (Antabuse) treatment
- Placement in drug-free community
- Aversion conditioning
- Referral to self-help groups, *e.g.*, Alcoholics Anonymous

Medical Treatment

Heavy consumption of alcohol adversely affects most body systems. Medical conditions that may need treatment include:

Gastrointestinal problems (*e.g.*, gastritis, ulcers)

Acute or chronic pancreatitis

Esophagitis

Alcohol cardiomyopathy

Alcoholic liver disease (reversible)

Alcoholic hepatitis (more serious but reversible)

Cirrhosis (irreversible; 90% of deaths from cirrhosis associated with chronic alcoholism)

Mouth, pharynx, larynx, and esophageal cancer

Drug Therapy

Short-term

Sodium luminal 100 mg subcutaneous (SQ) or amobarbital sodium (Amytal) 500 mg IM repeated $\times$ 1 in 30 to 40 minutes for agitation and combativeness associated with pathological intoxication

5% glucose IV to reduce hypoglycemia with alcoholic coma

Diazepam or chlordiazepoxide to promote relaxation and increase seizure threshold during withdrawal

Diazepam and chlordiazepoxide may be given during detoxification period in step-down dosage: 300 mg of diazepam/12 ounce of alcohol for day 1; dose decreased by half for 5 days (never by more than half in any 24-hour period)

Thiamin 100 mg IM stat and then followed by po doses of 50 mg tid for 4 days to prevent cardiovascular and nervous system complications caused by extreme vitamin deficiency

Long-term

Disulfiram (Antabuse) 250 mg/day as deterrent to drinking

Disulfiram-induced reactions to alcohol occur within 2 weeks after last dose

Reactions include nausea, vomiting, flushing, dizziness, tachycardia, and potential for cardiovascular collapse and death

Contraindicated for clients with myocardial disease and clients receiving metronidazole (Flagyl)

Clients must be instructed verbally and in writing against using alcoholic beverages, paraldehyde, or commercial medicines or preparations that contain alcohol

Nutrition Therapy

- Well-balanced meals including daily servings of four food groups
- Foods high in thiamin such as lean pork, beef, liver, whole grains, and legumes

Client/Family Teaching

Help alcohol-dependent client to:

Attain intellectual comprehension of the disorder

Accept dependency as an illness and not as a moral problem

Accept that disorder is chronic and is not cured

Accept disorder on an emotional level

View recovery as long term, but occurring on day-by-day basis

Evaluation

Treatment for withdrawal is successful if:

- Vital signs are stable
- Client is oriented to here and now
- Appetite improves

Long-term evaluation of abstinence is difficult; treatment is evaluated one day at a time.

Barbiturate and Similar Sedative/Hypnotic Organic Mental Disorders

Abuse of barbiturates or similar acting sedatives and hypnotics is characterized by a pathological use that causes impairment in social or occupational functioning and lasts at least 1 month.

Dependence is recognized by tolerance or withdrawal.

Assessment

Health Status

- Signs and symptoms of intoxication are similar to those of alcoholic intoxication
- Disinhibition of behavior is one of the first symptoms
- Withdrawal can occur with decrease or cessation of use for prolonged heavy users
- Abrupt withdrawal can be fatal (requires medical supervision)
- Signs and symptoms of withdrawal delirium are the same as those of alcohol delirium
- Withdrawal delirium usually occurs within 1 week of cessation of drug use
- Some clients experience delirium without seizures, some have seizures only and some have both
- Withdrawal delirium is medical emergency (client requires hospitalization)

Diagnostic Factors

Toxicologic screen of 100 mL of urine and 20 mL of blood may indicate presence of a variety of drugs of abuse

Tolerance can be evaluated with test dose of pentobarbital (Nembutal) 200 mg orally for the drug-free, fasting client, followed by exam in 1 hour

No tolerance produces sound sleep with response to arousal

Client tolerant to less than 500 mg will show course nystagmus, Romberg's sign, gross ataxia, and somnolence

If there is no effect with 200 mg, test is repeated with larger dose until tolerance has been established; that dose is then given qid. and decreased at rate of 10% per day

Psychosocial/Cultural Assessment

- Frequently used to commit suicide
- Have synergistic action with other drugs,

narrowing margin between maximum and lethal dose
- Death is frequently caused by accidental overdose or drug interaction
- Individuals usually use a variety of these drugs plus alcohol
- Often used to counteract effects of other drugs, *e.g.*, symptoms of heroin withdrawal, flashbacks from LSD

Two types of abusers are:

- Persons who obtain drugs legally (prescription) for medical problems and increase dosage and frequency of use (typically middle-class woman between ages of 30 and 60)
- Persons who obtain drugs illegally to get high or to relieve stimulant effect of amphetamines (usually persons in late teens or early twenties)

Nursing Plans and Interventions

Goals

Client undergoing withdrawal under medical supervision will:

- Not die or experience serious complications related to withdrawal
- Keep use of other chemical agents to a minimum
- Understand withdrawal experience as the result of substance abuse

Nursing Measures

- Find out what drugs are being used, in what quantity per day
- Determine frequency and duration of use and establish whether alcohol is also used
- Ask family and friends and check blood and urine tests for accuracy of client's report
- Attend to accompanying physical problems
- Give verbal reassurance and orient client to reality

Medical Aspects

Serious complications resulting from IV barbiturate use include:

- Cellulitis when drug infiltrates to subcutaneous tissue
- Vascular complications if drug is inadvertently injected into artery
- Serum hepatitis, endocarditis, pneumonia, tetanus

Client/Family Teaching

Like all substance abusers, client must attain intellectual comprehension of the disorder

Evaluation

- Withdrawal and detoxification take 2 to 3 weeks
- Gradual withdrawal is essential for abusers of barbiturates and similar sedatives and hypnotics

Opioid Organic Mental Disorders

Opioid abuse implies a pattern of pathological use of the substance for a duration of at least 1 month. Dependence is recognized by tolerance or withdrawal. Opioids include opium, morphine, codeine, and the synthetics heroin, meperidine, and methadone.

Assessment

Health Status

- Intoxication is marked by pupillary constriction, drowsiness, slurred speech, impairment in attention or memory, euphoria, dysphoria, apathy, and psychomotor retardation
- Physical symptoms of withdrawal include tearing, runny nose, dilated pupils, "gooseflesh" sweating, diarrhea, yawning, mild hypertension, tachycardia, fever, and insomnia
- Physical symptoms of withdrawal resemble flu symptoms: weakness, nausea, vomiting, muscle and joint pains
- Behavioral symptoms include irritability, depression, restlessness

Diagnostic Factors

Withdrawal begins 8 to 12 hours after last dose

Symptoms most intense for 36 to 48 hours

Acute phase lasts 10 to 14 days

Opioids cross placental barrier and result in physically dependent infants (signs of heroin withdrawal in infants appear within 24 hours of birth)

Withdrawal is usually not life threatening

Psychosocial/Cultural Assessment

- Prolonged use results in decreased motivation
- Quality of life is diminished
- Social and personal deterioration that usually involves problems with police and law enforcement agencies are common
- Family and interpersonal problems develop
- All narcotics create psychological and physical dependence
- Dependence occurs in persons who take drugs as a way of life rather than in those who use drugs during a specific traumatic time or for short-term medical reasons
- Health professionals live and work in an environment conducive to developing substance abuse problems
- Heroin is abused by persons from all socioeconomic and ethnic segments of the population

Medical Aspects

Heroin users are at high risk for hepatitis; abusers of opioids are at high risk for:

Acquired Immunodeficiency Syndrome (AIDS)

Poisoning or inflammation because drug often contains impurities

Chronic undernutrition

Death from overdose

Abscesses, tetanus, malaria, liver disease, gastric ulcers, endocarditis, heart arrhythmias, anemia, pneumonia, tuberculosis, lung abscesses, and kidney failure

Impaired sexual functioning due to low testosterone levels

Drug Therapy

Methadone (Dolophine) is most frequent treatment for heroin addiction in US

Evaluation

Treatment is successful if client shows:
- Stable vital signs
- Orientation to here and now
- Improved appetite
- Successful grieving over loss of use of drug
- Enhanced coping skills that allow for participation in work and play

Amphetamine and Similar Sympathomimetic Organic Mental Disorders

Abuse is defined by three criteria: a pattern of pathological use; impairment of social and occupational functioning; and duration of use of 1 month. Amphetamines are sympathomimetic amines that act on the cerebral cortex and reticular activating system to elevate mood and decrease fatigue and appetite. They do not create physical dependence, but produce a strong psychological dependence.

Assessment

Health Status

- *Intoxication:* elation, talkativeness, pacing, hypervigilance, pupil dilation, tachycardia, elevated blood pressure, GI symptoms, chills, perspiration, sometimes persistent delusions or hallucinations
- *Amphetamine delirium:* delirium, changing affect, frequent aggressive and violent behavior, panic states, hallucinations
- *Withdrawal:* depression, anxiety, prolonged fatigue, disorientation, irritability, muscle spasms, GI symptoms, headache

Psychosocial/Cultural Assessment

- Stimulants are most popular with student population (age 18 to 25)
- Used by many people to combat fatigue, elevate mood, increase alertness, and suppress appetite

Nursing Plans and Interventions

Goals

Immediate goal for client is to avoid harming self and others. During withdrawal, goals include:

- Minimize physical discomfort
- Decrease fear and anxiety
- Decrease hostile behavior
- Increase self-esteem
- Establish trusting relationships

Nursing Measures

- Seclude client experiencing amphetamine delirium (use physical restraints for safety if necessary)
- Follow seclusion guidelines of institution
- Stay with client if physical restraints are needed
- Remain aware of client's body space or territory; do not trap, crowd, or surprise client
- Talk in low, calm voice; reorient if needed
- Tell client what you are doing and what you are going to do
- Do not threaten, but state limits and expectations
- Administer medications safely
- Be sure of dosage and correct IM sites
- Monitor for effects of medicines, intervene as appropriate
- Position client on stomach or side, *not on back* if mechanical restraints are used
- Check extremities distal to restraints frequently for color, temperature, pulse
- Perform passive ROM exercises, reposition every 2 hours
- Remain aware of client's feelings of fear, need for dignity, and rights
- Assess nutrition, hygiene, and elimination needs

Evaluation

Reassess need for continued seclusion or restraints: release as soon as it is safe and therapeutic; base actions on client's needs, not staff's

Cocaine Organic Mental Disorders

Cocaine abuse may take up to 8 months to develop. Abuse is indicated by a pattern of pathological use that causes impairment in social or occupational functioning for at least 1 month.

Assessment

Health Status

Maladaptive Behavior

- Fighting
- Impaired judgment
- Problems functioning socially or occupationally

Psychological Symptoms

- Increased sense of wellbeing and confidence
- Increased awareness of sensory input
- Psychomotor agitation
- Elation
- Talkativeness
- Pressured speech

Physical Symptoms

- Increased heart rate, blood pressure
- Dilated pupils
- Sweating, chills, nausea, vomiting
- Client experiences characteristic "rush"
- "Crashing" is accompanied by anxiety, tremulousness, irritability, depression, and fatigue

Diagnostic Factors

Recovery from intoxication occurs in 24 hours

There is no apparent withdrawal syndrome

Severe skin ulcerations may result from client's attempting to dig out "insects" as result of tactile hallucinations

Tissue ulcerations in nasal septum are common in users who snort

Psychosocial/Cultural Assessment

- Cocaine is considered a "social drug" by its users, who believe that it facilitates social interaction

- Many users believe that cocaine is a safe drug, free from side-effects, because they see no evidence of physical dependence and experience intense psychological effects and a strong urge to continue use

Nursing Plans and Interventions*

- Provide for physical requirements
- Assist client to maintain emotional stability
- Reduce and eventually eliminate use of pathological defense mechanisms
- Help client understand and accept substance abuse/dependency disorder
- Help client identify with peers
- Help client develop hope for recovery
- Help client learn to socialize and develop interpersonal skills
- Help client develop increased self-worth and self-esteem
- Help client establish alternative coping skills
- Help client improve motivation to continue treatment and comply with therapy
- Involve family and significant others in treatment and recovery process

Mental Retardation

The American Association of Mental Deficiency defines mental retardation as subaverage general intellectual functioning that originates in the developmental period. Classifications include:

Custodial 0–25 IQ
Trainable 25–55 IQ
Educable 55–70 IQ
Borderline 70–85 IQ

Diagnosis is usually independent of the diagnosis of other medical problems. Causes include:

Inherited defects in metabolism
Chromosomal abnormalities (Down's Syndrome)
Developmental deficits
Prematurity

Assessment

Health Status

Mentally retarded children undergo the same developmental process as other children but at a slower rate. Deficits may be apparent in the child's ability to:

- Group new ideas
- Handle frustrations
- Deal with others socially
- Achieve educational goals

Nursing Plans and Interventions

Goals

- Child will achieve highest possible level of functioning (professionals and family must recognize limits and learn not to pressure child beyond his or her capabilities)

Nursing Measures

- Involve whole family in decisions
- Promote bonding
- Help parents with providing affection, security, and guidance to child

Client/Family Teaching

Educational programs are essential to provide a retarded adult with the basic skills for semi-independent or independent life. Types of programs include:

Sheltered workshops
Community programs
Group homes

Behavioral modification programs are helpful in training and improving coping skills.

---

* Johnson, 1986.

19

Nursing Care of the Client with a Mental Disorder from Psychological Causes

Schizophrenia

Schizophrenia is a cluster of symptoms characterized by disintegrative life patterns that cause disturbances in verbal and motor behavior, and in perception, thought, affect, and motivation. It can be defined personally, socially, legally, statistically, and medically.

Types as defined by a cross-sectional clinical picture include:

- Disorganized: essential features are incoherence, marked loosening of associations, grossly disorganized behavior
- Catatonic: psychomotor disturbance involving stupor, rigidity, posturing, waxy flexibility
- Paranoid: preoccupation with one or more systematized delusions
- Undifferentiated: prominent psychiatric symptoms that cannot be classified in any other category
- Residual: label used when there has been at least one previous episode of schizophrenia (DSM III-R)*

*DSM III-R (Diagnostic and Statistical Manual of Mental Disorders, 3rd ed, rev, Washington, DC, American Psychiatric Association, 1987) is a diagnostic publication developed and researched by members of the American Psychiatric Association. Its purpose is to provide standardized criteria for a comprehensive evaluation and understanding of mental disorders. It is widely accepted in the U.S. as the common language of mental health clinicians and researchers for communicating about the disorders for which they have professional responsibility. It has had considerable impact and influence internationally.

Assessment

Health Status

Auditory hallucinations are the most common perceptual disturbance.

Major disturbances in thought content disturbance are called *delusions*; types include:

- Persecutory: client believes others are spying or spreading false rumors about him or her
- Ideas of reference: client assigns particular and unusual significance to specific events, objects, people, for no apparent reason
- Somatic delusions, delusions of grandeur, religious or nihilistic delusions (less common types)
- Over-valued ideas: client is excessively or irrationally preoccupied with specific idea

Client's form of thought disintegrates, and is characterized by:

- Loosening of associations
- Poverty of thought (vagueness, abstractness, overly concrete thinking, repetitive thoughts, stereotyped thoughts)

Disturbances in affect include:

- Blunted or flat affect (monotone voice, immobile face)
- Affect inappropriate or incongruent with content of speech
- Sudden unexplainable changes, usually involving anger (especially associated with paranoia)

Motivation disintegrates; client experiences:

- Loss of sense of self or loss of ego boundaries
- Inability to perform self-initiated, goal-directed activity

Developmental Assessment

Onset usually during adolescence or early adulthood

Family history may reveal difficulties caused by a dominating caregiving parent

Course of disorder is long term

Active phase: symptoms very prominent

Residual phase: rarely involves complete return to premorbid functioning

Common pattern is acute exacerbations with increasing residual impairment between episodes

Psychosocial/Cultural Assessment

- Ambivalence interferes with decision making in school, work, social relations
- Regression to earlier developmental stage, even to infantile adaptive patterns, is common
- Withdrawal severely limits interaction with others
- Social history indicates the development of few or no friends, difficulty in school, and asocial behavior or clashes with legal authorities
- Social skills are severely limited

Nursing Plans and Interventions

Goals

Short-term (Acute Phase)

- Client will decrease withdrawn behavior
- Client will maintain contact with reality
- Client will respond to safe, protective environment
- Client will maintain adequate hygiene, grooming, and other activities of daily living (ADL)
- Paranoid client will decrease hostile behavior

Intermediate (Working Phase)

- Client will increase autonomous functioning
- Client will increase goal-structured activity
- Client will develop self-motivation and avoid regressive behavior

Long Term (Rehabilitation Phase)

- Client will take direct action to prepare for discharge and independence
- Client will maintain optimal level of functioning, understand illness and importance of continuing to take medication
- Family will participate in care plan
- Client will function with help of outside support systems (halfway house, residential homes, Veterans Administration, community mental health clinic)

Nursing Measures

- Establish one-to-one relationship
- Provide reality orientation
- Give clear, short, simple, concrete messages
- Tell client expectations directly; do not ask
- Do not ask client to make unnecessary choices
- Assist with ADL
- Be consistent and firm but gentle when confronting aggressive behavior

- Do not argue, become personally insulted, or defensive
- Protect client from harming self or others
- Support others who are targets of verbal and physical abuse, rather than giving attention to client
- Direct activities to help client remain in contact with reality and to increase social skills—refer to recreational therapy (RT), occupational therapy (OT)
- Support client's efforts to do things for self but do not expect all efforts to be successful
- Maintain empathy with clients and recognize their human rights—avoid becoming a caretaker

Drug Therapy (See Table 17-2)

Antipsychotics

Antiparkinsonian drugs

Fluphenazine decanoate (Prolixin Decanoate)

Evaluation

Short Term (Acute Phase)
- Client has contact with reality
- Client is oriented to time, place, person, self
- Client is able to establish trusting relationship with nurse
- Client maintains adequate hygiene and nutrition
- Client can assist with ADL
- Client is free of anxiety and fear associated with hallucinations
- Client's self-esteem increases

Intermediate (Working Phase)
- Client initiates interaction with nurse or at least one other person
- Client increases level of independence
- Client is responsible for own ADL
- Client maintains good personal hygiene

Long Term (Rehabilitation Phase)
- Client is able to function independently in society with occupation, school or vocation, family and friends

Bipolar Disorders

Bipolar disorders are characterized by one or more manic episodes usually accompanied by one or more major depressive episodes.

DSM III-R Classification
- Bipolar disorder, mixed
- Bipolar disorder, manic
- Bipolar disorder, depressed

Assessment

Health Status

Behavioral Effects of Mania
- Hyperactivity
- Inappropriate sexual behavior
- Pressured speech
- Inflated self-esteem
- Decreased need for sleep
- Involvement in activities that have high potential for painful consequences

Physical Effects of Mania
- Nutritional deficits (hyperactive behavior does not allow client time to eat)
- Exhaustion
- Self-inflicted injury

Developmental Assessment

"Bipolar disorder has clearly been shown to occur at much higher rates in first-degree biologic relatives of people with bipolar disorder than in the general population" (DSM III-R)

Usually begins in adolescence or early adult life

Nursing Plans and Interventions

Goals

During acute manic episodes, client will:
- Maintain physical health and safety
- Channel physical and psychic energy
- Perceive reality accurately

Nursing Measures

- Establish one-to-one relationship
- Promote expression of feelings
- Assist with hygiene and grooming (monitor for inappropriate make-up, encourage bathing)
- Channel physical energy (encourage overactive client to keep a diary or write autobiography)
- Decrease environmental stimulation

Drug Therapy

Chlorpromazine hydrochloride (Thorazine) for extreme agitation

Lithium carbonate for acute and maintenance therapy (see Table 17-6)

Nutrition Therapy

- High-carbohydrate, high-protein diets to increase metabolic rate during manic stage; low-sodium diet while on lithium
- Finger foods or foods easy to eat "on the go"
- Fluids to combat dehydration
- No caffeine

Evaluation

- Acute manic episodes are usually under control and abating within 2 to 3 weeks after initiation of lithium therapy
- Frequently a manic or major depressive episode is immediately followed by a short episode of the other kind
- There is evidence that cases of bipolar disorder with a mixed or rapid cycling episode have a much more chronic course

Depressive Disorders

- Major depression, single episode
- Major depression, recurrent
- Characterized by depressed mood for at least 2 weeks

Assessment

Health Status

- Sadness, loneliness, apathy
- Extreme guilt feelings common
- Low self-esteem
- Self-deprecatory feelings that may lead to suicidal ideation
- Physical effects: decreased sexual performance, difficulty sleeping, weight loss, decreased GI mobility, menstrual irregularities, and self-inflicted injury

Developmental Assessment

Twice as common in females as in males

1½ to 3 times more common among first-degree biologic relatives of persons suffering depression

Average age of onset in later 20s

Psychosocial/Cultural Assessment

- There is always some interference in social and occupational functioning
- Frequently major depressions follow a psychosocial stressor such as death of a loved one, marital separation, divorce, childbirth

Nursing Plans and Interventions

Goals

- Client will maintain physical health and safety
- Client will not commit suicide
- Client's isolation will be minimized
- Client will maintain nutritional status
- Client will increase feelings of self-esteem

Nursing Measures

- Establish one-to-one relationship
- Promote expression of feelings
- Assist with hygiene, grooming
- Encourage physical activity

Drug Therapy

Antidepressants (see Table 17-4)

Evaluation

Duration is variable (untreated lasts 6 months or longer)

Treatment is successful if remission of symptoms is complete and general functioning returns to premorbid level

Anxiety Disorders: Panic

- Panic disorder with agoraphobia*
- Panic disorder without agoraphobia
- Essential features are recurrent panic attacks (periods of intense fear or discomfort usually lasting minutes or more, rarely hours; initially unexpected and not connected with specific situation)

Assessment

Health Status

- Sudden onset of intense apprehension, fear, or terror
- Feeling of impending doom common
- Physical symptoms: dyspnea, dizziness, faintness, choking, palpitations, accelerated heart rate, shaking, sweating, nausea
- Depersonalization
- Fear of dying, going crazy, or doing something uncontrolled
- Symptoms of agoraphobia usually present

Developmental Assessment

Onset is in late 20s

The disorder is common

Panic disorder with agoraphobia is much more common than panic disorder without agoraphobia

---

* Agoraphobia is "the fear of being in places or situations from which escape might be difficult" (DSM III-R)—or from situations which might be embarrassing.

Nursing Plans and Interventions

Goals

- Client's anxiety will decrease

Nursing Measures

- Use calm, unhurried manner in approaching client
- Reduce environmental stimuli (may have to move client to quieter area)
- Speak in clear, short, concrete sentences
- Do not make demands or threaten client

Drug Therapy

Imipramine hydrochloride (Tofranil) drug of choice for panic attacks (see Table 17-4)

Evaluation

- Prognosis is good with therapeutic intervention
- May be limited to single brief period lasting several weeks or months or may recur several times
- Panic disorder with agoraphobia may last for years with varying periods of partial or full remission

General Anxiety Disorder

A general anxiety disorder involves unrealistic or excessive anxiety and worry about two or more life circumstances.

Assessment

Health Status

- Unrealistic, unrelenting worry (*e.g.*, worrying about possible danger to one's child when no danger is present)
- Constant vigilance and scanning (feeling keyed up or on edge, experiencing exaggerated startle response)
- Motor tension when anxious (twitching or feeling shaky, muscle tension, restlessness, easy fatigability)

Nursing Plans and Interventions

Goals

- Client will improve coping patterns to improve social or occupational functioning

Nursing Measures

- Establish one-to-one relationship
- Convey positive regard for client
- Help client use anxiety to learn about self to promote change
- Use confrontation as necessary after therapeutic relationship established
- Encourage activities therapies such as OT and RT to build self-esteem

Drug Therapy

Antianxiety drugs (see Table 17-7)

Evaluation

The disorder is usually chronic and difficult to overcome. Treatment is successful if:

- Client is free of motor symptoms and symptoms associated with autonomic hyperactivity
- Client has insight into underlying dynamics that prevent positive coping strategies

Obsessive Compulsive Disorder

The essential characteristic of an obsessive compulsive disorder is recurrent obsessions or compulsions sufficiently severe to cause marked distress and to interfere with normal routine, occupation, or usual social activities.

Assessment

Health Status

- Obsessions are persistent ideas, thoughts, impulses, or images that are experienced as intrusive and senseless
- Repetitive thoughts of violence and doubt are the most common obsessions
- Compulsions are repetitive, purposeful, and intentional behaviors that are performed in response to an obsession (client believes he or she must follow certain rules or a stereotyped pattern)
- Purpose of compulsive behavior is to neutralize or to prevent discomfort from the obsession

It is difficult to establish goals for these clients, whose personality traits make them poor candidates for change—traits include:

- Rigidity in thinking and behavior
- Tendency to form immature, dependent relationships
- Poor ability to tolerate anxiety
- Limited ability to express emotion
- Inability to be insightful and introspective

Nursing Measures

- Assess own feelings of frustration and anger when interacting with client
- Avoid confrontation and making demands
- Do not deny client his or her compulsion without substituting a behavior to release anxiety
- Give positive feedback for direct expression of feelings and self-assertion

Somatoform Disorders

The essential features of somatoform disorders are physical symptoms that suggest physical disorder but for which there are no demonstrable organic findings or known physiologic causes. Disorders include:

- Dysmorphic disorder
- Conversion disorder
- Hypochondriasis
- Somatization disorder

Assessment

Health Status

Dysmorphic Disorder

- Preoccupation with some imagined defect in appearance in a normal-appearing person (most commonly involve facial flaws, excessive hair, shape of nose, mouth, wrinkles, spots on skin)

Conversion Disorder
- Classic symptoms of conversion disorders involve neurologic system and include paralysis, blindness, tunnel vision, anesthesia

Hypochondriasis
- Preoccupation with fear of serious illness
- Client cannot be dissuaded by medical reassurance
- Social and occupational functioning are impaired

Somatization Disorder
- Recurrent and multiple somatic complaints of several years duration
- Symptoms suggest physical disorder but other evidence suggests psychological cause
- No demonstrable organic findings are present
- No physiological functions are abnormal or atypical according to medical examination, laboratory or x-ray studies
- Client presents complicated medical history with dramatic symptoms that are usually vague and exaggerated
- Client becomes "doctor shopper," often seeing several at once
- Client may undergo frequent and unnecessary surgery
- Client runs risk of substance abuse involving a variety of prescribed medications

Psychosocial/Cultural Assessment
- Frustrating people to work with
- Form few social relationships
- Antagonize and distance family, friends, and helping professionals

Nursing Plans and Interventions

Goals
- Client will resolve underlying conflicts and avoid focusing on physical symptoms
- Client will give up secondary gains and learn adaptive coping skills

Nursing Measures
- Assess all somatic complaints (must have baseline data for physical assessment; unsafe to assume that all physical complaints are related to somatoform illness)
- Minimize time and attention given to complaints
- Withdraw attention if client insists on making complaints the only topic of conversation
- Allow specific time period (minutes per hour or minutes per conversation) for physical complaints
- Do not argue about somatic complaints
- Give minimal objective reassurance to minimize physical complaints
- Encourage expression of feelings
- Give positive feedback for direct expression of feelings, self-assertion, and verbal expression of anger
- Relieve anxiety by expressing the positive attitude that you expect improvement in physical symptom
- Avoid making demands
- Restrict or limit visits if stress is strongly related to visits

Evaluation

Treatment is successful if:
- Client is able to express anger verbally
- Client's self-esteem is elevated
- Client can verbalize underlying emotional problems

Sexual Disorders

Paraphilias are characterized by arousal in response to sexual objects or situations that are not part of normative arousal activity.

Sexual dysfunctions are characterized by inhibitions of sexual desire or of the psychophysiologic changes that characterize the sexual response cycle.

Other sexual disorders include extreme feelings of inadequacy concerning body habitus, size and shape of sex organs, sexual performance, or other traits related to self-imposed standards of masculinity or femininity; distress about a pattern of repeated sexual conquests or other forms of nonparaphilic sexual addiction, involving a succession of people who exist only as things to be used; and persistent and extreme distress about sexual orientation.

Assessment

Health Status

Paraphilias

- Exhibitionism: exposure of one's genitals to a stranger
- Fetishism: sexually arousing fantasies involving use of nonliving objects
- Frotteurism: touching and rubbing against a nonconsenting person
- Pedophilia: sexual activity with a prepubescent child
- Sexual masochism: intense sexual urges and fantasies that result in sexual activity involving being humiliated, beaten, bound, or otherwise made to suffer
- Sexual sadism: intense sexual urges that result in sexual activity involving inflicting psychological or physical suffering on another person
- Transvestic fetishism: sexual urges and fantasies involving cross dressing
- Voyeurism: observing unsuspecting people who are either naked, in the process of undressing, or engaged in sexual activity

Sexual Dysfunctions

- Inhibition preventing enjoyment or experience of psychophysiological changes that characterize the complete sexual arousal cycle: appetitive, excitement, orgasm, resolution

Psychosocial/Cultural Assessment

- Human sexuality best understood holistically
- Nurses must be aware of their own personal attitudes toward sex to intervene helpfully
- Sexual normality is a changing concept and is defined by society's norms, values, ideals, ideology
- Key concept in American culture is consent
- There is a growing trend in contemporary society to accept alternative sexual styles rather than labeling them pathological
- Sexual assessment is an important part of total assessment but is generally short changed or inappropriately conducted (Wilson and Kneisl, 1983)

Psychological Factors Affecting Physical Diseases

A group of illnesses that involve life-threatening symptoms resulting from underlying emotional stress or creating intense emotional stress has been identified. Examples (classified by body systems) include:

GI: peptic ulcer, ulcerative colitis
Cardiovascular: MI, migraine headaches
Respiratory: asthma
Integumentary: rashes, hives, herpes zoster
Musculoskeletal: rheumatoid arthritis

Nursing Plans and Interventions

Nursing Measures

- Be aware of secondary gains resulting for client from dysfunctional emotional responses to these illnesses, and minimize their effects
- Always skillfully meet client's physical needs
- *Dependency:* allow client some control over environment and do not be too willing to do what client can do for himself or herself
- *Withdrawal/depressive reaction:* increase self-esteem
- *Hostility:* encourage verbalization of feelings

- *Denial, ambivalence:* minimize anxiety and keep conversation clear, simple, concrete
- *Loneliness/rejection:* use nonjudgmental, nonconfrontive approach
- *Regression:* involve family in understanding of emotional needs and importance of client being as independent as possible

Anorexia Nervosa

Anorexia nervosa is a condition characterized by severe emaciation due to an intense fear of becoming obese and a distorted body image, and by a weight loss of at least 25% of original body weight.

Assessment

Health Status

- No known physical illness to account for loss
- Intense fear of becoming obese that does not abate as weight loss progresses
- Disturbances in body image
- Refusal to maintain body weight over minimum standard
- Compromised nutritional status
- Vitamin and mineral deficiencies
- Hypokalemia may result in fatigue, seizures, cardiac dysrhythmias, nephropathy from chronically low potassium levels
- Muscle wasting
- GI intolerance to food
- Abdominal bloating
- Constipation
- Edema
- Bradycardia
- Susceptibility to infection
- Loss of hair
- Amenorrhea, infertility, hormonal imbalance

Developmental Assessment

Primarily affects adolescent girls and young women; an increasing number of adolescent boys affected also

More common among mothers and sisters of persons with the disorder than in general population

Clients often described as overly perfectionist, "model" children

May be precipitated by stressful life situation

Clients have strong need to maintain control of life

Preoccupation with dieting and exercising common

Clients become expert at counting calories and analyzing nutritional content of food

Nursing Plans and Interventions

Goals are reached using behavior modification and psychotherapy in an interdisciplinary approach. Nursing measures for hospitalized clients are directed initially toward alleviating malnutrition:

- Assist with hyperalimentation
- Assist with tube feedings
- Monitor vascular status, electrolytes, I and O, weight, elimination patterns
- Establish trusting relationship
- Avoid conflict, judgmental interactions, and punitive behavior
- Set consistent limits to avoid manipulation
- Promote sharing of feelings, build positive self-image, and provide positive reinforcement

Bulimia

Bulimia is a condition characterized by episodes of rapid consumption of large amounts of food within a discrete period of time, followed by self-induced vomiting.

Assessment

Health Status

- Frequent weight fluctuations varying from 10–15 pounds in either direction at any given time

- Physiologic symptoms: dehydration, hypokalemia, constipation, hormone imbalances, difficulty retaining food in even small amounts
- Effects of vomiting: esophageal irritation; swelling, pain, and tenderness in salivary glands; excessive tooth decay and erosion of tooth enamel; gum disorders; erosion of stomach lining

Psychosocial/Cultural Assessment

- Client aware of abnormal eating pattern and fears not being able to stop voluntarily
- Depression and self-deprecating thoughts follow binges
- Client feels extreme humiliation from loss of control with binging (unlike anorexic client who prides self on discipline and control)
- Symptoms become complicated blend of pleasure and pain and are difficult to give up
- Binging to ease tension creates sense of euphoria similar to that in substance abuse

Nursing Plans and Interventions

Nursing Measures

- Bulimic clients most often treated as outpatients with cognitive therapy aimed at education
- Psychotherapy emphasizes increasing self-esteem, positive body image

20

Nursing Care of the Client with an Adjustment Disorder

All adjustment disorders are characterized by a maladaptive reaction to an identifiable psychosocial stressor(s). The reaction occurs within 3 months of the onset of the stressor and persists for no longer than 6 months. Types identified by DSM III-R* include:

Adjustment with anxious mood

Adjustment with depressed mood

Adjustment with disturbances of conduct

Adjustment with mixed disturbances of emotions and conduct

Adjustment with mixed emotional features

Adjustment with physical complaints

Adjustment with withdrawal (social)

Adjustment with work or academic inhibition

---

*DSM III-R (Diagnostic and Statistical Manual of Mental Disorders, 3rd ed, rev, Washington, DC, American Psychiatric Association, 1987) is a diagnostic publication developed and researched by members of the American Psychiatric Association. Its purpose is to provide standardized criteria for a comprehensive evaluation and understanding of mental disorders. It is widely accepted in the U.S. as the common language of mental health clinicians and researchers for communicating about the disorders for which they have professional responsibility. It has had considerable impact and influence internationally.

Adjustment not otherwise specified (example: an immediate reaction to a diagnosis of physical illness that is characterized by maladaptive denial and noncompliance)

Assessment

Health Status

- Maladaptive nature of client's reaction is in excess of normal and expected reaction to stressor
- Severity of reaction is not completely predictable from intensity of stressor
- Vulnerable people may have more severe reaction following only mild or moderate stressor
- Others may have mild reaction in response to severe and continuing stressor

Developmental Assessment

May begin at any age

Common disorder

Diagnostic Factors

Adjustment disorders are short-term maladaptive responses and are not used as diag-

nostic catagories for disturbances that meet criteria for other, specific mental disorders
- Reaction should not be confused with uncomplicated bereavement (expected loss-grief response)
- Reactions occur within 3 months of precipitating stressor
- Stressors may be single or multiple: divorce, extreme business difficulties, marital problems, rape
- Stressors may be recurrent or continuous: seasonal business crisis, residence in deteriorating neighborhood, chronic illness
- Can occur with individuals, families, groups, or communities
- May accompany specific developmental events: going away to school, leaving home, getting married, becoming a parent, facing retirement

Psychosocial/Cultural Assessment

- Affects occupational, school, and social functioning
- Conduct disturbances result in truancy, vandalism, reckless driving, fighting, defaulting on legal responsibilities
- Situations in which an individual is subjected to chronic criticism and devaluation contribute to low self-esteem and sense of worthlessness
- Event that causes sudden change in self-concept (*e.g.*, disfigurement from accident) is especially stressful because client does not have time to adapt
- Role stress occurs when a social structure creates difficult, conflicting, or impossible demands for the position that individual holds within structure (students at risk at time of evaluation, *e.g.*, final exam week, paper due)
- Experiences that threaten sexual identity or interfere with sexual role behaviors may be stressful: rape, ego dystonic homosexual reaction
- Life events may be rated according to how stressful they are according to the Holmes and Rahe scale: death of a spouse or divorce are rated as very stressful while retirement, pregnancy, and occupational change are rated as less stressful; events rated as less stressful include a child leaving home and outstanding personal achievement

Nursing Plans and Interventions

Goal

- Client will reestablish level of functioning equal to or better than level preceding the crisis or stressful event that caused the maladaptive behavior(s)

Nursing Measures

Use crisis management techniques (phases parallel to nursing process):

- Assess
- Diagnose
- Plan
- Implement
- Evaluate

Use principles of anxiety management if necessary:

- Reduce environmental stimuli
- Speak in firm, clear, concrete terms
- Avoid invading client's territorial space if he or she feels threatened
- Give information in small doses and repeat as often as necessary
- Help client identify precipitating event or events leading to the anxiety

If necessary, manipulate client's environment and directly intervene to change physical or interpersonal situations (examples: arrange for substitute, short-term lodging in the case of natural disaster or abuse; restrict interaction with friends, family if necessary).

Provide anticipatory guidance to assist client with future stressors.

Drug Therapy

Haloperidol (Haldol) 2–5 mg IM for extreme aggravation

Antianxiety drugs (see Tables 17-7 and 17-8)

Client/Family Teaching

Crisis therapy involves instructing client in problem-solving techniques:

1. Identify stressors in one's life—may be major events or everyday occurrences, may be external (difficult boss) or internal (self-critical thought, lack of assertiveness)
2. Examine how one reacts to what occurs in a particular situation—identify physical and emotional responses that routinely are associated with unpleasant situations
3. Determine if one wants to eliminate, reduce contact with, or diminish one's response to each stressor
4. A positive attitude and willingness to cope in healthful ways with stressors are more critical than the quantity of stressors one encounters—in some cases, removing a stressor is impractical or would deprive one of challenge and personal growth opportunities
5. Develop effective coping mechanisms—recognize that emotional health is an evolving process; learn to recognize and accept feelings and to use emotional energy to enhance life situations

Evaluation

Treatment and client teaching are successful if client:

- Experiences decrease in distress
- Returns to his or her precrisis level of functioning, or increases coping skills from precrisis level
- Identifies source of distress and initiates positive changes (internally and externally)

Bibliography for Unit V
Care of the Client with a Mental Health Problem

American Psychiatric Association: Diagnostic and Statistical Manual of Mental Disorders, 3rd ed, rev. Washington DC, American Psychiatric Association, 1987

Beck C, Rawlins R, Williams S: Mental Health–Psychiatric Nursing: A Holistic Life-Cycle Approach, 2nd ed. St Louis, CV Mosby, 1988

Duldt B, Griffin K, Patton B: Interpersonal Communication in Nursing. Philadelphia, FA Davis, 1984

Johnson B: Psychiatric–Mental Health Nursing: Adaptation and Growth. Philadelphia, JB Lippincott, 1986

Kneisl C, Ames S: Adult Health Nursing: A Biopsychosocial Approach. Menlo Park, CA, Addison-Wesley, 1986

Mathewson K: Pharmacotherapeutics: A Nursing Process Approach. Philadelphia, FA Davis, 1986

Murray R, Hullskoelter M: Psychiatric Mental Health Nursing: Giving Emotional Care. Englewood Cliffs, NJ, Prentice-Hall, 1983

McFarland G, Wasli, E: Nursing Diagnosis and Process in Psychiatric Mental Health Nursing. Philadelphia, JB Lippincott, 1986

Pasquali E, Alesi E, Arnold H, DeBasio N: Mental Health Nursing: A Bio-Psycho-Cultural Approach, 2nd ed. St Louis, CV Mosby, 1985

Robinson L: Psychiatric Nursing as a Human Experience, 3rd ed. Philadelphia, WB Saunders, 1983

Schultz J, Dark S: Manual of Psychiatric Nursing Care Plans, 2nd ed. Boston, Little, Brown & Co, 1986

Stuart G, Sundeen S: Principles and Practice of Psychiatric Nursing, 3rd ed. St Louis, CV Mosby, 1987

Williams S: Nutrition and Diet Therapy, 5th ed. St Louis, Times/Mirror/Mosby, 1985

Wilson H, Kneisl C: Psychiatric Nursing, 2nd ed. Menlo Park, CA, Addison-Wesley, 1983

VI

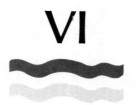

Practice Tests

How to Use the Practice Tests

This Practice Tests section is designed to help you practice taking standardized or teacher-made tests in four major content areas: care of the adult client, care of the client during childbearing, care of the child, and care of the client with a mental health problem. Practice test tools, including practice tests, answer sheets, answers with rationale and item code, and diagnostic grids, are included for your use. A summary sheet is placed at the end of the section to help you identify priority review topics.

The practice tests have been developed to represent content similar to that of the NLN Mobility Profile II examination and other standardized or teacher-made examinations. The questions sample your knowledge of both nursing content and the process of giving nursing care. The questions are written to determine that you have knowledge in these areas and are able to apply it in specific client situations.

Content Questions

The questions in each of the practice tests in this section have been written to test your understanding of the signs and symptoms that indicate a client's health status; nursing actions and nursing measures; and your ability to apply your knowledge of pharmacology, nutrition, and communication skills. Questions about the client's health status ask you to determine the stage of illness or wellness the client's behavior represents. Questions about nursing actions or nursing measures test your knowledge about the appropriate nursing measures to modify the client's health status. These questions may ask for a priority judgement about the severity of the health problem and nursing actions needed to intervene. Since many nursing actions are based on an understanding of pharmacology, nutrition, and interpersonal communications, questions have also been developed for these specific content areas. Questions here will ask about use of drugs, diets, or communication skills, or will ask you to evaluate the client's understanding of this information.

Process Questions

The test questions have also been written to test your understanding of the nursing process. Although most tests do not ask specific questions about the nursing process or formulation of nursing diagnoses, questions may test your ability to use a systematic approach to providing nursing care. For example, a question may be written to determine that you have gathered information (assessment) about the client's health status before planning interventions. Questions could also ask you to draw conclusions about the information (analyze data and identify nursing diagnoses and problems), make a plan and set priorities (planning), choose appropriate nursing actions (implementation/intervention), and note the effects of your actions (evaluation). Review the information about the particular validation examination you will be taking to determine how nursing process will be tested.

Answer Sheets

Practice answer sheets are provided to give you an opportunity to simulate test taking. If you wish to take a practice test more than once, reproduce the answer sheets before you use them.

Answers with Rationale and Item Code

Answers with the rationale for the correct answer are given for each practice examination. Each question is also coded according to the nursing content of the question and the step of the nursing process. Some questions may have more than one content code. The item code is as follows:

Nursing content:

H = Health status
O = Nursing actions/interventions
D = Drugs/pharmacology
N = Nutrition
C = Communication skills

Nursing process:

A = Assessment
R = Analysis/nursing diagnosis
P = Planning
I = Implementation/intervention
E = Evaluation

Diagnostic Grid

Use the diagnostic grid to identify nursing content and nursing process areas in which you need additional study. By determining the percentage of questions answered incorrectly in any one area, you will note a pattern of a content or process area in which you are consistently responding incorrectly. Since each question tests both content and process, you will need to decide if you answered the question incorrectly because you did not know the nursing content or because you misunderstood the step of the nursing process. If a pattern of incorrect responses exists in one or both of these areas, you will be better able to focus your review.

Practice Test Summary

A practice test summary sheet is included at the end of the unit. The sheet can be used to summarize the results of your use of all of the practice tests. Broad areas for study concentration could emerge as you identify your strengths and weaknesses in nursing content and nursing process.

Using the Practice Tests

The practice tests and diagnostic grids can be used in several ways. They can be used (1) to assess current knowledge prior to review, (2) to identify content needing further study, (3) as a self-test after review, and (4) to simulate testing conditions and practice test-taking skills. Although each learner has preferred ways of studying, many nurses find the following procedures useful:

1. Take the practice test before reviewing the content.
   - Take the test using the answer sheet. Do not worry about time or your score.
   - Review the answers, rationale, and item code for each question.
   - As you use the review book, make a note of the questions you answered incorrectly and direct additional attention to that content area.
2. Take the practice test after you have studied the review chapters, audiotapes, notes, or other study materials.
   - Take the test using the answer sheet.

Simulate test conditions by sitting at a desk, assuring quiet, and noting the time spent taking the entire test. (Remember that most tests are planned to allow the test-taker 1 minute per question.)
- Score the test. Using the answer sheet, total the number of questions answered incorrectly. A score of 70% to 80% is considered passing for most tests, but you should find out the passing score for the particular validation test you will be taking.
- Review the rationale for the answers you have answered incorrectly. If you need further information about a particular question refer to the appropriate unit in this book or to the bibliography for that unit.
- Use the diagnostic grid to note the type of questions you missed frequently. The grid will reveal patterns of nursing content and nursing process questions, but remember you will need to determine if you missed the question because you misunderstood the nursing content or the nursing process.
- When you have completed study and practice tests for all content areas, enter your test results on the summary sheet.
- Concentrate your final review in content areas where your skills are weakest as revealed by the summary sheet.

Practice Test 1: Care of the Adult Client

Read each question carefully and select the best answer from the choices presented. Mark your answers on the answer sheet on page 315.

1. The risk of developing lung cancer is directly related to
   a. The ingestion of carcinogens
   b. Cigarette smoking and other forms of smoke inhalation
   c. Poor respiratory hygiene and frequent respiratory infections
   d. None of the above
2. Joe Marks, a 76-year-old man, comes to the ER complaining of sudden onset of severe pain in his back, flank, and abdomen. He reports feeling weak and his BP is 68/31. Urine output is absent. Bilateral leg pulses are weak although bruit and pulsation are noted at the umbilicus. Because the client needs immediate medical attention, the nurse should recognize that these findings strongly suggest
   a. A degenerative lumbar disc
   b. Raynaud's phenomenon
   c. Thrombophlebitis
   d. An enlarging abdominal aneurysm
3. (Questions 3–10 refer to this situation) Jim Strube's cardiac enzymes profile is reported on his chart. CPK-MB is an intracellular isoenzyme found predominantly in the myocardial cells. An elevated amount of this enzyme in the patient's serum or blood is useful in diagnosing myocardial infarction and
   a. Identifying the specific coronary vessel involved
   b. Replacing necessary enzymes
   c. Planning client activity level
   d. Estimating urinary excretion of enzyme
4. The ICU nurse continues to monitor Mr. Strube's EKG. At 2:20 a.m. the nurse notes ST segment changes typical of ischemia, and immediately assesses Mr. Strube's condition. He reports severe chest pain over his midepigastric area. The nurse's priority in this situation is to
   a. Check the EKG lead patches to confirm proper chest adhesion
   b. Check the O_2 flow rate to be sure O_2 is being delivered
   c. Tell the unit secretary to call the physician
   d. Give Mr. Strube a sublingual nitroglycerin tablet and assess for pain relief
5. Mr. Strube reports relief from pain after taking one 1/150 grain tablet of sublingual nitroglycerin. However, he is quite agitated, fearful, and short of breath. The nurse should *first*

a. Administer a second nitroglycerin tablet to reduce his anxiety
b. Position Mr. Strube in a high semi-Fowler's position to improve ventilation
c. Check the bedside cardioscope to assess for EKG changes
d. Check the medication orders for sedative orders

6. Mr. Strube's diagnosis is angina pectoris. He states that he does not understand his problem, but knows he has chest pain. Which of the following statements best explains the pathophysiologic changes associated with angina?
   a. Chest pain occurs when too much blood is forced into the ventricles
   b. Chest pain occurs when too much blood is forced into the myocardial tissue
   c. Chest pain occurs when too little oxygen is available to heart muscle cells
   d. Chest pain occurs when the muscles of the blood vessels of the heart muscles dilate suddenly

7. The nurse continues to monitor Mr. Strube's cardiac electrical activity. Other nursing care goals during the acute period include all the following *except*
   a. Promoting comfort by positioning the client and providing medications
   b. Assessing vital functions including temperature and blood pressure
   c. Assessing fluid and electrolyte status
   d. Maintaining adequate nutrition via a soft regular diet

8. Mr. Strube is given 1/150 grain tablet of nitroglycerin sublingually at the onset of angina pain. Shortly afterward, he reports a throbbing headache and tingling under his tongue. The nurse should
   a. Report these findings to the physician immediately
   b. Recognize these findings as probable indicators of stress
   c. Provide mouthwash and oral hygiene to relieve these sensations
   d. Tell Mr. Strube that these are transient effects and indicate the medication potency

9. Mr. Strube is soon to return home. He expresses concern about returning to his normal pace of activity. The nurse should ask Mr. Strube what activities are permitted by the physician, and also reinforce that
   a. Activity, as permitted, will not result in chest pain
   b. Nitroglycerin should be taken prior to situations that are known to precipitate angina
   c. Some angina pain is expected now but should not slow him down
   d. Extremely vigorous exercise should only be undertaken in the morning hours

10. Mr. Strube is instructed to follow a low-sodium, low-cholesterol diet. Which of the following breakfast selections provides the lowest amounts of sodium and cholesterol?
    a. 1 egg poached, 1 cup lowfat (1%) milk, ½ grapefruit, 2 slices whole wheat toast with 1 teaspoon butter
    b. 1 cup oatmeal, ½ cup lowfat (1%) milk, 1 teaspoon sugar, ½ cantaloupe, 1 slice crisp fried bacon
    c. 2 pork links, 1 egg poached, 8 ounces orange juice (frozen), 1 slice raisin bran bread with 1 teaspoon strawberry preserves
    d. 8 ounces raspberry yogurt, 1 egg bagel with 1 ounce cream cheese, 8 ounces cranberry juice cocktail (canned)

11. Jack Thompson is admitted to the hospital with a diagnosis of myocardial infarction. He says to the nurse, "My father died of a heart attack and I probably will too." Which of the following responses is most appropriate?
    a. "Remember that because your father

died that way doesn't mean you will too."
b. "Try to relax. You'll get the best care possible while you're here."
c. "Are you afraid you'll die soon?"
d. "You sound fearful that you too might die."

12. Ed Taylor is recovering well following cardiac surgery 2 days ago. His wife, who is assisting with his care, says, "He is doing too much. I told him to let me help him but he won't let me." The nurse says, "It sounds like Mrs. Taylor needs to feel more helpful." The nurse's response would be supported by the nurse
    a. Directing her eyes at Mr. Taylor
    b. Directing her position and eyes at Mrs. Taylor
    c. Avoiding direct eye contact with both Mr. and Mrs. Taylor
    d. Shifting her eyes back and forth between Mr. and Mrs. Taylor

13. (Questions 13–22 refer to this situation) Tom Smith has a long history of COPD. He reports a weight loss of 10 pounds over the last 9 months. The nurse should recognize that weight loss in a client with COPD most likely is related to all of the following *except*
    a. Carbon monoxide intoxication of the appetite center
    b. Hypermetabolic state
    c. Dyspnea with eating
    d. Alteration of taste sensations related to sputum expectoration and nebulization medications

14. Mr. Smith is receiving 0.5 mL (500 mg) saturated solution of potassium iodide 3 times daily. In Mr. Smith's case, the goal of administering SSKI is to
    a. Reduce thyroid function by trapping thyroid hormone in the thyroid gland
    b. Provide replacement potassium to maintain muscle tone
    c. Arrest the destruction of respiratory bronchioles and alveoli associated with emphysema
    d. Liquify respiratory secretions and facilitate expectoration

15. Mr. Smith continues to receive SSKI as ordered. The nurse should recognize that to safely administer the drug
    a. SSKI should be taken only on an empty stomach
    b. SSKI should be taken in its liquid form, but not followed by water or food for at least 30 minutes
    c. SSKI should be diluted in 8 ounces of water, milk, or juice
    d. SSKI should be diluted only in 4 ounces of orange juice to enhance proper absorption

16. Mr. Smith will receive an expectorant to promote removal of sputum. Important related assessment data to chart include all of the following *except*
    a. Color, odor, viscosity, and amount of sputum
    b. Changes in bowel sounds
    c. Auscultated breath sounds
    d. Skin and mucous membrane color changes
    e. Blood gas findings

17. Mr. Smith continues experiencing shortness of breath and difficulty expectorating sputum. The nurse should assess Mr. Smith's understanding of effective coughing technique and reinforce which of the following efforts?
    a. Taking a deep inhalation and exhaling forcefully
    b. Taking several diaphragmatic inhalations and pursed-lip exhalations before initiating a cough
    c. Taking a deep inspiration and holding the volume as long as possible before coughing
    d. Taking short shallow inspirations before one rapid forceful exhalation

18. The physician has ordered that Mr. Smith receive oxygen prn for comfort at 2 L/min. The nurse should recognize that the rationale for administering low flow O_2 is that

a. Low flow O₂ protects against excessive drying of mucous membranes
b. High flow O₂ should be avoided because it has addictive properties
c. High flow O₂ might inhibit the client's respiratory center
d. There is no special rationale for administering low flow O₂; the nurse should seek permission to adjust the flow rate according to client comfort

19. Because of Mr. Smith's long history of COPD, he receives isoproterenol (Isuprel) per nebulizer. He reports nervousness, nausea, headache, and palpitations, and asks if something is wrong. The nurse should recognize that these symptoms are
    a. Serious toxic effects of Isuprel
    b. Side-effects of Isuprel
    c. Caused by interactions between Isuprel and antibiotic drugs
    d. Typical clinical features of COPD

20. After Mr. Smith's nebulizer treatment, the nurse should instruct him to
    a. Relax and breathe normally
    b. Inhale deeply and exhale quickly
    c. Practice effective coughing techniques
    d. Breathe shallowly to retain nebulized Isuprel

21. Mr. Smith is breathing rapidly in a tripod body position. He appears short of breath and anxious. The nurse should encourage him to use pursed-lip breathing exercises which he has been previously taught. Pursed-lip breathing will
    a. Slow and lengthen expiration and decrease alveolar air trapping
    b. Distract him and lower his anxiety
    c. Increase the force of inspiration to increase inhaled O₂ concentration in the alveoli
    d. Decrease the amount of sputum in the major airways

22. Mr. Smith received 0.1 mL of PPD intradermally. After 72 hours, the nurse reads the area of induration at the injection site as 13 mm. This means that Mr. Smith has
    a. A negative Mantoux test reaction, and is free of pulmonary disease
    b. Tuberculosis of the lung
    c. A positive Mantoux test reaction
    d. A questionable test result (test should be repeated)

23. The usual mode of transmission of the mycobacterium tuberculosis organism is
    a. Via fomites
    b. Via airborne droplet nuclei
    c. Hand to mouth
    d. Via insect vectors

24. For a client with diagnosed active pulmonary tuberculosis, the medication most likely ordered for treatment would be
    a. Penicillin
    b. BCG (bacillus-Calmette-Guérin)
    c. Solumedrol
    d. INH (isoniazid)

25. Medication treatment time with first-line antitubercular drugs is a minimum of
    a. 2 weeks of intravenous administration
    b. 1 month or until Mantoux test reaction reverts to negative
    c. 6 months or until weight gain occurs
    d. 9 months or until 6 months after the client's sputum has converted to negative for the myobacterium

26. (Questions 26–32 refer to this situation) Jason Evert, a client with congestive heart failure, will be treated with a cardiac glycoside such as digoxin (Lanoxin). The desired effect of digoxin is to
    a. Increase the heart rate to increase cardiac output
    b. Decrease the heart rate to improve cardiac output
    c. Alter the conduction impulse rate from the sinoatrial node
    d. Block out ventricular ectopic myocardial foci to prevent premature ventricular contractions

27. Mr. Evert has stat electrolytes drawn. Electrolytes most closely associated with the conductile and contractile properties of the heart are
    a. Sodium, magnesium, and chloride

b. Potassium, magnesium, and sulfates
c. Calcium, sodium, and potassium
d. Phosphates, sulfates, and potassium

28. Mr. Evert continues to receive digoxin (Lanoxin) as ordered. A report of his electrolytes returns showing hypokalemia. The nurse should recognize that this is a (an)
   a. Typical finding in severe CHF, but no action is necessary
   b. Significant finding in severe CHF because it puts Mr. Evert at greater risk for digitalis toxicity
   c. Important abnormality because it demonstrates myocardial cell damage
   d. Typical finding expected when digitalis preparations are administered

29. In assessing Mr. Evert's cardiac sounds, the nurse would expect to hear which abnormal heart sound associated with congestive heart failure?
   a. Heart sound 1 (S_1)
   b. Heart sound 2 (S_2)
   c. Heart sound 3 (S_3)
   d. Heart sound 4 (S_4)

30. Mr. Evert has a chest AP x-ray. Chest x-ray can provide information relative to congestive heart failure, including
   a. Cardiac size and infiltrates in lungs
   b. Direct measures of cardiac output
   c. Visualization of cardiac valves
   d. Perfusion of coronary vessels

31. Mr. Evert has been prescribed digoxin (Lanoxin) 0.25 mg po qod on *odd* days and Lanoxin 0.125 mg po qod on *even* days. The nurse should recognize the physician's rationale for these orders to be that
   a. (An error has been made: the nurse should clarify the dosage with the physician)
   b. The variation of the dosage of digoxin (Lanoxin) is too small to make a difference for the client
   c. The appropriate maintenance dosage is achieved in this fashion based on urinary excretion rates
   d. The physician wants to provide emotional support for the client, by making him think he is getting two different medications

32. Mr. Evert is admitted to the CICU with severe left-sided congestive heart failure and early pulmonary edema. The nurse institutes the standing rotating-tourniquet order stat. Rotating tourniquets are used to
   a. Maintain circulation to the heart and other core structures
   b. Reduce arterial circulation to the extremities
   c. Reduce venous blood return to the heart
   d. Increase peripheral vascular resistance in the extremities to maintain adequate blood pressure

33. First-degree heart block is associated with
   a. Atrial depolarizations for each ventricular depolarization
   b. One atrial depolarization for each ventricular depolarization
   c. Prolonged PR intervals leading to eventual dropped ventricular response
   d. Ventricular depolarizations dissociated from atrial depolarization

34. Third-degree heart block is defined as
   a. Complete loss of the conduction link between the atrial depolarization and ventricular depolarization
   b. Complete loss of sinoatrial node impulse formation
   c. Complete loss of atrial ectopic impulse formation
   d. Complete nonresponsiveness of ventricles to ventricular ectopic impulse formation

35. Wilma Stone is admitted with third-degree heart block. The nurse should recognize which of the following?
   a. Intravenous digitalis preparations will be needed to correct the block
   b. Intravenous atropine must be administered to correct the block and slow the conduction through the AV node

c. A temporary or permanent pacemaker is the treatment of choice
d. Intravenous lidocaine bolus and continuous drip will improve escape rhythms of the ventricle

36. Janie Ward is an 11 year old admitted with a diagnosis of rheumatic heart disease. Rheumatic heart disease is associated with which of the following risk factors?
  a. Type A blood
  b. Urinary tract defects
  c. Obesity
  d. Recent infection with group A β-hemolytic streptococcal organisms

37. Signs and symptoms of rheumatic heart disease are *primarily* associated with
  a. Conduction abnormalities of the atria
  b. Conduction deficits of the ventricles
  c. Valvular deformities of the heart
  d. Thrombosis of one or more branches of the coronary artery system

38. (Questions 38 and 39 refer to this situation) Marge Wilson is admitted with pulmonary embolism. The most common source of emboli is
  a. Intramural thrombi of the left ventricle
  b. Thrombi from the bifurcation of the hypogastric or femoral arteries
  c. Thrombi from the bronchial veins
  d. Thrombi in the deep veins of the legs

39. Ms. Wilson is immediately started on continuous intravenous heparin therapy. While assessing the infusion; however, the nurse notices that the intravenous drip has infiltrated. The nurse should
  a. Restart the infusion again in a different site
  b. Restart the infusion and attempt to "catch up" the infusion to the amount that should already have been infused
  c. Restart the infusion and run the rate as ordered
  d. Call the physician to see if the infusion needs to be restarted

40. (Questions 40–42 refer to this situation) Karen Zimmer is admitted to the hospital after an automobile accident. Two chest tubes are positioned through the left chest wall. The main purpose of chest tubes is to
  a. Restore positive pressure to the intrapleural space
  b. Provide route for irrigation of pleural space
  c. Restore negative pressure to the intrapleural space
  d. Allow atmospheric pressure to enter the pleural space to equalize pressures

41. Ms. Zimmer's chest tubes are attached to underwater seal drainage bottles. The purpose of the water in the water seal drainage system is to
  a. Provide a sterile media to prevent bacterial growth
  b. Prevent bacteria from the chest drainage from entering the air
  c. Prevent air at atmospheric pressure from entering the chest tube system
  d. Establish the level of positive pressure in the chest tube system

42. While monitoring the client's water seal drainage system, the nurse notes that air bubbles rise continuously through the water. This occurs because
  a. Inspiration causes changes in air pressure in the system, which forces air out of the intrapleural space
  b. Exhalation causes changes in air pressure in the system, which forces air out of the intrapleural space
  c. The lung is totally reexpanded
  d. There is an air leak in the chest tube/water seal system

43. Tina Neff is a 28-year-old mail delivery driver with diagnosed Raynaud's phenomenon. Raynaud's phenomenon is associated with young women predominantly and is
  a. An inflammatory intravascular thrombotic disorder of the medium-sized veins of the lower extremities
  b. A problem of medial necrosis of the vein wall
  c. A chronically dilated venous channel

d. An episodic vasospastic disorder of small cutaneous arteries

44. Raynaud's phenomenon is associated with
   a. Ingestion of chemical allergens, for example, red food dye
   b. Amenorrhea or dysmenorrhea in young women
   c. Exposure of skin surfaces to low temperatures
   d. Latent symptoms from childhood scarlet fever

45. Of the following clients, which one should be referred to a physician for treatment for hypertension?
   a. A 40-year-old man with a blood pressure of 160/90, recorded during a one-stop shopping center screening
   b. A 51-year-old woman with four serial morning blood pressure readings of 140/89, 148/96, 144/94, and 150/90, who also reports headaches
   c. An 80-year-old woman with six serial weekly blood pressure readings between 150/85 and 162/89
   d. A 16-year-old boy with an initial blood pressure of 154/82 recorded at his sports physical examination

46. (Questions 46–49 refer to this situation) Mrs. Maxwell is watching her grandson's basketball game when she suddenly falls to the floor and lies inert, comatose, face flushed, and with cheeks puffing ipsilaterally on respiration. Priority nursing care is to
   a. Quickly gather a health history from her family
   b. Cover her and elevate her legs to prevent shock
   c. Loosen her clothing at neck and position her on her side
   d. Shake her, smell her breath for acetone, and give her caloric liquid

47. Mrs. Maxwell's physician diagnoses left intracerebral hemorrhagic CVA. Based on this medical diagnosis, the nurse should challenge which of the following medical orders?
   a. Methylprednisolone sodium succinate (Solu-Medrol) 15 mg IV q 6 hours
   b. Heparin 40 units/mL continuous IV drip
   c. Elevate head of bed 30°
   d. Phenytoin sodium (Dilantin) 300 mg IV at 50 mg/minute tid; then 100 mg IV q 8 hours

48. Mrs. Maxwell survives the acute phase of stroke and needs help adjusting to residual deficits resulting from her left intercerebral hemorrhagic CVA. Mrs. Maxwell is right-handed. All of the following nursing interventions are necessary *except*
   a. Providing passive range of motion exercises or teaching joint range of motion exercises, using unaffected limbs to move affected limbs
   b. Using an alphabet board or picture/words device to aid communication
   c. Teaching medication purpose, dose, schedule, side-effects, and interactions
   d. Teaching about a liquid diet to prevent swallowing difficulty

49. Mrs. Maxwell is placed on a post-stroke medication program that includes methyldopa (Aldomet). The primary therapeutic effect of Aldomet is
   a. Increased urinary output
   b. Decreased blood volume
   c. More stable blood vessel membranes
   d. More stable blood pressure at a lower level

50. (Questions 50–52 refer to this situation) Barbara Lease is receiving heparin hourly per continuous IV drip for diagnosed deep vein thrombosis in her left calf. Assessment of the effectiveness of heparin therapy is a nursing responsibility. Which of the following nursing measures is most appropriate for monitoring heparin therapy?
   a. Comparing and recording calf circumference measurements each shift

b. Monitoring the report of the prothrombin time
c. Monitoring calf pain on dorsiflexion in the affected leg (Homans' sign)
d. Teaching active range of motion exercises for the lower extremities

51. Ms. Lease continues on heparin therapy and begins coumarin (Coumadin) therapy as well. The nurse should teach Ms. Lease to avoid which of the following foods while on this regimen?
    a. Oranges, bananas, and plums
    b. Whole grain cereals and breads
    c. Lettuce, cabbage, and greens
    d. Beef and other red meats

52. Ms. Lease reports classic symptoms of deep vein thrombosis in her lower left leg. Application of local heat is ordered. In order to correctly apply local heat, the nurse should
    a. Palpate the affected leg veins for firmness and location
    b. Apply loosely an elastic bandage to affected leg from heel to groin
    c. Position the lower leg in a slightly dependent position to maintain arterial circulation
    d. Apply loosely a gauze dressing under the warming water circulation pad (K pad)

53. Debbie Short is preparing for home care of her left calf deep vein thrombosis. She is discharged on coumarin (Coumadin) 5 mg po daily. The most important information to teach Ms. Short about Coumadin therapy is that
    a. Headache and blurred vision are usual side-effects
    b. Diet and over-the-counter drugs do not alter the effects of coumarin (Coumadin) therapy
    c. Any bleeding should be reported immediately
    d. Hirsutism (unusual hair growth) is a transient side-effect

54. (Questions 54–56 refer to this situation) Ms. Forgey is 3 hours post right saphenous vein ligation and stripping. Appropriate nursing goals for Ms. Forgey's care include
    a. Maintaining firm elastic pressure evenly over the entire limb
    b. Maintaining the immobility of the operated limb for 8 hours
    c. Removing elastic dressing materials every 2 hours to assess for hemorrhage and swelling
    d. Maintaining the limb no higher than heart level to promote venous return

55. While preparing to discharge, Ms. Forgey states that she is worried about varicosities returning in the future because of her excess weight. Which of the following is the *most* appropriate response?
    a. "Ms. Forgey, the doctor was pleased with the results of your surgery."
    b. "Ms. Forgey, gradual weight reduction would help lessen the risk of future varicosities."
    c. "Ms. Forgey, you should not diet after surgery."
    d. "Ms. Forgey, there is nothing you can do to prevent varicosities."

56. Ms. Forgey is instructed to wear measured support stockings at home. Until her support stockings arrive, she will wear elastic wrapping. The most important principle for the nurse to teach her regarding application of elastic wrappings is that
    a. Brisk leg exercise should precede application of the wrap
    b. The toes and heel should be enclosed in the wrap
    c. Uniform pressure over the entire limb should result from the wrap
    d. The wrap should never terminate below the knee

57. Which of the following statements is *not* true regarding effective communication skills?
    a. The degree of both persons' involve-

ment in a relationship has a direct impact on the emotional tone
  b. An effective interpersonal relationship is one in which only positive interactions occur
  c. In an interpersonal relationship, a submissive person allows the other person to dominate
  d. Health professionals can improve the quality of their interactions by becoming more sensitive to the dynamics of communication
58. Inherent in the concept of care is
  a. Effective communication
  b. Being a good listener
  c. Telling clients what is important for them to know
  d. Communicating your feelings
59. Confrontation is best described as
  a. A way of asserting yourself
  b. Being aggressive when it is necessary
  c. The only way to handle a hostile client
  d. Fighting fire with fire
60. Mary Tate has just learned that the heartburn she has been experiencing at night is due to a hiatal hernia. When she asks for recommendations to alleviate heartburn, the nurse should suggest
  a. Sleeping on two pillows
  b. Placing 6-inch blocks under the head of the bed
  c. Taking antacids regularly
  d. Eating a snack at bedtime
61. The purpose of administering cimetidine preoperatively is to
  a. Decrease the volume of gastric secretions
  b. Decrease the pH of gastric secretions
  c. Reduce the amount of anesthetic needed
  d. Dispel the memory of unpleasant events associated with surgery
62. Following a partial gastrectomy, it is important to maintain patency of the NG tube in order to
  a. Assess characteristics of drainage at the anastomosis
  b. Delay peristalsis until initial healing takes place
  c. Remove stomach contents
  d. Assess the pH of gastric secretions
63. Alice Green is recovering from abdominal surgery. She persists in shouting for the nurse instead of using the call light, as she has been repeatedly asked to do. The other clients are disturbed by her shouting. Which of the following responses is most appropriate for the nurse to make?
  a. "Ms. Green, please stop shouting for me instead of using your light."
  b. "You must stop shouting, Ms. Green, because you are disturbing others."
  c. "Ms. Green, when you shout for me instead of using your light, I feel very frustrated because I want to take care of you as well as the other clients."
  d. "I'm sorry that I can't get to your room as soon as I'd like, Ms. Green. Please try to use the light instead of shouting for me."
64. Before administering medication to a client who will have an oral cholecystogram, the nurse should assess the client's condition for
  a. Adequate hydration
  b. Intolerance to fatty foods
  c. Diarrhea
  d. Allergy to iodine
65. Ellen Smith has taken six dye tablets in preparation for an oral cholecystogram tomorrow. Which of the following symptoms should be reported so the test can be rescheduled?
  a. Diarrhea
  b. Abdominal pain
  c. Temperature 99.6°
  d. Vomiting
66. Your client is experiencing abdominal pain 3 days after a cholecystectomy and states, "I feel like my stomach is going to

burst." After determining that her vital signs are stable and that the prn pain medication is not due for an hour, the nurse should
a. Call a physician
b. Tell the client to lie quietly in bed
c. Give the client a pillow to splint the abdomen
d. Assist the client to ambulate

67. To decrease the risk of colon cancer, appropriate dietary choices include
a. Organ meats and citrus fruits
b. Fried fish fillet, french fries, and asparagus
c. Baked chicken, broccoli, and apples
d. Roast beef, mashed potatoes, and peas

68. Which of the following would be appropriate menu choices for a client being discharged following a hemorrhoidectomy?
a. Meat loaf, boiled potatoes, and apple sauce
b. Peanut butter and jelly on white bread
c. Cottage cheese and canned peaches
d. Shredded wheat cereal and one half grapefruit

69. When a client experiences pain the day after a hemorrhoidectomy, an appropriate intervention would be
a. Giving the client a sitz bath
b. Turning the client on his or her side
c. Providing a "donut" to sit on
d. Having the client lie on his or her stomach

70. In the early postoperative period following a hemorrhoidectomy, the client may
a. Become dehydrated
b. Develop paralytic ileus
c. Have difficulty voiding
d. Develop pneumonia

71. When giving cleansing enemas, the nurse should
a. Temporarily stop solution flow if cramping occurs
b. Instruct the client to retain the solution for 30 minutes
c. Position the client on his or her right side
d. Insert the rectal tube 6 inches

72. (Questions 72–74 refer to this situation) Tina King, age 23, has symptoms of hepatitis, causative agent as yet undetermined. She may exhibit all of the following symptoms *except*
a. Mahogany colored urine
b. Clay colored stools
c. Lethargy
d. Insatiable thirst

73. Nursing measures for Ms. King would include
a. Wearing mask, gown, and gloves during direct client contact
b. Placing contaminated needles and syringes in plastic bags
c. Special handling of the client's eating utensils
d. Administering immune human serum globulin

74. Ms. King's cholestyramine has been effective if her
a. Temperature comes down
b. Itching is relieved
c. Nausea subsides
d. Pain decreases

75. (Questions 75–78 refer to this situation) Larry Jones is admitted with a diagnosis of cirrhosis. He has ascites and is receiving an infusion of salt-poor albumin. He complains that he is feeling short of breath. The nurse's *first* nursing action should be to
a. Stop the infusion
b. Observe for head of the bed elevation
c. Slow the infusion
d. Check his vital signs

76. After Mr. Jones' liver biopsy, the nurse should instruct him to
a. Lie quietly on his back for an hour
b. Remain npo for 4 hours
c. Force fluids

d. Report feelings of dampness on the sheets beneath him

77. To prepare Mr. Jones for paracentesis, the nurse should
    a. Raise the bed to mid-Fowler's position
    b. Have him empty his bladder
    c. Administer enemas until the excretion is clear
    d. Keep him npo

78. Upon Mr. Jones' discharge from the hospital, the nurse knows that client teaching has been successful if he states that
    a. He should report restlessness, insomnia, and loss of motor coordination to the physician
    b. He can eat poultry and fish but should avoid red meats
    c. He can skip one dose of lactulose if he experiences diarrhea
    d. He should take nothing stronger than ASA or acetaminophen (Tylenol) for headache

79. Norma Hall, a client with diabetes, received 20 units of lente Insulin at 7:30 a.m. She is most likely to become hypoglycemic at
    a. 10:00 a.m.
    b. 12:00 noon
    c. 4:00 p.m.
    d. 10:00 p.m.

80. (Questions 80–82 refer to this situation) Tim Gregory, age 16, is a client with newly diagnosed diabetes. He is an avid tennis player and is popular among his friends. He is afraid that his diabetes will make his friends think of him as "different" and less socially acceptable. The nurse should tell him that
    a. Playing tennis will increase his insulin requirements, but a less strenuous sport could be substituted
    b. He can continue to play tennis if he wears shoes designed to protect the wearer against foot injuries
    c. He can continue his activities as before and learn to regulate his insulin dosage each day based on his blood sugar readings
    d. His diet and insulin can be regulated so that he can continue his previous activities with some modifications

81. Tim can accept invitations to eat out with his friends if he
    a. Orders salad without dressing and drinks sugar-free beverages
    b. Avoids desserts
    c. Understands and applies the ADA exchange system
    d. Omits his bedtime snack for that day

82. Tim complains of feeling nervous and hungry. There are beads of perspiration on his forehead. The nurse should
    a. Have him drink 4 ounces of orange juice
    b. Check his urine for glucose and acetone
    c. Suspect that his insulin dose has been decreased
    d. Tell him these symptoms are not unusual and will subside shortly

83. Kussmaul respirations in a client with diabetes
    a. Are an attempt by the body to correct an acid-base imbalance
    b. Indicate hypoglycemia
    c. Indicate cerebral anoxia
    d. Are among the major diagnostic findings associated with diabetes

84. Edith Smith, a 45-year-old client with newly diagnosed diabetes, is told by her physician that she must watch her diet carefully in order to control her health problems. The nurse plans to assist Ms. Smith in changing her diet habits. Which of the following statements is *least* accurate regarding behavior change?
    a. Ms. Smith will change her eating habits if the nurse provides her with accurate and understandable written information
    b. The nurse and Ms. Smith should define and solve the problem together

c. Ms. Smith's beliefs, values, and behavior will influence her ability to make effective changes in her eating patterns
d. Ms. Smith will probably have difficulty changing her present eating habits regardless of what the nurse tells her

85. Clients with pernicious anemia should comply with the treatment regimen prescribed by the physician to avoid
    a. Loss of intrinsic factor
    b. Liver dysfunction
    c. Permanent neurological damage
    d. The need to receive injections of vitamin B_{12} for the remainder of their lives

86. Which of the following is contraindicated for clients with severely depressed WBCs and platelets?
    a. Visitors under age 5
    b. Taking of rectal temperatures
    c. Applying electric heating pads
    d. Bathroom privileges

87. To obtain an accurate CVP reading, the nurse should
    a. Take the reading when the water level on the manometer is at its lowest level during fluctuations with respiration
    b. Take readings with the client in sitting and reclining positions and average the results
    c. Make certain that the zero point on the manometer is at the level of the 4th intercostal space in the midaxillary line
    d. Make certain that the client is lying flat in bed

88. Accuracy in CVP readings is important because the readings
    a. Reflect cardiac output
    b. Directly measure the blood pressure
    c. Reveal the degree of pulmonary resistance
    d. Provide guidance to the physician in determining the amount of fluids needed for replacement

89. (Questions 89–92 refer to this situation) Carl Struthers suffered a ruptured spleen as a result of an auto accident and is scheduled to undergo a splenectomy. He is to receive meperidine (Demerol) 75 mg and atropine 0.7 mg on call to the OR. The vial of atropine is marked 1/120 grain per mL. How much atropine should the nurse administer?
    a. 0.5 mL
    b. 1.0 mL
    c. 1.4 mL
    d. 2 mL

90. While Mr. Struthers is in the recovery room following his splenectomy, the nurse should
    a. Monitor his vital signs every hour
    b. Measure his urine output every hour
    c. Raise the head of the bed if he becomes restless
    d. Run the IV fluids at a keep-open rate

91. In the immediate postoperative period, which of the following may indicate cerebral hypoxia?
    a. BP 100/60
    b. Pulse 110
    c. Projectile vomiting
    d. Restlessness

92. Prior to discharge Mr. Struthers should understand that
    a. No alteration in his health maintenance habits is necessary, because other organs can assume the functions of the spleen
    b. He may need to receive vitamin injections of B_{12} for about 6 months
    c. He is at increased risk of pneumococcal infections and should be immunized accordingly
    d. It is not unusual for a client to develop an intolerance to fatty foods after a splenectomy

93. First-aid treatment for burns includes
    a. Application of ice to the burned area
    b. Flushing the burned area with cool water

c. Application of Vaseline to the burned area
d. Removal of adherent clothing from the burned area

94. Ben Ferris sustained third-degree burns on his legs while he was burning leaves. In the ER the nurse should anticipate an order for
   a. Respiratory therapy
   b. Jobst stockings
   c. Tetanus prophylaxis
   d. Cortisone ointment application to the burned area

95. Plasmanate is administered to clients with severe burn injuries for the purpose of
   a. Expanding circulating blood volume
   b. Preventing infection
   c. Supplying clotting factors
   d. Providing electrolytes

96. The most appropriate foods for a client recovering from second- and third-degree burns would be
   a. Chicken and dumplings
   b. Macaroni and cheese
   c. Liver and spinach
   d. Fish and legumes

97. (Questions 97–99 refer to this situation) Mike Reardon has acute pancreatitis. Which of the following medical orders should the nurse question?
   a. Administer TPN at 125 mL per hour
   b. Keep the client npo
   c. Administer morphine 10 mg every 3 to 4 hours prn for pain
   d. Connect the NG tube at low constant suction

98. Mr. Reardon complains of an extremely dry mouth. The nurse should
   a. Provide lemon and glycerin swabs to relieve the dryness
   b. Give him ice chips in limited amounts
   c. Explain that this symptom is a side-effect of his medication
   d. Have him rinse his mouth with clear water

99. Mr. Reardon's TPN is to infuse at 125 mL per hour. The infusion equipment will deliver 15 gtts per mL. The nurse should set the drip rate at
   a. 32 gtts/min
   b. 125 gtts/min
   c. 60 gtts/min
   d. 50 gtts/min

100. (Questions 100 and 101 refer to this situation) Leona Thomas has just returned to the unit after undergoing a subtotal thyroidectomy for goiter. Which of the following medications should be kept at the bedside?
   a. Calcium gluconate
   b. Sodium levothyroxine (Synthroid)
   c. Potassium chloride
   d. Aminophylline

101. In monitoring Ms. Thomas for bleeding, the nurse should check the
   a. Dressing for bright red drainage
   b. Serum hematocrit every 6 hours
   c. Sheets under the patient's neck
   d. Blood pressure and pulse every shift

102. All of the following are appropriate precautions for a client experiencing exophthalmos *except*
   a. Wearing protective glasses while outside
   b. Avoiding watching TV for more than 1 hour at a time
   c. Sleeping with the head elevated
   d. Having the eyelids taped shut at night

103. Angela Bone is admitted to the hospital for a total hip replacement. She has been on prednisone therapy daily for the past 2 years for treatment of rheumatoid arthritis. Prior to surgery the nurse should be sure that
   a. Extra doses of cortisone have been ordered
   b. The dosage of prednisone has been cut in half
   c. The client discontinued prednisone therapy for at least 3 days prior to surgery

    d. Ms. Bone receives her regular daily dose of prednisone

104. Preoperative care for a client who will have a colon resection should include
  a. Shaving the abdomen the night before surgery
  b. Hexachlorophene scrubs of the operative site
  c. Maintaining npo status for 24 hours prior to surgery
  d. Administering IV antibiotics

105. (Questions 105–106 refer to this situation) Kevin McPherson underwent a resection of the sigmoid colon 3 days ago. He asks when he can have something to drink. The client's physician is likely to allow clear liquids when
  a. The client can expel flatus
  b. The client's gas pains subside
  c. The client's nausea subsides
  d. The NG tube is removed

106. Mr. McPherson will be ready to learn how to adjust to the effects of his colostomy when he
  a. Begins to expel fecal material
  b. Is ready to be discharged home
  c. Can cope with looking at his stoma
  d. Is able to get up and move around

107. A client is being discharged after treatment for diverticulitis. The nurse's client teaching has been successful if the client states
  a. "I should drink at least eight glasses of water per day."
  b. "From now on, I should avoid uncooked cereals and vegetables."
  c. "I should take a laxative on days that I do not have a bowel movement."
  d. "The next time I travel outside the U.S., I will not drink water unless it has been boiled."

108. A client with Crohn's disease is likely to experience
  a. Malnutrition
  b. Respiratory infections
  c. Periods of immobility
  d. Chronic constipation

109. Stan Allen is a 32-year-old man whose lymph node biopsy revealed Hodgkin's disease. CT scans confirmed enlarged nodes present on both sides of the diaphragm. The physician has explained the chemotherapy treatment regimen to Mr. Allen, but he asks the nurse for clarification. The nurse should explain
  a. The drugs used to treat Hodgkin's disease rarely cause severe side-effects
  b. The purpose of chemotherapy and its potential severe side-effects
  c. Chemotherapy has no permanent effect on fertility
  d. The treatment is likely to be curative since the disease was diagnosed early

110. Anna Hunt has been feeling nervous lately and has lost 10 pounds over the last 2 months. She complains of feeling hot when others in a room seem to feel comfortable. She should see her physician because these are symptoms of
  a. A malignant condition
  b. Addison's disease
  c. Hyperthyroidism
  d. Diabetes

111. Which of the following symptoms should be medically evaluated as quickly as possible?
  a. A painful mouth lesion
  b. A weight loss of 10 pounds over 2 months
  c. An enlarged, painless axillary lymph node
  d. Menstrual irregularities

112. Client teaching of parents of children with sickle cell disease should include stressing the importance of
  a. A diet high in iron and vitamin C
  b. Restricting participation in physical education and sports
  c. Blood transfusions
  d. Maintaining a high fluid intake

113. (Questions 113–117 refer to this situation) Donna North is a 66-year-old woman recently admitted to a community hospital for evaluation and treatment of glaucoma. Which of the following signs and symptoms would you expect Mrs. North to experience?
    a. Loss of peripheral vision
    b. Color blindness
    c. Photophobia
    d. Ptosis
114. The most common diagnostic test for assessment of intraocular pressure in glaucoma is the
    a. Visual fields examination
    b. Pupillary reflex examination
    c. Ophthalmoscopic examination
    d. Tonometer examination
115. Mrs. North is to receive eye medication in both eyes for the treatment of glaucoma. The nurse should instruct Ms. North to
    a. Spread her eyelids apart and instill the drops in the center of each eye
    b. Instill the drops at the inner area of each eye
    c. Instill the drops in a "pouch" of the lower lid of each eye
    d. Instill the drops at the outer area of each eye
116. The ophthalmic solution Mrs. North is receiving is pilocarpine. The therapeutic effect of pilocarpine is to
    a. Reduce intraocular pressure
    b. Decrease pupillary constriction
    c. Decrease the production of aqueous humor
    d. Increase the blood flow to the damaged retina
117. Client teaching is an important part of Mrs. North's care. Which of the following statements is an essential component of the nurse's teaching plan?
    a. "Decrease your fluid intake."
    b. "Report any eye pain to your physician."
    c. "Maintain a low-sodium diet."
    d. "Wear darkened glasses at all times."
118. (Questions 118–122 refer to this situation) Jake Walters, a 23-year-old white man, is admitted to the hospital with a head injury and possible temporal skull fracture he sustained in a motorcycle accident. Upon admission he was conscious but lethargic; vital signs were temperature 99°F, pulse 100, respirations 18, BP 140/70. Primary neurological nursing assessments should focus on the potential for increased intracranial pressure. Which of the following is an indicator of increased intracranial pressure?
    a. Decreasing urinary output, decreasing blood pressure
    b. Changing level of consciousness, widening pulse pressure
    c. Bulging eyeballs, decreasing pulse pressure
    d. Increasing cranial bleeding, increasing pulse
119. A nursing intervention to prevent further increases in intracranial pressure is
    a. Position the client on his side
    b. Position the client flat with a 90° angle at the knees
    c. Position the client with the head of the bed flat
    d. Position the client with the head of the bed at a 30–45° angle
120. While assisting Mr. Walters into bed, the nurse notices a clear substance exuding from his nose. Which of the following interventions should the nurse perform?
    a. Testing the drainage for the presence of glucose
    b. Packing his nose with sterile gauze
    c. Suctioning his nose and mouth
    d. Instructing Mr. Jake to blow his nose
121. Mr. Walters is at risk for developing posttraumatic seizures. Which of the following nursing interventions should be instituted?

a. Placement of an NG tube to prevent aspiration
b. Adjusting the bed to a low position and placing a padded tongue blade by the bedside
c. Moving the client to a room near the nurses' station and placing a tracheotomy set by the bedside
d. Adjusting the bed to a low position and wrapping the client's head with gauze to prevent injury

122. Mr. Walters is receiving multiple medications for his condition. One of the medications is dexamethasone (Decadron). The major therapeutic effect of this drug is to
a. Promote vasodilation of the blood vessels in the brain
b. Prevent the formation of blood clots in the brain
c. Decrease cerebral edema
d. Increase venous drainage

123. Which of the following scales assists the nurse in evaluating a client's neurological status in response to medical and nursing therapy?
a. Neurological scale
b. Consciousness rating
c. Motor/sensory sensitivity scale
d. Glasgow Coma Scale

124. Joyce Carson has diagnosed rheumatoid arthritis. Her physician has prescribed aspirin 600 mg every 4 hours. As part of the nurse's client teaching, Ms. Carson should be advised of which of the following precautions?
a. To avoid driving until the dosage effect is established
b. To take the medication with food, milk, or antacid
c. To report any dermatitis or lesions occurring in her mouth to her physician
d. To take the medication on an empty stomach to avoid delay in absorption

125. (Questions 125–128 refer to this situation) Jenny Kay is a 60-year-old, 200-pound, 5-foot 4-inch woman, who was admitted to a community hospital for evaluation of joint pain. Upon examination, a diagnosis of osteoarthritis was made. In performing a physical assessment of Mrs. Kay's condition, the nurse should expect to find which of the following signs and symptoms in the joints of her affected hands?
a. Pain, swelling, redness, and warmth
b. Pain, asymmetry of joints, and warmth
c. Pain, stiffness, and Heberden's nodes
d. Pain, stiffness, deformities, and redness

126. Further nursing assessment of Mrs. Kay's condition should concentrate on
a. The pelvic joints
b. The weight-bearing joints of the lower extremities
c. The joints of the shoulder and the elbows
d. The joints of the cervical and thoracic vertebrae

127. Mrs. Kay is experiencing pain in the joints of her hands. To relieve the pain and make the client comfortable, the nurse should
a. Provide a heat pack as prescribed
b. Encourage activity to lessen rigidity of the joints
c. Encourage active range of motion in the joints
d. Provide hand splints to restrict movement of the joints

128. Client teaching for Mrs. Kay includes education regarding her diet and nutritional state. Which of the following statements reflects the information necessary to help Mrs. Kay maintain a healthy nutritional status?
a. "You need to have six or seven small meals per day."
b. "You need to eat a well-balanced, low-calorie diet."

c. "You need to increase your consumption of red meat."
d. "You need to eat a low-protein, low-carbohydrate diet."

129. (Questions 129–131 refer to this situation) Dave McDermott, a 69-year-old man, has been a heavy smoker and drinker for the past 50 years. His physician has recently confirmed a diagnosis of tumor of the larynx. He is to undergo a laryngectomy in the morning. Which of the following postoperative nursing observations will be most important?
    a. Monitoring for cranial nerve damage and bleeding
    b. Monitoring for edema and peristaltic waves
    c. Assessing the urinary output and bleeding
    d. Monitoring for bleeding and subcutaneous emphysema

130. Upon his return from surgery, the most suitable position for Mr. McDermott is
    a. Bed flat, client positioned on his right or left side
    b. Bed flat, client positioned supine
    c. Head of bed at 30° angle, client positioned supine
    d. Foot of the bed elevated at 15° angle, client positioned supine

131. The physician has inserted an NG tube in the client, and has ordered tube feedings to begin later in the week. The reason for placing the NG tube is
    a. To prevent aspiration
    b. To prevent laryngeal edema and spasms
    c. To prevent contamination of the suture line
    d. To prevent the formation of subcutaneous emphysema

132. (Questions 132–135 refer to this situation) Al Foster is a 35-year-old black man with insulin-dependent diabetes, hypertension, and arterosclerotic heart disease. He has been admitted to the hospital for a diagnostic work up for "gouty arthritis." Gout differs from other diseases of the joints in a number of ways. Which of the following signs or symptoms is more diagnostic of gout than of any other disease of the joints?
    a. No pain in affected joint upon palpation
    b. Pain usually occurs in the joint of the great toe
    c. Swan neck deformities in affected joints
    d. Appearance of nodules in affected joints of the toes

133. A variety of diagnostic tests are performed on Mr. Foster. Which of the following test results is most diagnostic of gout?
    a. Increased sedimentation rate, increased serum uric acid level
    b. Decreased sedimentation rate, increased serum calcium level
    c. Increased sedimentation rate, increased serum sodium level
    d. Decreased sedimentation rate, increased serum potassium level

134. The nurse, in consultation with the dietician, is planning an appropriate diet for Mr. Foster. Which of the following foods should be restricted in his diet?
    a. Red meats, carrots, onions
    b. Chicken, beans, mushrooms
    c. Shellfish, roe, sardines
    d. Pork, tomatoes, peppers

135. In evaluating client teaching with Mr. Foster, the nurse knows he or she has succeeded in communicating important drug therapy information when Mr. Foster states
    a. "I will refrain from taking antihistamines while on my medications."
    b. "I will refrain from taking aspirin while on my medications."
    c. "I will avoid people with active infectious processes."
    d. "I will limit my fluid consumption during the evening."

136. (Questions 136–139 refer to this situation) Lydia Diaz is a 57-year-old Hispanic woman admitted to the hospital complaining of severe headaches. She is scheduled for a variety of diagnostic tests in the morning. Her physician diagnoses her complaint as a rule-out pituitary adenoma (brain tumor). On admission her vital signs are temperature 98°F, pulse 70, respirations 12, and BP 130/74. She is alert and oriented but does not understand why she is in the hospital. Ms. Diaz does not understand why her physician reached his diagnosis. The nurse continues to question Ms. Diaz regarding her health status. The physician's tentative diagnosis of a dysfunction/tumor of the pituitary gland was based on the client's symptoms of
    a. Visual disturbances, pulsating frontal headaches
    b. Frontal headaches, dysfunctions of the adrenal glands
    c. Visual disturbances, thyroid disturbances
    d. Bulging eyeballs, personality changes

137. Following an extensive diagnostic workup, Ms. Diaz undergoes surgery to remove the adenoma. Postoperatively, the nurse must be alert for
    a. A decrease in temperature
    b. Leakage of cerebrospinal fluid
    c. An increase in mental alertness
    d. An increase in urine output

138. Ms. Diaz is placed on a variety of medications to prevent an increase in intracranial pressure. Which of the following signs would indicate that the medications are probably producing the appropriate effect?
    a. A decrease in urine specific gravity
    b. An increase in urine specific gravity
    c. A decrease in respirations
    d. A decrease in blood pressure

139. Postoperatively, Ms. Diaz is experiencing a great deal of "dull, constant, aching pain." The nurse contacts the physician, who orders a drug to help relieve the pain. Which of the following drug orders should the nurse question?
    a. Acetaminophen (Tylenol) 10 grains po every 3 to 4 hours prn pain
    b. Morphine sulfate 1 mg every 3 to 4 hours prn pain
    c. Propoxyphene (Darvocet) 1 or 2 tablets po every 3 to 4 hours prn pain
    d. Acetaminophen elixir 1 to 2 teaspoons every 3 to 4 hours prn pain

140. When assessing a client with possible aseptic meningitis, the nurse should be alert for which of the following as a sign of meningeal irritation?
    a. Projectile vomiting
    b. Pulsating frontal headaches
    c. Nuchal rigidity
    d. Photophobia

141. Which of the following nursing strategies should be implemented with a client with aseptic meningitis?
    a. Placing the client in respiratory isolation
    b. Taking precautionary measures to limit contact with the client's blood and body fluids
    c. Placing the client in reverse isolation
    d. Raising the head of the bed

142. (Questions 142–144 refer to this situation) Mickey Brown has been diagnosed with a convulsive disorder as a sequela to a head injury he sustained some years ago. The frequency and intensity of his seizures have increased in the past few weeks, prompting him to seek medical attention. His seizures are of a generalized nature. The nurse is assessing Mr. Brown's condition and having a pleasant conversation with him when he suddenly asks if there are always strange odors in the hospital. The nurse asks him to describe the odor, when he begins to enter the tonic-clonic phase of his seizure. What

other signs should the nurse look for to define the origin of the seizure?
a. Automatisms
b. Spread of seizure activity
c. Asymmetry of body movements
d. Level of consciousness

143. Mr. Brown's physician has arranged for him to undergo extensive diagnostic testing. He is scheduled for an electroencephalogram (EEG) in the morning. Mr. Brown asks the nurse to explain to him why this test is necessary. Which of the following responses best answers the question?
a. "An EEG indicates lack of increased brain activity."
b. "An EEG indicates to your physician the best way to treat your seizures."
c. "An EEG indicates the presence of scar tissue in the brain."
d. "An EEG indicates brain wave activity in various parts of your brain."

144. Which of the following information should be included in the nurse's teaching plan for Mr. Brown?
a. To avoid water sports
b. To avoid over-the-counter antihistamines
c. To understand his medical inability to drive a motor vehicle
d. The necessity for carrying a "bite block"

145. Nursing care of a client with Parkinson's disease includes a cooperative effort of the nurse and the physical therapy team aimed at assisting the client to perform the prescribed exercises. Indications that the exercises have been helpful include
a. Increased circulation to hands and feet
b. Increased range of motion
c. Decreased muscle rigidity
d. Decreased disequilibrium

146. A client is undergoing an edrophonium chloride (Tensilon) test to confirm a diagnosis of myasthenia gravis. Which of the following responses indicates a positive Tensilon test reaction?
a. An increase in signs and symptoms of myasthenia gravis
b. A decrease in amount of pain experienced
c. A decrease in signs and symptoms of myasthenia gravis
d. An increase in amount of pain experienced

147. The client with myasthenia gravis is scheduled for minor surgery in the morning. The nurse is aware that increased stress enhances the severity of symptoms of myasthenia. Which of the following vital signs is crucial for the nurse to measure?
a. Temperature
b. Blood pressure
c. Pulse
d. Respirations

148. The nurse is dispensing medications on the nursing unit. All medications are ordered for 8:00 a.m. It is now 8:00 a.m. and there are still 15 clients who must receive medications. The nurse should first administer medications to
a. A client with myasthenia gravis
b. A client with a convulsive disorder
c. A client with meningitis
d. A client with a cerebrovascular accident

149. (Questions 149–150 refer to this situation) Cathy Wallace is a 23-year-old client with multiple sclerosis. The nurse planning her care decides to place all the items she needs within easy reach. The nurse's reason for doing this is
a. To reduce her intention tremors
b. To reduce her activity and provide rest
c. To encourage her independence
d. To assist her in ADL despite blurred vision

150. The nurse is evaluating Ms. Wallace's understanding of what she has been taught.

Teaching has been successful if Ms. Wallace states
  a. "I am planning to eat a diet low in fiber and fat."
  b. "I will exercise regularly and schedule regular rest periods."
  c. "I understand that there is no muscle atrophy with this disease."
  d. "I will take my prescribed medications exactly on time."

151. (Questions 151–152 refer to this situation) Raymond Johns is a 19-year-old man who suffered a cervical spine injury while playing football earlier in the afternoon. His spine was stabilized and an IV of D_5 1/2 N/S was begun in his left hand. IV methylprednisolone sodium succinate (Solu-medrol) was also ordered. A #16 French Foley catheter was anchored. The physician will insert Crutchfield tongs several hours later. The nurse's assessment of Mr. Johns's condition is of the utmost importance during the acute phase of his cervical spine injury. Which of the following assessments is the most critical in the acute phase?
  a. The presence or lack of pain below the injury
  b. The absence of perspiration below the level of injury
  c. Any blood pressure changes
  d. The respiratory pattern

152. Crutchfield tongs have been inserted by the physician, and 10 pounds of cervical traction have been applied to the client. Which of the following nursing strategies will help to maintain skeletal traction?
  a. Maintaining body alignment
  b. Checking the patency of the Foley catheter
  c. Turning off the IV infusion
  d. Waiting 10 minutes and rechecking the client's vital signs

153. (Questions 153–156 refer to this situation) Georgia Davis is a frail, 78-year-old grandmother of 10. She was babysitting yesterday and slipped on a toy left on the floor by one of her grandchildren, and fractured her right hip. Mrs. Davis, who lives alone in her two-storey house, frequently babysits her grandchildren. Her son is very distraught and feels guilty about the accident. He has stated his intention to remain with his mother throughout the night. Which of the following symptoms indicates that Mrs. Davis's hip was fractured?
  a. The affected hip is abducted and internally rotated
  b. The affected hip is adducted and externally rotated
  c. The affected hip is adducted and internally rotated
  d. The affected hip is abducted and externally rotated

154. To help correct the above problem, the physician orders implementation of
  a. Buck's extension
  b. Balkan traction
  c. Russell traction
  d. Robert's extension

155. Postsurgery nursing measures for Mrs. Davis are numerous. Which of the following nursing strategies should be instituted to prevent postoperative complications?
  a. Providing trochanter rolls to maintain external rotation
  b. Regular monitoring of neurovascular function
  c. Providing ROM exercises to affected extremities
  d. Monitoring the client's elimination pattern

156. Mrs. Davis will soon be discharged from the hospital. Which of the following factors needs to be evaluated prior to discharging her to her own home?
  a. Her degree of independence in ADL

b. The degree of mobility in her affected hip
c. The degree of mobility in her unaffected hip
d. Her expertise in self-catheterization

157. (Questions 157–158 refer to this situation) Ed Connell has bilateral cataracts. He is to have his (R) cataract (lens) surgically removed in the morning. Which classification of eye drops would be appropriate for the physician to prescribe preoperatively?
    a. Mydriatics
    b. Miotics
    c. Ophthalmic
    d. Photo-ophthalmic

158. Following the removal of the cataract, Mr. Connell is discharged. Before leaving, he repeats some of his discharge instructions to the nurse to illustrate his understanding of them. Which of the following instructions is most correct?
    a. Avoid sexual relations for 6–8 weeks
    b. Avoid salty foods
    c. Avoid dark rooms
    d. Avoid the Valsalva maneuver

159. (Questions 159–160 refer to this situation) Which of the following drugs would most likely be prescribed for a client with Meniere's syndrome?
    a. Anticonvulsants
    b. Antivertiginous agents
    c. Antibiotics
    d. Cholinergics

160. The nurse encourages the client with Meniere's syndrome to maintain an appropriate diet. Which of the following food choices indicates the client's understanding of dietary guidelines suggested by the nurse?
    a. Fish
    b. American cheese
    c. Unsalted popcorn
    d. Chicken teriyaki

161. (Questions 161–164 refer to this situation) Julie Smith is a 41-year-old white woman admitted to a community hospital complaining of progressive loss of vision. Her admitting diagnosis is detached retina. Which of the following signs or symptoms revealed during the nursing assessment also relates to a detached retina?
    a. Extreme pain behind the bulbus oculi and photosensitivity
    b. Blind spots and flashes of light
    c. Redness of bulbus oculi and nystagmus
    d. Lack of pupil accommodation and aching

162. So as not to disturb Ms. Smith's bedrest, the nurse encourages the client to use the call light if she needs assistance. Which of the following strategies is also necessary to prevent injury or trauma to the client?
    a. Keeping the head of bed in a flat position
    b. Having the client lie on the unaffected side
    c. Having the client lie on the affected side
    d. Having the client maintain her head in a neutral position

163. The physician applies bilateral eye patches preoperatively to prevent further retinal detachment. Which of the following nursing strategies would be most useful in preventing further injury?
    a. Placing the client in a brightly lit room
    b. Adjusting the bed to a low position and raising the side rails
    c. Placing the client in a room near the nurses' station
    d. Placing the client in a dark room

164. Ms. Smith has undergone surgery to repair the retinal damage. She has suffered no complications and is to be discharged shortly. Client teaching has been successful if Ms. Smith remembers which of the following points?
    a. "No water sports"
    b. "No beverages containing caffeine."

c. "No warm compresses to the affected eye."
d. "No heavy lifting or active sports for 6 weeks."

165. Nurse A asks Nurse B to administer a pain-relieving injection to Nurse A's client, because Nurse A thinks that the client does not like Nurse A. Which of the following responses from Nurse B is most appropriate to promote behavioral change in Nurse A?
    a. "OK. He doesn't give me any problems."
    b. "I'd like to, but I'm behind on my meds."
    c. "Let me see if I can first finish two dressing changes."
    d. "I'd like to help, but I think it is important for you to deal with him. He's done this to others because he has been allowed to."

166. (Questions 166–171 refer to this situation) Sharon Bloom is a 43-year-old woman who has been an insulin-dependent diabetic for more than 30 years. She has had a number of health problems related to her diabetes, including glaucoma, hypertension, and an amputation of her right foot because of gangrene. During the past 6 months, she has had multiple recurrent urinary tract infections. Her physician admitted her to the hospital last evening with a tentative diagnosis of acute renal failure.

    The physician has ordered that Ms. Bloom have an indwelling catheter inserted. Given the client's diagnosis, the nurse assessing Ms. Bloom's I and O might expect to see which of the following conditions?
    a. Increased urinary output
    b. Increased sediment in the urine
    c. Hematuria
    d. Decreased urinary output

167. Ms. Bloom has exhibited increasing mental confusion over the past several shifts. Because the client's glucose level has remained within normal limits, the nurse is confident that her confusion is due to uremia. Which of the following laboratory tests may confirm the nurse's suspicion?
    a. BUN determination
    b. Creatinine kinase determination
    c. Coagulation studies
    d. Electrolyte studies

168. Both the nurse and the physician are concerned about fluid retention in Ms. Bloom. Which of the following nursing measures provides the best indication of changes in fluid status?
    a. Measuring urine specific gravity
    b. Assessing for peripheral edema
    c. Obtaining daily weights
    d. Assessing respiratory status

169. Mrs. Bloom's fluid intake has been restricted, and sodium polystyrene sulfonate (Kayexalate) enemas have been ordered. Because of the potential for electrolyte imbalances accompanying these measures, which of the following is a vital nursing measure?
    a. Assessing for cardiac arrhythmias
    b. Assessing for muscle pain and cramping
    c. Assessing for dry mucous membranes
    d. Assessing for orthostatic hypotension

170. The nurse who is preparing a care plan for Ms. Bloom understands that nutrition therapy is an integral part of therapy for acute renal failure, and consults with the dietician to plan a diet for Ms. Bloom. Which of the following diets would be appropriate?
    a. Low fat, low carbohydrate
    b. High protein, high carbohydrate
    c. High carbohydrate, high fat
    d. Low-protein, low carbohydrate

171. The nurse is evaluating the client teaching provided to Ms. Bloom. Which of the following statements indicates that client teaching is successful and that Ms. Bloom

understands and can incorporate the important points about her diet?
   a. "I will stay away from eating popcorn, potato chips, and pretzels."
   b. "I will not eat any more red meat, only white meat."
   c. "I will eat more leafy green vegetables and less fresh fruit."
   d. "I will decrease my consumption of red meat, but increase my consumption of cheese."

172. (Questions 172–174 refer to this situation) Amy Forrest was admitted to the hospital complaining of "severe left flank pain." Her admitting diagnosis is renal calculi. Ms. Forrest states that the pain is becoming increasingly severe. The nurse administers the pain-relieving medication prescribed by the physician. Which of the following strategies is also important in Ms. Forrest's nursing care plan?
   a. Restrict fluid intake during the night shift
   b. Encourage a diet with few acid-producing foods
   c. Strain all her urine
   d. Place her in a high-Fowler's position

173. In assessing Ms. Forrest's physical condition, the nurse should not be surprised to see which of the following physical symptoms?
   a. Abdominal distention
   b. Periorbital edema
   c. Clubbed fingers
   d. Periorbital ecchymosis

174. To further ascertain a definitive diagnosis of Ms. Forrest's symptoms, the physician would order which of the following diagnostic tests?
   a. Retinal arteriography
   b. Intravenous pyelogram
   c. Cystograms
   d. Urine cultures and sensitivity tests

175. The nurse is evaluating the client teaching Steve Donovan received regarding his glomerulonephritis medications. Which of the following statements reflects Mr. Donovan's understanding of the important points about his medications?
   a. "I will take my antibiotic until I'm told to stop."
   b. "I will drink plenty of fluids to wash the medicine out."
   c. "I will take my pulse prior to taking my medicines."
   d. "I will take my medications with carbonated beverages."

176. (Questions 176–178 refer to this situation) Sheila Joyce has been rehospitalized with a diagnosis of cystitis. This is her third admission for cystitis in a relatively short period of time. In planning nursing care for Ms. Joyce, the nurse must consider the importance of
   a. Encouraging bed rest
   b. Straining all her urine
   c. Discussing self-care hygiene practices
   d. Explaining the necessary fluid restrictions

177. Ms. Joyce is receiving phenozapyridine hydrochloride (Pyridium) to relieve bladder pain. Prior to initiating the medication therapy, the nurse should alert Ms. Joyce to which of the following possible side-effects of the drug?
   a. Possible burning upon urination
   b. Cloudy particles in urine
   c. Foul-smelling urine
   d. Orange red urine

178. Which of the following signs or symptoms is the most diagnostic for an "early" bladder tumor or neoplasm?
   a. Intermittent pain with anuria
   b. Painless intermittent hematuria
   c. Constant pain with oliguria
   d. Sharp, severe pain with anuria

179. (Questions 179–181 refer to this situation) Tom Coates is a 22-year-old man who is admitted to the hospital with a diagnosis of gonorrhea. He appears to be embarrassed and has asked to be left alone. He will not make direct eye contact with any

member of the health care team. Gonorrhea is an inflammation of the genital mucous membranes. Signs or symptoms indicative of gonorrhea include
   a. Purulent, greenish yellow discharge from the penis
   b. A chancre (ulcer) on the penis
   c. Headache, malaise, fever, skin rash
   d. Abscesses on the penis and on the urethral tract

180. Which of the following nursing measures is necessary when caring for Mr. Coates?
   a. Maintaining respiratory isolation
   b. Saving all urinary output
   c. Wearing gloves when obtaining specimens
   d. Maintaining strict I and O

181. A variety of nursing strategies have been implemented to promote Mr. Coates' acceptance of his diagnosis. Which of the following communication strategies might facilitate the nursing goal?
   a. Conflict resolution
   b. Bargaining
   c. Direct listening
   d. Active listening

182. Genital herpes differs from other sexually transmitted diseases in that
   a. It masks the symptoms of syphilis
   b. There is no enlargement of lymph nodes
   c. There are no ulcers or skin rashes
   d. It is not a reportable disease

183. Clients with genital herpes may benefit from which of the following nursing interventions?
   a. Application of alcohol to the affected area to help dry lesions
   b. Application of ointments to soothe the affected area
   c. Application of topical steroids to the affected area to decrease the edema
   d. Application of topical antibiotics to the affected area to reduce the spread of the disease

184. Client teaching is important with clients with genital herpes. An important point for the nurse to include in client teaching is that
   a. Antiviral agents, when used appropriately, can cure the disease
   b. Herpes can be transmitted only during the primary stage of the disease
   c. For pregnant clients, prenatal care is essential to monitor for fetal complications
   d. Secondary infections occur when drug therapy has been initiated

185. (Questions 185–188 refer to this situation) Lisa Kohl is a 58-year-old woman who has been admitted to the hospital with a diagnosis of uterine cancer. She is 8 years past menopause. She is scheduled for a radium implant in the morning. An IV of D_5W at 100 mL per hour is begun. She now has an indwelling Foley catheter. The nurse conducts an admission nursing assessment. Which of the following pieces of information is most helpful in planning a teaching program for Mrs. Kohl and her family?
   a. She has three children
   b. Her husband is uncircumcised
   c. She is not on estrogen therapy
   d. She is a retired real estate agent

186. Mrs. Kohl asks the nurse to explain to her why the Foley catheter was placed. Which of the following reasons for catheter placement is the most accurate?
   a. To closely monitor urinary output
   b. To maintain sterility around the genital orifices
   c. To prevent dislodgment of the implant
   d. To monitor for complications of the implant

187. Mrs. Kohl has had the radium implanted. Safe post-implant nursing care includes
   a. Considering and treating all bowel and bladder discharges as contaminated
   b. Encouraging the client to be active within the confines of the private room

c. Maintaining protective isolation
d. Maintaining reverse isolation

188. The nurse is attempting to help Mrs. Kohl develop healthy coping skills to deal with her problems. Which of the following behaviors demonstrates the use of these skills?
    a. Directing anger at self instead of others
    b. Avoiding direct eye contact with nurse
    c. Crying frequently when alone
    d. Openly expressing feelings to the nurse or to significant others

189. (Questions 189–195 refer to this situation) Louis Dunn, a 67-year-old black man, is admitted to the hospital via the ER with the complaint that he has been unable to void for over 24 hours. He complains of extreme abdominal discomfort. A Foley catheter is inserted and 1,000 mL of urine is obtained. The catheter is clamped for 2 hours, then released. An additional 500 mL of urine is obtained. A tentative diagnosis of benign prostatic hypertrophy (BPH) is made. After completing the nursing assessment, the nurse discusses the client's past history, particularly regarding urinary elimination. Which of the following signs or symptoms is the client likely to report to the nurse?
    a. Difficulty in initiating a urinary stream
    b. Nocturia
    c. Hematuria
    d. Frequent voiding of large amounts

190. As assessment continues, the nurse asks questions about the client's nutritional intake and pattern. Which of the following questions indicates the nurse's knowledge of dietary influences on BPH?
    a. "Do you frequently consume fish and fish oil?"
    b. "Do you frequently consume spicy food?"
    c. "Do you frequently consume large quantities of salty products?"
    d. "Do you follow a vegetarian diet?"

191. Mr. Dunn is scheduled for surgery. The nurse responsible for his preoperative teaching should stress how important it is for Mr. Dunn to
    a. Maintain an active range of motion in all joints
    b. Maintain a low-sodium diet
    c. Maintain fluid restrictions
    d. Avoid the Valsalva maneuver

192. Mr. Dunn underwent a perineal prostatectomy. In providing postoperative care, the nurse should watch for which of the following indications that further action is necessary?
    a. Hematuria, consistent over 1 hour
    b. Decreasing urinary output over several hours
    c. Pain in the lower abdomen
    d. Urine specific gravity of 1.015

193. Mr. Dunn's care plan is posted on his chart. To maintain safe care it is vital for the nurse to
    a. Monitor orthostatic blood pressures
    b. Avoid taking rectal temperatures
    c. Prevent the client from turning on his stomach
    d. Take precautionary measures regarding body discharges

194. Mr. Dunn is receiving continuous bladder irrigations. Since complications can arise from implementation of this therapy, the nurse should monitor Mr. Dunn for development of
    a. Hematuria
    b. Renal calculi
    c. Water intoxication
    d. Pulmonary emboli

195. Mr. Dunn will soon be discharged from the hospital. One nurse has been active in providing in-hospital client teaching as well as discharge teaching. Teaching has been successful if Mr. Dunn states
    a. "I know that now I'm as good as new!"
    b. "I can't wait to get to the gym to lift my weights!"

c. "I'll ask my grandson to climb on my lap so I won't have to lift him."
d. "Well, I guess my sex life is over!"

196. (Questions 196–199 refer to this situation) Isaac Roy is a 30-year-old man who is admitted to the hospital after he discovered a nodular lump on his right testicle. He is admitted for a diagnostic work-up and, possibly, radiation therapy or surgery. He is alert and oriented and in no pain; however, he is pacing the floor in his room. He is apparently upset or worried about something. When questioned about his anxiety, Mr. Roy replies, "They're going to take away my manhood." The nurse should implement the nursing care plan and draw Mr. Roy into a discussion of
    a. His feelings about his sexuality
    b. His viewpoint about his health care thus far
    c. His feelings about complications from radiation
    d. His feelings about a prolonged hospitalization

197. If Mr. Roy has radiation therapy, which of the following nursing actions will assist in maintaining his skin integrity?
    a. Applying ice packs to the irradiated area to decrease edema
    b. Avoiding heat applications to the irradiated area
    c. Applying moisturizing creams to the irradiated area
    d. Avoiding washing the irradiated area

198. If Mr. Roy has an orchiectomy, the most effective postoperative nursing strategy to promote comfort would be to
    a. Elevate the foot of the bed for 24 hours
    b. Administer heat applications to the scrotum for 24 hours
    c. Apply ice packs to the scrotum for 24 hours
    d. Elevate the head of the bed for 24 hours

199. After an extensive diagnostic work-up, it is confirmed that Mr. Roy does *not* have testicular cancer as suspected. Mr. Roy is to be discharged this morning. Which of the following statements from Mr. Roy indicates that he has understood pertinent client teaching information?
    a. "I will practice good hygiene techniques."
    b. "I will avoid spicy foods."
    c. "I will watch for signs and symptoms of infection."
    d. "I will do a testicular self-exam every month."

200. The presenting signs and symptoms of cancer of the prostate are similar to the signs and symptoms of
    a. Bowel obstruction
    b. Kidney infection
    c. Urinary tract infections
    d. Urethral obstruction

201. Pharmacologic therapy for cancer of the prostate is sometimes not well received by the client. Which of the following therapeutic drugs induces gynecomastia as a side-effect?
    a. Diuretics
    b. Estrogen
    c. Steroids
    d. Progesterone

202. Gary Jones is hospitalized with terminal cancer. His wife, who spends many hours by his bedside, is seen in the hall looking out the window. The nurse approaches Mrs. Jones and finds her crying. She says, "I just don't know how I will live without him." The nurse should respond by saying
    a. "I know it's hard for you now, but things will work out."
    b. "We should probably talk about how you can best cope with your husband's death."
    c. "You seem sad and scared when you think about life without your husband."

d. "Maybe it would be helpful for you to spend less time here at the hospital."

203. Select the underlying feeling *best* reflected in this statement: "Young people today sure do have a lot more sexual freedom than we did when I was growing up!"
    a. Frustration
    b. Powerlessness
    c. Anger
    d. Confusion

204. (Questions 204–209 refer to this situation) Geri Fay, a 31-year-old woman, is admitted to the hospital for a hysterectomy following a prolonged course of endometriosis. She is married and has no children. She and her husband have stated that they have no desire to have children and therefore do not view the hysterectomy in a negative way. An IV of D_5W is begun in her right arm. Mrs. Fay tells the nurse that she really does not understand what it meant to have endometriosis, why it caused her so much pain, or why it caused menstrual abnormalities. She asks the nurse to explain endometriosis to her. The nurse should explain that
    a. "It results from a portion of the uterine lining functioning outside the uterus."
    b. "It results from an overproduction of hormones from the ovaries."
    c. "It results from an overabundance of endometrial tissue in the uterus."
    d. "It results from a tumor of the endometrial lining in the uterus."

205. The nurse asks Mrs. Fay about the details of her endometriosis. Which of the following signs or symptoms might Mrs. Fay have experienced?
    a. Urinary obstructions
    b. Sacral backache
    c. Hematuria
    d. Constipation

206. Mrs. Fay has undergone a total hysterectomy and bilateral salpingo-oophorectomy. Her lab work returns postoperatively, and she is found to have low hemoglobin and hematocrit levels. The physician orders 2 units of packed cells to be infused. Immediately prior to infusion, the nurse should
    a. Place the bed in a high-Fowler's position
    b. Monitor the client's apical pulse rate
    c. Take the client's baseline vital signs
    d. Monitor the client's blood pressure

207. Transfusion reactions usually occur within the first 15 minutes of receiving blood. Which of the following signs or symptoms indicates a transfusion reaction?
    a. Flank pain
    b. Rise in blood pressure
    c. Decrease in respirations
    d. Change in level of consciousness

208. If Mrs. Fay does have a transfusion reaction, the nurse should initiate action to
    a. Slow the transfusion and notify the physician
    b. Slow the transfusion and take vital signs
    c. Stop the transfusion and infuse a new blood transfusion
    d. Stop the transfusion and notify the physician

209. Three days postoperatively, Mrs. Fay is still complaining of abdominal pain. She has bowel sounds in all four quadrants. Her orders are "up ad lib." Which of the following nursing measures would assist Mrs. Fay in alleviating the *cause* of her pain?
    a. Providing a Sitz bath
    b. Applying warm abdominal compresses
    c. Increasing walking activity as tolerated
    d. Administering analgesics as prescribed

210. (Questions 210–214 refer to this situation) Rebecca Water is a 53-year-old black woman admitted to the hospital for a breast biopsy and possible lumpectomy or mastectomy. She admits to doing a breast self-examination on occasion. She

admits also to a family history of breast cancer. Her mother had bilateral radical mastectomies, and her sister had a lumpectomy, both for breast cancer.

Breast lump is only one sign of possible breast cancer. Which of the following signs might also indicate breast cancer?
   a. Menstrual abnormalities
   b. Severe pain in breast or nipple
   c. Edematous appearance of the affected breast
   d. Change of color of the affected breast

211. Several developmental factors influence the incidence of breast cancer. Developmental data can be obtained by ascertaining the
   a. Client's age at onset of menses and menopause
   b. Client's age at first pregnancy
   c. Number of children breastfed
   d. Client's characterization of her monthly menses

212. Following a breast biopsy, Ms. Water has a modified radical mastectomy. Postoperatively, the nurse elevates Ms. Water's arm on her affected side to
   a. Increase circulation
   b. Prevent edema
   c. Relieve pressure on her wound
   d. Decrease pain

213. Several days postoperatively the nurse reviews discharge teaching points for Ms. Water. One client teaching point that the nurse should reinforce is
   a. To avoid wearing tight clothing above the waist
   b. To avoid people with active infections
   c. That the client will have no active range of motion in the affected arm
   d. That the client should have no blood pressure or venipunctures in the affected arm

214. The nurse is evaluating Ms. Water's discharge teaching. Which of the following is a desired client outcome in the nurse's teaching plan?
   a. The client restates the steps of a breast self-examination
   b. The client correctly demonstrates effective coughing technique
   c. The client correctly demonstrates a breast self-examination
   d. The client restates the effects of an effective coughing technique

215. Linda Dove states, "I don't want my husband to see me like this. With only one breast I can't see how he can look at me." A facilitating response from the nurse is
   a. "I know how you feel; all women feel that way at first."
   b. "Don't let it bother you; you know he loves you."
   c. "You're worried because you think you won't be attractive anymore."
   d. "You'll have time to adjust; be patient."

216. In the above facilitating response, trust between the client and the nurse is promoted by the nurse
   a. Indicating an understanding for the client's feelings as well as for their cause
   b. Listening and encouraging the client to say more
   c. Acknowledging that he or she heard what the client said
   d. Maintaining close posture and eye contact with the client

217. (Questions 217–221 refer to this situation) Sofia Schul is a 26-year-old woman admitted to the hospital complaining of severe lower abdominal pain. Her vital signs are temperature 102°F, pulse 122, respirations 22, and BP 140/84. Her diagnosis is acute pelvic inflammatory disease (PID). Which of the following signs or symptoms is also indicative of acute PID?
   a. Foul-smelling vaginal discharge
   b. Hematuria

c. Low back pain
d. Sudden unexplained weight loss

218. The etiology of PID may vary. The nurse should ask about or assess Ms. Schul for
    a. Endometriosis
    b. Bladder infections
    c. Gonorrhea
    d. Cystitis

219. Which of the following nursing measures would help to promote Mrs. Schul's comfort?
    a. Applying a heating pad to her lower back
    b. Encouraging her to exercise (walking)
    c. Adjusting the bed to a flat position
    d. Applying a heating pad to her lower abdomen

220. One nursing measure for PID is to assess vaginal discharge. The nurse should assess these discharges for the
    a. Presence of protein
    b. Presence of blood
    c. Amount of discharge
    d. Presence of glucose

221. The nurse is evaluating her client teaching with Mrs. Schul. Teaching has been successful if the client states that she can best prevent a recurrence of PID by
    a. Avoiding the use of tampons
    b. Monitoring the amount and odor of discharge
    c. Using good handwashing techniques
    d. Avoiding the use of salicylates during menses

Answer Sheet—Test 1

1. a b c d
2. a b c d
3. a b c d
4. a b c d
5. a b c d
6. a b c d
7. a b c d
8. a b c d
9. a b c d
10. a b c d
11. a b c d
12. a b c d
13. a b c d
14. a b c d
15. a b c d
16. a b c d
17. a b c d
18. a b c d
19. a b c d
20. a b c d
21. a b c d
22. a b c d
23. a b c d
24. a b c d
25. a b c d
26. a b c d
27. a b c d
28. a b c d
29. a b c d
30. a b c d
31. a b c d
32. a b c d
33. a b c d
34. a b c d
35. a b c d
36. a b c d
37. a b c d
38. a b c d
39. a b c d
40. a b c d
41. a b c d
42. a b c d
43. a b c d
44. a b c d
45. a b c d
46. a b c d
47. a b c d
48. a b c d
49. a b c d
50. a b c d
51. a b c d
52. a b c d
53. a b c d
54. a b c d
55. a b c d
56. a b c d
57. a b c d
58. a b c d
59. a b c d
60. a b c d
61. a b c d
62. a b c d
63. a b c d
64. a b c d
65. a b c d
66. a b c d
67. a b c d
68. a b c d
69. a b c d
70. a b c d
71. a b c d
72. a b c d
73. a b c d
74. a b c d
75. a b c d
76. a b c d
77. a b c d
78. a b c d
79. a b c d
80. a b c d
81. a b c d
82. a b c d
83. a b c d
84. a b c d
85. a b c d
86. a b c d
87. a b c d
88. a b c d
89. a b c d
90. a b c d
91. a b c d
92. a b c d
93. a b c d
94. a b c d
95. a b c d
96. a b c d
97. a b c d
98. a b c d
99. a b c d
100. a b c d
101. a b c d
102. a b c d
103. a b c d
104. a b c d
105. a b c d
106. a b c d
107. a b c d
108. a b c d
109. a b c d
110. a b c d
111. a b c d
112. a b c d
113. a b c d
114. a b c d
115. a b c d
116. a b c d
117. a b c d
118. a b c d
119. a b c d
120. a b c d
121. a b c d
122. a b c d
123. a b c d
124. a b c d
125. a b c d

Answer Sheet—Test 1 (*Continued*)

126. a b c d
127. a b c d
128. a b c d
129. a b c d
130. a b c d
131. a b c d
132. a b c d
133. a b c d
134. a b c d
135. a b c d
136. a b c d
137. a b c d
138. a b c d
139. a b c d
140. a b c d
141. a b c d
142. a b c d
143. a b c d
144. a b c d

145. a b c d
146. a b c d
147. a b c d
148. a b c d
149. a b c d
150. a b c d
151. a b c d
152. a b c d
153. a b c d
154. a b c d
155. a b c d
156. a b c d
157. a b c d
158. a b c d
159. a b c d
160. a b c d
161. a b c d
162. a b c d
163. a b c d

164. a b c d
165. a b c d
166. a b c d
167. a b c d
168. a b c d
169. a b c d
170. a b c d
171. a b c d
172. a b c d
173. a b c d
174. a b c d
175. a b c d
176. a b c d
177. a b c d
178. a b c d
179. a b c d
180. a b c d
181. a b c d
182. a b c d

183. a b c d
184. a b c d
185. a b c d
186. a b c d
187. a b c d
188. a b c d
189. a b c d
190. a b c d
191. a b c d
192. a b c d
193. a b c d
194. a b c d
195. a b c d
196. a b c d
197. a b c d
198. a b c d
199. a b c d
200. a b c d
201. a b c d

202. a b c d
203. a b c d
204. a b c d
205. a b c d
206. a b c d
207. a b c d
208. a b c d
209. a b c d
210. a b c d
211. a b c d
212. a b c d
213. a b c d
214. a b c d
215. a b c d
216. a b c d
217. a b c d
218. a b c d
219. a b c d
220. a b c d
221. a b c d

Answers and Rationales for Test 1

1. b. Cigarette smoking causes a change in the bronchial epithelium that may lead to cancerous change. A, H
2. d. The symptoms noted are classic symptoms of abdominal aneurysm that should alert the nurse to obtain emergency surgical assessment. A, H
3. c. If the creatine phosphokine MB (CPK-MB) elevates in the typical pattern for myocardial infarction (MI), the client's activity level can be adjusted to maintain cardiac reserves. A, H
4. d. Pain relief in angina pectoris is of highest priority since pain is correlated with ischemic damage. P, O
5. b. Placing Mr. Strube in a high semi-Fowler's position to improve ventilation will be an immediately effective nursing intervention. I, O
6. c. Myocardial cell hypoxia alters myocardial cell metabolism in such a way that more acidic cellular waste materials trigger nerve endings. D, H
7. d. A client is placed on a clear or full liquid diet in the acute phase to minimize amount of circulation for digestion to the gastrointestinal tract and maximize the blood flow to the myocardium. P, O
8. d. Nitroglycerin is a potent vasodilator. Transient vasodilation of the vasculature of the brain and superficial facial structures are expected responses of the medication. E, D
9. b. Angina pain results from an imbalance of oxygen available to and oxygen needed by the myocardial cells. Taking nitroglycerin prior to activities that are known to provoke oxygen imbalance will prevent the imbalance and thus prevent the pain. The medication works through vasodilation of coronary vessels, which allows greater coronary blood flow. I, C
10. b. Even though bacon has high sodium and cholesterol content, it has less than that found in the other combinations. P, N
11. d. Active listening encourages clients to express their feelings. I, C
12. b. This body language would make the nurse's nonverbal message congruent with her verbal message. I, C
13. a. No research to date indicates any relationship between carbon monoxide intoxication and the appetite center. R, H
14. d. Although SSKI is an antithyroid drug, it is administered in Mr. Smith's case to liquify respiratory secretions and facilitate expectoration. E, D
15. c. SSKI has a very disagreeable taste which can be disguised by water, milk, or juice. Absorption is not affected by diluent. I, D
16. b. Expectorant preparations are not associated with change in peristalsis and therefore do not cause changes in bowel sounds. A, D
17. b. Taking several diaphragmatic inspirations and pursed-lip exhalations before initiating a cough helps mobilize secretions into the major airways. I, O
18. c. Retention of CO_2 in the client with chronic obstructive pulmonary disease (COPD) leads to high blood CO_2 levels, which over time cause the respiratory center to be unresponsive to CO_2. A low blood O_2 level, which normally is only a secondary stimulus to the respiratory center, becomes the primary stimulus. If high flow O_2 is given, the blood O_2 level rises, producing no respiratory center stimulus and no respiratory effort. R, H
19. b. Isuprel induces activation of sympathetic receptors in the vascular system. A, D
20. c. Isuprel is a bronchodilator. After nebulization treatment Mr. Smith should

be able to cough up sputum more easily because of reduced airway resistance. I, D

21. a. Air is trapped in the alveoli in clients with COPD, because of structural changes associated with the disease. Pursed-lip breathing maintains positive pressure in the alveolar duct and prevents collapse of the airway before alveolar air can be expired. R, H

22. c. A positive test reaction for purified protein derivative (PPD) occurs when the area of induration at the injection site is greater than 10 mm. A, H

23. b. Close, frequent, prolonged exposure to airborne droplet nuclei inhaled into the respiratory system is usually required for disease transmission. R, H

24. d. Isoniazid (INH) is thought to interfere with DNA metabolism of *Mycobacterium tuberculosis*. P, D

25. d. Long-term treatment is necessary to prevent relapse of the active disease process because the organism may become dormant and resist drug therapy. E, D

26. b. By slowing conduction through the atrioventricular (AV) node, greater ventricular filling occurs, allowing greater muscle fiber stretch of the ventricle. The greater the stretch, the greater the contractile recoil during systole, strengthening and increasing cardiac output. E, D

27. c. Sodium and potassium play a critical role in establishing the cell membrane action potential. Calcium has a predominant role in mechanical coupling within the muscle fibrils. R, H

28. b. Low potassium levels potentiate the effect of digitalis preparations as do low magnesium levels. R, D

29. c. Heart sound 3 (S_3) is associated with turbulent filling that occurs when ventricular end-diastolic pressure is high. A, H

30. a. Compensatory changes of the failing heart cause enlargement of the cardiac size and congested vasculature of the lungs. A, H

31. c. If 0.25 mg were administered daily the client would become digitalis toxic because the daily excretion rate is less than the daily dose. If 0.125 mg were administered daily, the desired therapeutic effect might be achieved, since urinary excretion is greater than the dose. Alternate day, alternate dose regimen affects excretion rates. R, D

32. c. Since congestive heart failure is characterized by the heart's inability to pump forward all the blood it receives, heart pumping efficiency is improved by reducing the volume of blood it receives to pump. Rotating tourniquets reduce the amount of blood the heart must pump by trapping blood in the periphery. I, O

33. b. Even though the PR interval prolongs beyond .20 seconds, the P-wave depolarizations are present each time with QRS ventricular depolarizations. A, H

34. a. Third-degree, or complete, heart block is an absolute loss of the atrial impulse transmission to the ventricular tissue. The atria are independent and the ventricles are independent. No progression of atrial impulses is conducted to the ventricles. A, H

35. c. In third-degree heart block, completely independent depolarization of the atria and ventricles occurs and results in loss of effective cardiac output. Temporary or permanent sequential pacing will restore cardiac output by reproducing cyclic depolarization of atria and ventricles. E, O

36. d. β-Hemolytic streptococci cause antibodies that produce characteristic lesions within the various tissues of the heart. A, H

37. c. Antibodies produced against streptococcal endotoxin materials cause valve leaflet swelling, deposits of platelet and fibrin on the margins of the valve. R, H
38. d. Thrombi develop in areas of venous stasis such as those that develop in deep leg veins in inactive clients. R, H
39. c. The infusion should be restarted and run at the ordered rate because otherwise extension of thrombi will occur. Increasing the drip rate might cause excessive bleeding. P, O
40. c. In order for reexpansion of lung tissue to occur, a negative pressure must be reestablished in the intrapleural space. R, H
41. c. Water provides a mechanical barrier to the entrance of air at atmospheric pressure into the chest tube system. R, H
42. d. Air should bubble into the water only when the client inspires, not continuously when the client is generating his or her own respiratory effort. R, H
43. d. Raynaud's phenomenon is an arterial problem. R, H
44. c. Exposure of skin surfaces to cold in a susceptible client usually triggers the vasospastic episode. A, H
45. b. Hypertension is diagnosed only when the average of at least two separate blood pressure readings is higher than 140/90. E, H
46. c. Maintenance of a patient airway is the most important concern. Recording other data is a secondary goal. A, O
47. b. Administering therapeutic levels of heparin to a client suffering a hemorrhagic stroke could promote continued hemorrhage into the cerebral tissue and worsen the neurologic damage and permanent deficits. R, D
48. d. Usually liquid diets intensify swallowing difficulties. Soft semisolid material placed in the unaffected side of the mouth is usually better manipulated by hemispheric stroke clients. P, O
49. d. The primary effect of methyldopa (Aldomet) is more stable blood pressure at a lower level. R, D
50. a. Since deep vein thrombosis (DVT) is characterized by redness, pain, and swelling in the affected part, measurement of changes in swelling is most helpful. Homans' sign is positive only 50% of the time with DVT. Prothrombin time (PT) is used for monitoring coumarin (Coumadin) therapy. A, O
51. c. The high vitamin K content of lettuce, cabbage, and greens (turnip) decreases the PT. The decreased PT puts the client at risk for thrombus reformation. I, N
52. d. A loosely applied gauze (wet or dry) protects the integrity of the skin and provides comfort. I, O
53. c. Because many factors (e.g., food, drugs) may alter the level of coumarin (Coumadin) in circulation and alter the effect on the prothrombin time, any bleeding should be reported to health personnel so further evaluation can be undertaken. P, C
54. a. Pressure evenly distributed over the entire limb promotes venous return, helps prevent pooling of venous blood in dependent areas, and lessens the risk of thrombus formation. R, H
55. b. Excess weight is a predominant predisposing factor in the development of varicosities. P, C
56. c. Pressure evenly distributed over the limb promotes venous return, helps prevent pooling of venous blood, and lessens the risk of thrombi formation. I, O
57. b. Both positive and negative interactions occur. The frequency of both types of interactions determines the quality of an interpersonal relationship. I, C

58. a. Effective communication is critical to quality nursing care and includes several interpersonal skills. I, C
59. a. Aggression is hostile and negates the effectiveness of confrontation. Confrontation is standing up for your rights without violating the rights of others. I, C
60. b. Gravity facilitates the passage of stomach contents and helps prevent reflux. P, O
61. a. Cimetidine (Tagamet) is administered preoperatively to decrease the likelihood of the client aspirating gastric secretions. P, D
62. c. Stomach contents, if not removed, put pressure on the suture line. R, H
63. c. Confrontation points out aggressive behavior. Indicating how the nurse feels about the client's aggressive behavior promotes a working relationship rather than a defensive reaction from the client. I, C
64. d. Dye tablets contain iodine. A, H
65. d. Vomiting eliminates the dye. A, O
66. d. Symptoms are those of excess flatus; ambulation stimulates peristalsis. I, O
67. c. Foods listed are low in fat, high in fiber. Broccoli belongs to the cruciferous group, which is thought to protect against cancer. P, N
68. d. These items are high in fiber and help prevent constipation. P, N
69. a. Sitz baths are soothing to the irritated area. P, O
70. c. Local edema may cause pressure on the urethra. A, H
71. a. Instilling solution stimulates peristalsis and discomfort. The patient usually experiences relief and is able to tolerate additional fluid if the flow is stopped temporarily, then infused at a slower rate. P, O
72. d. Lethargy, dark urine, and light stools are characteristic symptoms of hepatitis. A, H
73. c. The virus can be transmitted in saliva. It is not necessary to wear a mask to avoid contamination. P, O
74. b. Cholestyramine is given for pruritus associated with jaundice. E, D
75. b. Salt-poor albumin is hypertonic and will pull fluid from the peritoneal cavity and interstitial spaces into the vascular space, putting the client at risk for circulatory overload. The client will find it easier to breathe if the head of the bed is elevated. A, O
76. d. Blood can collect on the sheets beneath the client and feel damp. Bleeding is a possibility after liver biopsy because of the high vascularity of the liver. P, O
77. b. The bladder should be empty to avoid puncture during the procedure. P, O
78. a. These symptoms are indicative of high ammonia levels and impending hepatic coma. E, O
79. c. Lente Insulin reaches peak activity time in 8 hours. A, H
80. d. Activity level determines caloric and insulin needs. Physical exercise decreases insulin requirements. P, C
81. c. Appropriate foods can be substituted within each exchange group to meet the dietary requirements of the diabetic. P, O
82. a. Anxiety and hunger are symptoms of hypoglycemia. Tim needs glucose. P, C
83. a. The respiratory system is the first compensatory system activated in response to a decreasing blood pH. Carbon dioxide is "blown off" in an attempt to rid the body of excess acid. R, H
84. a. It cannot be assumed that acquisition of knowledge alone will induce the client to change her eating habits. P, C
85. c. A deficiency of vitamin B_{12} interferes with nerve regeneration. Permanent damage results if vitamin B_{12} stores are not replenished consistently and early in the course of the disease. P, H

86. b. Rectal temperatures are invasive and can puncture the mucous membrane lining of the rectum, predisposing the client to infection and bleeding. P, O
87. c. The area described is approximately at the level of the right atrium. A, O
88. d. Central venous pressure (CVP) reflects both the amount of fluid being returned to the right atrium and the ability of the right side of the heart to assume the pumping function. A, H
89. c. The ordered and available dosages must first be converted to the same unit of measure; 1/120 grain is equal to 0.5 mg. P, O
90. b. Adequate kidney perfusion is especially important after splenectomy, because blood loss is likely to be relatively high. I, O
91. d. Restlessness is a symptom of decreased oxygenation to the brain. A, H
92. c. Increased risk of pneumococcal infections is the only adverse effect resulting from absence of the spleen. I, O
93. b. Burn injuries should be flushed with cool water as quickly as possible. P, O
94. c. Contaminated wounds covering large areas of the body provide portals of entry for the tetanus bacillus, which is often present in soil. P, O
95. a. Plasmanate is a plasma volume expander. Protein exerts osmotic pull, causing fluids to shift from interstitial spaces into the vascular space. R, H
96. c. These foods contain high amounts of iron and protein, both of which are important for a client suffering from burn injuries. P, N
97. c. Morphine induces spasm of the sphincter of Oddi, and exacerbates pain. E, H
98. d. Maintaining strict npo orders is essential to provide rest for the client's pancreas. Lemon swabs stimulate salivation and are therefore inappropriate. P, O
99. a. Drops per minute = total volume/total minutes × drip factor; therefore, X = 125/60 × 15 = 31.5 gtts/min is the correct setting. P, O
100. a. The parathyroids may be accidentally removed during surgery, drastically affecting the client's serum calcium levels. P, D
101. c. Gravity causes the blood to pool under the neck. The dressing may appear clean and dry even though bleeding may have occurred. BP and pulse should be assessed more frequently than once every shift. A, O
102. c. Sleeping with the head elevated decreases edema in the fat pads behind the eyes. P, H
103. a. The client needs extra cortisone in stressful situations such as surgery. The adrenals are unable to respond when the client has been receiving exogenous steroids over a period of time. P, O
104. b. Shaving the client's abdomen immediately prior to making the incision decreases the bacterial population on the skin. P, O
105. a. The client may resume oral intake of fluids when peristalis returns, as evidenced by the client's ability to pass flatus. E, H
106. c. The client's willingness to view the stoma is one of the first signs that he has accepted his medical situation. E, H
107. a. A goal of therapy is to prevent constipation because it predisposes the client to future attacks of diverticulitis. Drinking water promotes this goal. E, O
108. a. The inflammatory process of Crohn's disease adversely affects the ability of the intestine to absorb nutrients. A, H
109. b. Chemotherapy produces severe side-effects, including the possibility of permanent infertility. Enlarged nodes on both sides of the diaphragm indi-

cate that disease has reached an advanced stage. I, C
110. c. Feeling of anxiety and unexplained weight loss are symptoms consistent with the hypermetabolic state associated with hyperthyroidism. A, H
111. c. An enlarged painless node is a symptom of lymphoma. Early diagnosis and treatment can result in cure; delay gives the tumor time to metastasize, diminishing the likelihood of cure. E, H
112. d. A high fluid intake decreases blood viscosity and the likelihood that sickled cells will logjam in the capillaries, precipitating sickle cell crisis. P, N
113. a. Loss of peripheral vision is the most common symptom of glaucoma, caused by the increased pressure of the aqueous humor and subsequent retinal damage. A, H
114. d. Tonometry is used to measure ocular pressure. A, H
115. c. Eye drops should be instilled in a pouch of the lower eyelid. I, D
116. a. Pilocarpine's action is to constrict the pupil, thus enhancing the drainage and circulation of the aqueous humor, which decreases intraocular pressure. I, D
117. b. Eye pain may indicate a medical emergency due to the potential for sudden and permanent loss of vision. P, O
118. b. A change in the client's level of consciousness is usually the first indication of increasing intracranial pressure. Widening pulse pressure also indicates increased cerebral edema or increased intracranial pressure. A, H
119. d. With the head of the bed at a 30° angle, maximum intracranial venous drainage is promoted, decreasing the potential for increasing intracranial pressure. P, O
120. a. Testing the drainage for glucose will indicate whether the drainage is spinal fluid. Spinal fluid contains a high amount of glucose. A, O

121. b. Precautionary measures against seizure include adjusting the bed to a low position and raising the side rails. A padded tongue blade should be readily available. I, O
122. c. Dexamethasone (Decadron) decreases the inflammatory response, which in turn decreases cerebral edema. I, D
123. d. The Glasgow Coma Scale is a standard scale developed for neurological assessments. E, H
124. b. Aspirin is a gastric irritant. Food, milk, or an antacid provides a protective "coat" to the stomach. R, D
125. c. Osteoarthritis is a noninflammatory degenerative disease of the joints, characterized by joint pain, stiffness, and Heberden's nodes (noted in finger). A, H
126. b. The weight-bearing joints, especially those of the lower extremities, are more prone to structural damage because of the increased stress and weight placed on them. A, H
127. a. Heat packs are prescribed to increase circulation to the affected area and to decrease pain. I, O
128. b. Mrs. Kay may need to lose extra pounds to reach her "ideal weight," but she needs to maintain a well-balanced diet while doing so. Extra weight places extra stress and strain on affected weight-bearing joints. P, N
129. d. Of the given observations, assessing for postoperative bleeding and subcutaneous emphysema is the most important because of the danger to the client of respiratory compromise from the fluid or subcutaneous emphysema. P, O
130. c. Elevating the head of the bed facilitates drainage and helps to maintain the patency of the client's airway. R, O
131. c. The function of the nasogastric tube is to protect the client from possible contamination of food or liquid. R, O

132. b. Gout is a metabolic disorder whereby uric acid crystals are deposited in joints, causing pain. The joint most commonly affected is the joint at the great toe. A, H
133. a. Gout is a metabolic disorder resulting from an increase in circulating uric acid causing an increase in sedimentation rate and an increase in serum uric acid levels. A, H
134. c. Foods such as glandular meats, shellfish, sardines, and fish roe are high in purine (nitrogenous compound) and should be avoided by the client. P, N
135. b. Aspirin counteracts the effects of uricosuric agents, thereby decreasing the efficacy of drug therapy for gout. E, D
136. c. The pituitary gland is the master gland of the body and affects the functioning of the thyroid gland. The pituitary gland is also located near the optic chiasm, and thyroid dysfunction can cause visual disturbances. A, H
137. b. A transphenoidal approach may be used to remove the adenoma. As with any cranial surgery, assessing for leakage of cerebrospinal fluid is important. A, O
138. a. Osmotic diuretics decrease cerebral edema, which increases the urinary output without increasing the concentration of the urine; the result is diluted urine and decreased specific gravity. E, D
139. b. In a client being assessed for increasing intracranial pressure, evaluation of mental status is critical. Morphine sulfate can mask the signs of an altered mental state. I, D
140. c. Nuchal rigidity indicates meningeal irritation. A, H
141. d. Aseptic meningitis is not contagious. The major strategy here is to treat for increasing pressure by raising the head of the bed to enhance venous return. I, O
142. b. The sequence of the spread of seizure activity in the client can assist the physician in locating the source of seizure activity. A, H
143. d. The electroencephalogram indicates the electrical activity in various parts of the brain. A, H
144. a. A client with a convulsive disorder should avoid water sports so that if a generalized seizure does occur, the client will not be in danger of drowning. P, O
145. c. Muscle rigidity, a classic symptom of Parkinson's disease, can be decreased by physical therapy. E, O
146. c. Edrophonium chloride (Tensilon) is a short-acting anticholinergic medication that temporarily alleviates the signs and symptoms of myasthenia gravis. A, H
147. d. Under stress, fatigue in muscles increases, including the muscles involved in respiration. A, H
148. a. It is crucial that clients with myasthenia gravis receive their medication on time so that their muscle strength does not deteriorate to the point where swallowing becomes difficult or impossible. P, O
149. a. Placing personal effects within the client's reach will limit exertion which induces the intention tremors that are a symptom of multiple sclerosis. P, O
150. b. To maintain a high level of wellness, clients with multiple sclerosis need to have scheduled exercise as well as rest periods. E, O
151. d. Muscles of the respiratory system are frequently affected by injuries to the cervical spine. A, H
152. a. Maintaining body alignment reduces the potential of further cord injury. P, O
153. d. A classic symptom of a fractured hip is the finding that the affected limb is abducted and externally rotated. A, H

154. a. Buck's extension is a method of traction used to maintain the alignment of the hip joint. P, O
155. b. Postoperative edema may compromise neurologic as well as vascular systems in the affected leg. Urinary retention is a common complication experienced by clients with fractured hips. A, O
156. a. For the client to return to her own home, she needs to be as independent as possible in performing activities of daily living (ADL). E, O
157. a. Mydriatrics cause pupillary dilation, thus allowing a larger opening for the surgical procedure. P, D
158. d. The Valsalva maneuver can cause an increase in intraocular pressure. E, O
159. b. Meniere's syndrome is characterized by vertigo. Appropriate pharmacologic therapy is the administration of antivertiginous medication. P, D
160. c. One of the suggested dietary therapies to treat Meniere's syndrome is a low-sodium diet. Unsalted popcorn is appropriate in this diet. E, N
161. b. Retinal detachment is characterized by visual disturbances such as blind spots and flashes of light. A, H
162. d. A neutral head position with the retinal tear at the lowest part of the eye helps prevent further retinal detachment. P, O
163. b. To prevent serious injury to any client, the bed should be adjusted to a low position with the side rails raised. P, O
164. d. Heavy lifting may increase intraocular pressure, increasing the strain on the surgical site after retinal repair. Participation in active sports may increase the potential for further eye trauma or injury. E, O
165. d. The nurse can encourage behavioral change in his or her coworker by expressing support for the coworker's feelings and providing information about the client. I, C
166. d. Oliguria (decreased urinary output) is common in early stages of acute renal failure. A, H
167. a. A rise in circulating blood urea nitrogen (BUN) causes mental confusion. A, H
168. c. The client's weight is one of the best indicators of changes in fluid volume. A, H
169. a. Sodium polystyrene sulfonate (Kayexalate) enemas are used to lower serum potassium levels; cardiac arrhythmias are associated with hypokalemia. A, H
170. d. A low-protein diet maintains a positive nitrogen balance, but reduces gluconeogenesis and eliminates ketones from fat metabolism. P, N
171. a. The statement reflects the client's understanding of a low-sodium diet. E, O
172. c. Straining the client's urine aids in diagnosing the type of calculi and the subsequent therapeutic measures to be employed. P, O
173. b. Facial edema occurs because of water and sodium retention resulting from glomerular damage. A, H
174. b. The intravenous pyelogram provides information regarding the structure and function of the kidneys, ureters, and bladder. A, H
175. a. Drug therapy for glomerulonephritis involves antibiotics. The client follows the regimen for a prescribed length of time. E, D
176. c. Cystitis is commonly caused by improper hygienic techniques, particularly those used after a bowel movement. P, O
177. d. Phenazopyridine hydrochloride (Pyridium) turns the urine an orange red color. P, O
178. b. An early sign of a bladder tumor is painless hematuria. A, H

179. a. The gonorrhea bacteria cause a greenish yellow discharge from the penis. A, H
180. c. It is necessary for the nurse to wear gloves when obtaining specimens to avoid contact between the organism and the nurse's skin. P, O
181. d. Active listening involves verbally reflecting back to the client the thoughts and feelings he or she expresses. E, O
182. d. Genital herpes is not a reportable sexually transmitted disease (STD). R, H
183. a. Genital herpes lesions are best treated with alcohol. I, O
184. c. In pregnant clients with genital herpes, prenatal care is essential to prevent fetal complications. P, O
185. c. Many cancers are related to estrogen therapy, which the client is *not* receiving. A, O
186. c. A Foley catheter is placed to prevent dislodgment of the implant by pressure and by movement associated with urinary elimination. R, H
187. a. All products of elimination have been in close contact with the implant and should be considered contaminated. I, O
188. d. A client who can openly express feelings to the nurse or significant others is coping in a healthy way. E, O
189. a. Many men with an enlarged prostate have difficulty initiating a urinary stream. A, H
190. b. Ingestion of spicy foods and alcohol seems to precipitate acute prostatic congestion. A, H
191. d. The Valsalva maneuver may put unnecessary strain on the surgical site. P, O
192. b. Decreasing urinary output may indicate an obstruction in the Foley catheter or obstructions or complications of the urinary tract. A, H
193. b. Inserting a rectal thermometer may cause vagal stimulation (increased BP, decreased pulse) and also stimulate a Valsalva manuever. P, O
194. c. Water intoxication may be due to retention of the irrigating fluid the patient is receiving. P, O
195. c. The client should avoid lifting heavy objects for at least 3 weeks postoperatively. E, O
196. a. The client is probably referring to his sexuality. The nurse should initiate communication regarding his feelings about his sexuality. I, O
197. c. Moisturizing cream helps prevent infection of irradiated (compromised) skin. P, O
198. c. Applying ice to the scrotal area helps decreasing edema, which in turn decreases postoperative discomfort. P, O
199. d. Monthly testicular self-examinations help to identify abnormalities in the early stages. E, O
200. d. An enlarged prostate may cause some urinary stasis and, consequently, infections. A, H
201. b. Estrogen is prescribed to reduce the symptoms of prostatic cancer, and because it is a "female hormone," a side-effect is gynecomastia. E, D
202. c. Active listening is a helping response that communicates caring and understanding. I, C
203. c. Anger is often expressed as annoyance or irritation and can be used to mask fear. R, C
204. a. The definition of endometriosis is the presence of functioning endometrial tissue outside the uterus. I, H
205. b. Much of the pain of endometriosis is referred pain to the sacral area of the back. A, H
206. c. Baseline vital signs are critical for the assessment of changes after surgery. I, O
207. a. Flank pain may indicate a hemolytic reaction to the blood transfusion, if intravascular clotting is occurring. R, H

208. d. The blood transfusion should be stopped to prevent further reactions, and the physician must be notified before further therapy can be initiated. I, O
209. c. Her pain is partly caused by flatulence. Increasing activity stimulates peristalsis, thereby relieving the "gas pains." I, O
210. c. Depending on the location of the growth, venous return may be inhibited, causing venous congestion and edema. A, H
211. a. Early or late onset of menses or menopause increase the risk of breast cancer. A, H
212. b. Elevating the affected extremity enhances venous return and decreases or prevents edema formation. P, O
213. d. Blood pressures or venipunctures in the affected arm could be harmful to the circulation and increase the risk of infection. A, H
214. c. If the client can correctly demonstrate a breast self-examination the nurse's learning outcome has been met. E, O
215. c. The client's feelings and the underlying cause are acknowledged. I, C
216. a. Use of active listening facilitates trust. Active listening means that the nurse indicates in his or her own words an understanding of what the client said and of the feelings underlying what she said. It involves recognizing both the content and the feeling of what was said. I, C
217. a. A foul-smelling vaginal discharge indicates the presence of an infectious process. A, H
218. c. Pelvic inflammatory disease (PID) is a common complication of venereal disease, either gonorrhea or chlamydia infection. A, H
219. d. Heat promotes vasodilation and enhances circulation and comfort. I, O
220. c. An increasing or a decreasing amount of vaginal discharge may be helpful in assessing the efficacy of the prescribed medical therapy. A, H
221. c. Pelvic inflammatory disease (PID) may be caused by improper handwashing or poor hygienic techniques. E, O

DIAGNOSTIC GRID
Test 1

Directions: The diagnostic grid is used to reveal deficiencies in nursing content and nursing process knowledge. Determine which questions you answered incorrectly and circle the corresponding codes. Total each column and note the percentage of incorrect answers.

Nursing Process
A = Assessment
R = Analysis/nursing diagnosis
P = Planning
I = Implementation/intervention
E = Evaluation

Nursing Content
H = Health status
O = Nursing actions/interventions
D = Drugs/pharmacology
N = Nutrition
C = Communication skills

Question	\	Nursing Process					Nursing Content				
		A	R	P	I	E	H	O	D	N	C
1.		A					H				
2.		A					H				
3.		A					H				
4.				P				O			
5.					I			O			
6.			R				H				
7.				P				O			
8.						E			D		
9.					I						C
10.				P						N	
11.					I						C
12.					I						C
13.			R				H				
14.						E			D		
15.					I				D		

DIAGNOSTIC GRID (Continued)

Question	Nursing Process					Nursing Content				
	A	R	P	I	E	H	O	D	N	C
16.	A							D		
17.				I			O			
18.		R				H				
19.	A							D		
20.				I				D		
21.		R				H				
22.	A					H				
23.		R				H				
24.			P					D		
25.					E			D		
26.					E			D		
27.		R				H				
28.		R						D		
29.	A					H				
30.	A					H				
31.		R						D		
32.				I			O			
33.	A					H				
34.	A					H				
35.					E		O			
36.	A					H				
37.		R				H				

DIAGNOSTIC GRID (*Continued*)

Question	Nursing Process					Nursing Content				
	A	R	P	I	E	H	O	D	N	C
38.		R				H				
39.			P				O			
40.		R				H				
41.		R				H				
42.		R				H				
43.		R				H				
44.	A					H				
45.					E	H				
46.	A						O			
47.		R						D		
48.			P				O			
49.		R						D		
50.	A						O			
51.				I					N	
52.				I			O			
53.			P							C
54.		R				H				
55.			P							C
56.				I			O			
57.				I						C
58.				I						C
59.				I						C

DIAGNOSTIC GRID (*Continued*)

Question	Nursing Process					Nursing Content				
	A	R	P	I	E	H	O	D	N	C
60.			P				O			
61.			P					D		
62.		R				H				
63.				I						C
64.	A					H				
65.	A						O			
66.				I			O			
67.			P						N	
68.			P						N	
69.			P				O			
70.	A					H				
71.			P				O			
72.	A					H				
73.			P				O			
74.					E			D		
75.	A						O			
76.			P				O			
77.			P				O			
78.					E		O			
79.	A					H				
80.			P							C
81.			P				O			

330

DIAGNOSTIC GRID (Continued)

Question	Nursing Process					Nursing Content				
	A	R	P	I	E	H	O	D	N	C
82.			P							C
83.		R				H				
84.			P							C
85.			P			H				
86.			P				O			
87.	A						O			
88.	A					H				
89.			P					D		
90.				I			O			
91.	A					H				
92.				I			O			
93.			P				O			
94.			P				O			
95.		R				H				
96.			P						N	
97.					E	H				
98.			P				O			
99.				I			O			
100.			P					D		
101.	A						O			
102.			P			H				
103.			P				O			

DIAGNOSTIC GRID (Continued)

Question	Nursing Process					Nursing Content				
	A	R	P	I	E	H	O	D	N	C
104.			P				O			
105.					E	H				
106.					E	H				
107.					E		O			
108.	A					H				
109.				I						C
110.	A					H				
111.					E	H				
112.			P						N	
113.	A					H				
114.	A					H				
115.				I				D		
116.				I				D		
117.			P				O			
118.	A					H				
119.			P				O			
120.	A						O			
121.				I			O			
122.				I				D		
123.					E	H				
124.		R						D		
125.	A					H				

DIAGNOSTIC GRID (Continued)

Question	Nursing Process					Nursing Content				
	A	R	P	I	E	H	O	D	N	C
126.	A					H				
127.				I			O			
128.			P						N	
129.			P				O			
130.		R					O			
131.		R					O			
132.	A					H				
133.	A					H				
134.			P						N	
135.					E			D		
136.	A					H				
137.	A						O			
138.					E			D		
139.				I				D		
140.	A					H				
141.				I			O			
142.	A					H				
143.	A					H				
144.			P				O			
145.					E		O			
146.	A					H				
147.	A					H				

DIAGNOSTIC GRID (Continued)

Question	Nursing Process					Nursing Content				
	A	R	P	I	E	H	O	D	N	C
148.			P				O			
149.			P				O			
150.					E		O			
151.	A					H				
152.			P				O			
153.	A					H				
154.			P				O			
155.	A						O			
156.					E	H				
157.			P					D		
158.					E		O			
159.			P					D		
160.					E				N	
161.	A					H				
162.			P				O			
163.			P				O			
164.					E		O			
165.				I						C
166.	A					H				
167.	A					H				
168.	A					H				
169.	A					H				

DIAGNOSTIC GRID (Continued)

Question	Nursing Process					Nursing Content				
	A	R	P	I	E	H	O	D	N	C
170.			P						N	
171.					E		O			
172.			P				O			
173.	A					H				
174.	A					H				
175.					E			D		
176.			P				O			
177.			P					D		
178.	A					H				
179.	A					H				
180.			P				O			
181.					E		O			
182.		R				H				
183.				I			O			
184.			P				O			
185.	A						O			
186.		R				H				
187.				I			O			
188.					E		O			
189.	A					H				
190.	A					H				
191.			P				O			

DIAGNOSTIC GRID (Continued)

Question	Nursing Process					Nursing Content				
	A	R	P	I	E	H	O	D	N	C
192.	A					H				
193.			P				O			
194.			P				O			
195.					E		O			
196.				I			O			
197.			P				O			
198.			P				O			
199.					E		O			
200.	A					H				
201.					E			D		
202.				I						C
203.		R								C
204.				I		H				
205.	A					H				
206.				I			O			
207.		R				H				
208.				I			O			
209.				I			O			
210.	A					H				
211.	A					H				
212.			P				O			
213.	A					H				

DIAGNOSTIC GRID (Continued)

Question	Nursing Process					Nursing Content				
	A	R	P	I	E	H	O	D	N	C
214.					E		O			
215.				I						C
216.				I						C
217.	A					H				
218.	A					H				
219.				I			O			
220.	A					H				
221.					E		O			
Total items this test	65	27	59	39	31	82	92	29	10	18
Your total										
Percent Incorrect										

337

Practice Test 2: Care of the Client During Childbearing

Read each question carefully and select the best answer from the choices presented. Mark your answers on the answer sheet provided on page 351.

1. Maggie Brown is pregnant for the fourth time and is due to deliver her baby next week. Six years ago she gave birth to twins at term, and 3 years ago delivered a stillborn fetus at 8 months of gestation. She has also had a spontaneous abortion at 8 weeks of gestation. Which of the following is correct regarding her gravida and para status?
   a. Gravida 4, para 4
   b. Gravida 3, para 4
   c. Gravida 4, para 3
   d. Gravida 4, para 2

2. Judy Baker visits her obstetrician because she suspects she is pregnant. Her last *normal* menstrual period started on January 12th. Calculated according to Nägele's rule, her EDC is
   a. September 19th
   b. October 12th
   c. October 19th
   d. November 19th

3. The nurse is obtaining a client's prenatal history. It is important to teach the client that
   a. Weight gain should not be curtailed during pregnancy unless it exceeds 40 pounds
   b. Bathtub bathing during pregnancy is not recommended
   c. Drinking in moderation during pregnancy is acceptable since alcohol molecules do not cross the placenta
   d. The client should check with the obstetrician or family physician before taking medications during pregnancy

4. At the prenatal clinic, the nurse is interviewing a client about her previous pregnancies and deliveries. Which of the following comments would indicate that the client is at high risk of developing complications of pregnancy?
   a. "With my last baby, I delivered a week early."
   b. "My first baby was stillborn at 8 months."
   c. "My second babies were twins weighing 5½ pounds each."
   d. "I gained 30 pounds during my first

pregnancy. Nobody talked to me about my diet."

5. In the prenatal clinic, the nurse is interviewing a primigravida client, who is very frightened and tense about her upcoming pelvic examination. The nurse should have the client practice which of the following exercises to relax the perineum before the examination?
   a. Huffing briskly
   b. Kegel's exercise
   c. Pelvic rocking
   d. Pelvic tilt

6. According to current thinking concerning weight gain during pregnancy, a pregnant client should be advised to gain
   a. At least 10 pounds
   b. Between 12 and 14 pounds
   c. Between 22 and 32 pounds
   d. As much as results from satisfying a normal appetite

7. Of the following food constituents, the one which *most* pregnant women need in supplementary amounts is
   a. Iron
   b. Calcium
   c. Potassium
   d. Vitamin C

8. In the prenatal clinic, the nurse is testing a client's urine for protein content. The normal protein level during pregnancy is
   a. Negative
   b. A trace
   c. Less than 1 g
   d. 1 g

9. Regarding travel during pregnancy, the client should be advised that
   a. Air travel is the safest mode of transportation
   b. Strenuous travel should be postponed
   c. If traveling by car, fastening the seatbelt is recommended
   d. All of the above

10. In assessing the condition of an expectant mother in her first trimester, the nurse might expect to find which of the following symptoms?
    a. Ankle edema
    b. Bursts of energy
    c. Increased appetite
    d. Urinary frequency

11. In assessing a prenatal client's condition, an objective sign of pregnancy is
    a. Weight gain
    b. Braxton Hicks contractions
    c. Presence of fetal heart beat
    d. Nausea, vomiting

12. One of the major psychological tasks of the expectant parents during the first trimester of pregnancy is to
    a. Accept the diagnosis and implications of the pregnancy
    b. Concentrate their interest on the unborn child
    c. Focus introspectively
    d. Recognize their respective roles in the birth process and recognize the reality of parenthood

13. Pregnancy is viewed as a maturational crisis. Which of the following statements is correct regarding the psychosocial changes of pregnancy and is therefore appropriate to share with the parents?
    a. Only the woman experiences emotional stress during the first trimester
    b. Often, these changes can weaken the couple's relationship
    c. Sharing their thoughts and feelings about the changes they are experiencing is of primary importance
    d. It is a time of emotional upheaval only for the man

14. The nurse's effective use of communication skills
    a. Increases the nurse's control over the client
    b. Determines for the client what is expected regarding health care procedures
    c. Enhances the quality of nursing care

d. Determines the outcome of nursing care
15. The nurse should suggest to the expectant father that he can be *most* helpful to his partner during the prenatal period by
    a. Monitoring her activities and shielding her from any problems during her pregnancy
    b. Paying critical attention to her diet and activities
    c. Keeping her so busy that she doesn't have time to think about herself and their baby
    d. Realizing and accepting that her attention is now centered on herself and their baby
16. The *most* critical time in the physical and mental development of a fetus is
    a. The first trimester
    b. The second trimester
    c. The third trimester
    d. Birth
17. Which of the following would *not* be good advice to offer a client who has just missed a menstrual period and may be pregnant?
    a. Do not take any drugs that are not prescribed by a physician
    b. Avoid exposure to radiation whether for diagnostic or therapeutic purposes
    c. Obtain a vaccination against rubella infection
    d. Eat a good quality diet and do not smoke
18. Nurse/client communication is affected by
    a. The emotional climate of a given situation
    b. The reasonableness of the participants involved
    c. The time they can devote to their interaction
    d. The circumstances, physical disposition, and atmosphere prevailing at the time
19. A couple has just completed an infertility work-up that revealed that the woman has no identifiable abnormalities other than anovulation. The man has an adequate sperm count and sperm mobility. Pregnancy for this couple is more likely to occur
    a. After they have been carefully instructed in coitus
    b. After therapy with clomiphene (Clomid) or menotropins (Pergonal)
    c. By a homologous insemination
    d. Within the next year
20. The nurse is reviewing a pregnant client's chart in clinic before interviewing her. The nurse knows that the woman is classified as a client at high risk because she
    a. Is 5 feet, 3 inches tall with a prepregnancy weight of 118 pounds
    b. Is 14 years of age
    c. Has had four previous pregnancies
    d. Had nausea with occasional vomiting with her first two pregnancies
21. Linda Jones is a vegetarian. Nutritional counseling for this client should include advising her to
    a. Include meat in her diet at least twice a week
    b. Seek the advice of a nutritionist
    c. Eat a variety of plant foods (particularly legumes, nuts, and seeds) to meet her nutritional needs
    d. Discontinue the vegetarian diet during her second and third trimesters
22. (Questions 22 and 23 refer to this situation) Sally Turner mentions that her sister's use of salt was restricted when she was pregnant and asks, "Will I have to do that, too?" The nurse's *best* response is
    a. "If you develop pregnancy-induced hypertension, salt will be eliminated from your diet."
    b. "During a normal pregnancy there is a slight increase in the need for sodium."
    c. "If your legs start swelling, you will need to limit your salt."

d. "It would be best to add salt to your food neither when cooking nor at the table."

23. In further discussing the client's nutritional needs, the nurse should advise Ms. Turner that she can satisfy her increased need for iron by eating more
    a. Oranges
    b. Cheese and other dairy products
    c. Whole or enriched grain products
    d. Seafood

24. The nurse should teach the expectant mother to make certain her diet includes foods that contain considerable residue (fiber) to
    a. Meet developmental needs of the fetus
    b. Minimize heartburn during pregnancy
    c. Overcome the tendency toward constipation
    d. Prevent nausea in early pregnancy

25. Caroline Johnson plans to breast-feed her infant. Her prenatal rubella titer was 1:4. The nurse plans for Mrs. Johnson to
    a. Receive gamma globulin
    b. Be vaccinated against rubella after she has weaned her infant
    c. Not receive further treatment since she has immunity to rubella
    d. Be vaccinated against rubella while on the postpartum unit

26. A pregnant woman has just been diagnosed with moniliasis. Client teaching in regard to this infection should include the fact that
    a. This is a serious infection that contraindicates vaginal delivery
    b. The only treatment is proper hygienic practices
    c. It is a sexually transmitted disease, and abstention from intercourse is recommended until treatment is completed
    d. The fetus may contract ophthalmia neonatorum through an infected birth canal

27. One of the major psychological tasks of expectant parents during the third trimester is to
    a. Accept the diagnosis and implications of the pregnancy
    b. Prepare for the birth and their parental role
    c. Make sure the father's role in relationship to the mother remains static
    d. Accept the reality of the baby

28. Backaches during pregnancy are common. The *most* helpful exercise to relieve this problem is
    a. Sit-ups
    b. Leg lifts
    c. Pelvic rock
    d. Knee bends

29. Maria Brown is advised to undergo amniocentesis. Amniocentesis is used to obtain information about
    a. The possibility of multiple birth
    b. The presence of Down's syndrome and other chromosome abnormalities
    c. Rh factor and blood type of the fetus
    d. The total amount of amniotic fluid present

30. Which one of the following findings relating to estriol levels would warrant the *most* immediate nursing response?
    a. A fluctuation of estriol levels
    b. A significant rise in estriol levels
    c. No change in the estriol level on the estimated date of confinement
    d. An abrupt fall in estriol levels

31. Pregnant clients with Rh-negative blood factor require a laboratory work-up to identify their candidacy for RhoGam. RhoGam should be administered to an Rh-negative nonsensitized mother
    a. Within 48 hours following delivery
    b. After delivery of an Rh-negative baby and after every miscarriage or abortion
    c. After delivery of an Rh-positive baby and after every miscarriage or abortion
    d. Only after the client's first delivery

32. The nurse is planning care for a woman with hyperemesis gravidarum. Nursing management of this condition includes
    a. Feeding by gavage
    b. Parenteral fluid administration
    c. Establishing a high-fat diet
    d. Establishing a high-protein diet
33. Elaine Graves, a woman in her 12th week of gestation, presents with persistent headache, ankle edema, some visual disturbances, intermittent brownish vaginal discharge, and larger than normal fundal measurement. These signs indicate
    a. Threatened abortion
    b. Ectopic pregnancy
    c. Hydatidiform mole
    d. Placenta previa
34. Nursing management of a ruptured tubal pregnancy should include
    a. Bedrest until vital signs stabilize
    b. Measures to prevent shock, and prepare the client for surgery
    c. Monitoring for shock, blood replacement, and waiting for expulsion of conceptus
    d. Measures to prevent shock and to prepare the client for delivery by a cesarean section
35. Arlene Rogers is a 28-year-old client with diabetes. Which of the following statements is true regarding pregnancy in this client?
    a. The stress of pregnancy may deplete pancreas reserve of insulin, in which case the client will exhibit gestational diabetes
    b. Uteroplacental insufficiency in clients with gestational diabetes results in their delivering small-for-gestational-age babies
    c. Insulin requirements tend to increase during the first trimester of pregnancy
    d. Infants must be monitored carefully postdelivery for signs of hypercalcemia
36. Frances Carson, g1p0, had rheumatic fever as a child, and has residual valvular damage which causes her to suffer shortness of breath during strenuous exercise. The nurse should be concerned about cardiac reserve status and assess the client's condition closely for cardiac decompensation
    a. During the immediate postdelivery period
    b. A week before she goes into labor
    c. When her membranes have been ruptured for 12 hours
    d. When she feels nauseated during her first trimester
37. In a small antepartal clinic, the nurse routinely interviews clients before they see the physician. The client who is showing signs of pregnancy-induced hypertension (PIH) is the one on whose chart the nurse has written
    a. "2 months pregnant—abdominal discomfort, at times accompanied by vaginal spotting."
    b. "7 months pregnant—BP 150/110, gained 10 pounds in last 2 weeks."
    c. "4 months pregnant—BP 160/70—occasional headache after using eyes for fine work."
    d. "6 months pregnant—epigastric discomfort after meals—complains of progressive constipation."
38. On the high-risk labor unit, a preeclamptic patient is receiving magnesium sulfate therapy. Repeat dosage is safe if
    a. Deep tendon reflexes are absent
    b. Urine output is 20 mL per hour
    c. Serum $MgSO_4$ levels are 15 mg/dL or more
    d. Respirations are 12 or more per minute
39. Magnesium sulfate constitutes effective therapy for pre-eclampsia
    a. If combined with a low protein diet
    b. If combined with dehydrating the client to prevent cerebral edema
    c. Because there is no danger that the mother may convulse after delivery
    d. Because it decreases irritability by act-

ing directly on the CNS and by causing vasodilation, which lowers the BP

40. In abruptio placenta, shock
    a. Seldom occurs when a cesarean delivery is accomplished
    b. Occurs to a lesser degree than the amount of bleeding would indicate
    c. Occurs to a greater degree than the amount of bleeding would indicate
    d. Occurs when vaginal delivery is attempted

41. Sign(s) indicative of placenta previa are
    a. Dark bleeding from the vagina and tenderness of the uterus during the midtrimester
    b. History of habitual abortions in midtrimester
    c. Severe abdominal pain and irregular fetal heart tones
    d. Painless, bright red bleeding from the vagina occurring in the third trimester

42. A client is in triage to learn whether she is in true labor. False labor is indicated by
    a. Progressive dilation of the cervix
    b. Increased frequency, duration, and intensity of contractions
    c. Contractions of variable frequency that are relieved by walking
    d. Increased frequency, duration, and intensity of contractions, intensified by walking

43. It is generally accepted that three significant elements of a helping relationship are
    a. Sensitivity, understanding, and a desire to help
    b. A desire to help, a need to be helped, and congruence between both
    c. Empathy, sensitivity, and respect
    d. Understanding, sensitivity, and respect

44. (Questions 44 and 45 refer to this situation) A woman in active labor is admitted to OBICU. While preparing for a manual assessment of cervical dilation, the nurse notices a lesion on the client's vulva. The nurse's initial question should be
    a. "Did you know you have a sore down here?"
    b. "I notice you have a sore down here. How long have you had this?"
    c. "Does this hurt when I touch you?"
    d. "Do you get these sores down here frequently?"

45. The client admits that it hurts, but that the sore erupted only this past week. The nurse's next question should be
    a. "Have you ever had these before?"
    b. "Have you found it to be painful?"
    c. "It looks sore. Have you ever had anything like this before?"
    d. "This could be a problem. Have you had intercourse this week?"

46. Katy Plant is in the first stage of labor. During this stage
    a. Effacement and dilation of the cervix occur
    b. "Pushing" is necessary
    c. Crowning occurs
    d. Thinning of the perineum occurs

47. During labor, a client's FHR is 130 beats/minute. The nurse should
    a. Reassess the FHR in 5 minutes because it is too low
    b. Inform the client that the FHR is normal
    c. Inform the client that her baby will be a girl because the FHR is slow
    d. Immediately report the FHR to the physician

48. Fetal tachycardia is indicated by a baseline FHR
    a. Below 100 beats/minute
    b. Between 100 and 130 beats/minute
    c. Between 130 and 160 beats/minute
    d. Over 160 beats/minute

49. The fetal monitor records early deceleration patterns that are usually related to
    a. Compression of the umbilical cord
    b. Compression of the head
    c. Uteroplacental insufficiency
    d. Maternal hypotension

50. Donna Black was admitted to the labor and delivery suite at 7:00 a.m. after experiencing contractions for 3 hours. Labor assessments revealed dilation of 2 cm, 0 station, and contractions every 5 minutes lasting 40 seconds. Based on these assessments Ms. Black is in the
    a. Descent phase of the second stage of labor
    b. Active phase of the first stage of labor
    c. Transition phase of the first stage of labor
    d. Latent phase of the first stage of labor

51. During induction of labor with intravenous oxytocin, the nurse determines the appropriate rate of administration by
    a. A predetermined calculation of the flow rate
    b. The concentration of the oxytocin solution
    c. The amount of intravenous fluids the client has received
    d. The response of the uterus to the oxytocin solution

52. While caring for the client in labor who is receiving oxytocin (Pitocin), the nurse should watch for signs and symptoms that may indicate a complete uterine rupture, including
    a. Outpouring of blood into the abdominal cavity and sometimes into the vagina, while contractions continue
    b. Pain and abdominal tenderness, while contractions continue
    c. Cessation of regular contractions, presence of pain, and abdominal tenderness
    d. Abdominally palpated uterus presenting as a hard mass lying alongside the fetus while contractions continue

53. Although Laura Rouse has attended classes in prenatal care, she still feels tense and apprehensive about labor and delivery. Administration of agents from which of the following drug categories might relieve her apprehension and tension?
    a. Amnesics
    b. Antihypertensives
    c. Narcotics
    d. Tranquilizers

54. Expression of pain by the client in labor may be *most* influenced by
    a. The ambience and surrounding physical environment
    b. Her cultural and ethnic background
    c. Her education and financial status
    d. The size and position of the fetus

55. A major consideration when administering analgesic agents to a woman in labor is the
    a. Age and parity of the parturient
    b. Degree of discomfort exhibited
    c. Duration of contractions
    d. Status and stage of labor

56. When the uterine membranes rupture in a breech presentation, classified as footling, the nurse should observe carefully for
    a. An arm prolapse
    b. Presenting buttocks
    c. Prolapse of the umbilical cord
    d. Rupture of the uterus

57. (Questions 57 and 58 refer to this situation) Susan Locke's cervix has dilated 8 cm, and the nurse recognizes, from her facial expression, that she is pushing. The proper breathing technique for the nurse to suggest is
    a. Slow abdominal breathing
    b. Brisk blowing (panting)
    c. Shelf breathing
    d. Slow, shallow chest breathing

58. The nurse's verbal instruction to Ms. Locke during the second stage of labor is directed toward
    a. Encouraging her to pant to avoid lacerating her cervix
    b. Encouraging expulsive efforts, using specific statements
    c. Having her anticipate each contraction
    d. Having her tighten perineal muscles

59. A significant problem common to lumbar, epidural and caudal block is
    a. A fall in maternal blood pressure
    b. An increase in the frequency of uterine contractions
    c. A rise in maternal blood pressure
    d. Stimulation of rapid and forceful labor

60. Ruth Sours' labor is being induced with IV oxytocin (Pitocin). She is now in active labor. For 3 contraction cycles, the fetal monitor has shown a decreased FHR baseline variability and bradycardia with late decelerations during uterine contractions. Appropriate nursing intervention is to
    a. Wait to see if the pattern continues
    b. Increase administration of oxytocic drugs
    c. Change maternal position, administer 6–9 L of oxygen per face mask, and notify the physician
    d. Change maternal position, administer oxygen, stop oxytocic drug, and notify the physician

61. Secondary uterine inertia may result in prolongation of all of the following *except* the
    a. Active phase of the first stage of labor
    b. Descent of the fetus
    c. Latent phase of the first stage of labor
    d. Placental expulsion phase of the third stage of labor

62. A young woman in labor says, "I told the doctor I wanted my tubes tied after this delivery. Will they do that before I go home?" The nurse's response should be
    a. "Tubals are done after delivery but you're quite young to have that."
    b. "The doctor didn't tell us that. You'll have to ask her."
    c. "I'm not sure what your doctor's plans are. What did she tell you?"
    d. "Your doctor didn't plan for that. She likes to wait until your 6-week check up."

63. It has been decided that a client in labor, g1p0, should have delivery by cesarean section. The leading indication for performing a primary cesarean section is
    a. Bleeding disorders
    b. Diabetes
    c. Cephalopelvic disproportion
    d. Uterine dysfunction

64. Labor that is prolonged and characterized by increased discomfort in the sacral area is usually the result of a
    a. Cephalic presentation with the occiput in the transverse position
    b. Breech presentation with the sacrum in the anterior position
    c. Cephalic presentation with the occiput in the posterior position
    d. Breech presentation with the sacrum in a transverse position

65. Anne Gray is experiencing a labor typical of a posterior position. Her distress can be *most* effectively relieved by
    a. Applying counterpressure to her back
    b. Massaging her shoulders
    c. Placing her in a semi-Fowler's position
    d. Lowering the head of her bed

66. During the labor and delivery of a client with class III heart disease, all of the following nursing care measures would be supportive *except*
    a. Placing the client in a semi-Fowler's or side-lying position to assure cardiac emptying and proper oxygenation
    b. Limiting the client's contact with the newborn following delivery, to alleviate anxiety
    c. Using a low-forceps delivery to reduce the stress of pushing
    d. Administering penicillin to prevent infection

67. The priority objective of emergency care when a prolapse of the umbilical cord occurs is
    a. To prepare the parents for potential loss of the infant

b. To prevent or relieve pressure on the cord
c. To allow quick repositioning of the cord
d. To effect delivery as soon as possible

68. After delivery of the placenta, an oxytocic drug was administered IV to Jane Crosse to
    a. Control postdelivery bleeding
    b. Ensure adequate lactation
    c. Relieve hypotension
    d. Prevent contractions

69. The *most* critical nursing measure in the immediate care of the newborn is
    a. To assess gestational age
    b. To establish a clear airway
    c. To protect from injury and infection
    d. To provide care for dry skin

70. Baby Sara had a 1 minute Apgar score of 8. This suggests to the nurse that the infant
    a. Was severely depressed and needed rigorous resuscitation
    b. Was moderately depressed and needed minimal resuscitation
    c. Needed intubation and tactile stimulation
    d. Was considered in good condition and needed minimal stimulation

71. Vitamin K is administered routinely to most newborns because
    a. They lack the intestinal flora at birth that are necessary for synthesizing vitamin K
    b. Vitamin K synthesis can occur only in a sterile intestine
    c. Prothrombin time in newborns is insufficient for several months
    d. An external source of vitamin K is necessary for humans

72. During the fourth stage of labor, the *most* appropriate assessments for the nurse to obtain are
    a. Blood pressure, pulse, fundal status, lochial characteristics, status of bowel elimination
    b. Vital signs, oral intake, level of comfort, nutritional status, perineal status
    c. Elimination status, vital signs, characteristics of lochial discharge
    d. Vital signs, fundal status, characteristics of lochial discharge, perineal and urinary status

73. (Questions 73 and 74 refer to this situation) Jane Jones, a 16 year old, is at the family planning clinic for assistance in planning a birth control program. After discussing the available options, she indicates her preference for birth control pills and asks, "Since I'm only 16, will these pills mess me up?" Which of the following nurse responses reflects a communication error by the nurse in decoding or translating the message received from Jane?
    a. "This type has been proven safe for all ages."
    b. "How do you think they'll mess you up?"
    c. "You seem to have some concern about taking these pills."
    d. "If the pill worries you, perhaps you'd like to reconsider another option."

74. In the above situation, the nurse should demonstrate empathy toward the client by saying
    a. "This type has been proven safe for all ages."
    b. "How do you think they'll mess you up?"
    c. "You seem to have some concern about taking these."
    d. "If the pill worries you, perhaps you'd like to reconsider another option."

75. (Questions 75–84 refer to this situation) Gloria Bates, g2p2, delivered a 7-pound, 4-ounce girl 12 hours ago. She is on the postpartum unit. Ms. Bates's fundus is "boggy." The appropriate nursing action would be to
    a. Notify the physician
    b. Elevate the foot of the bed

c. Massage the client's fundus
d. Administer the prescribed analgesic
76. Ms. Bates's perineal discomfort during the first 12 hours after delivery may be relieved by
    a. Applying moist heat to the area
    b. Administering diazepam (Valium) 10 mg tid
    c. Applying ice packs to the area
    d. Having her sit up in a chair for 1 hour
77. When the nurse checks Ms. Bates's fundus about 24 hours after delivery, the fundus is to the right of the midline. The condition that most likely caused this is
    a. Constipation
    b. Uterine atony
    c. A full bladder
    d. Retention of blood clots
78. On the first day postpartum, Ms. Bates's baby nurses for only 1 minute before falling asleep. The nurse should instruct the mother
    a. To allow the baby to continue sleeping
    b. That using a nipple shield will make it easier for the baby to nurse
    c. To interrupt the feeding and attempt to awaken the infant
    d. To massage her breast
79. The nurse teaches Ms. Bates about breast-feeding. Since her nipples are becoming irritated, the nurse should instruct her to
    a. Massage lotion into the nipple area
    b. Expose her breasts to the air after each feeding for 20–30 minutes
    c. Limit nursing time to 12–15 minutes
    d. Discontinue nursing for 24 hours
80. Ms. Bates asks how she will know if her baby is getting enough breast milk. The nurse's best response is
    a. "Weigh her before and after each feeding."
    b. "Nurse the baby 20–30 minutes on each breast every feeding."
    c. "Offer the baby water between feedings. If she refuses, she is getting enough breast milk."
    d. "She is getting enough milk if she sleeps 2–4 hours between feedings."
81. In discussing dietary requirements for Ms. Bates, the nurse should teach her that caloric requirements during lactation increase over nonpregnant requirements by
    a. 300 calories
    b. 500 calories
    c. 700 calories
    d. 800 calories
82. Ms. Bates asks about the safety of using oral contraceptives while she is breast-feeding her baby. Oral contraceptives are contraindicated for breast-feeding mothers, especially in the early lactating period. Other contraindications for OCs are
    a. A client or family history of diabetes
    b. A client or family history of stroke
    c. A client or family history of thromboembolic disease
    d. All of the above
83. Ms. Bates complains of abdominal pains while nursing the baby. The nurse should explain to Ms. Bates that these pains are uterine contractions caused by
    a. Blood loss during delivery
    b. Retention of small placental tags
    c. Excessive stretching of the uterus during pregnancy
    d. Release of oxytocin during nursing
84. If progress is normal, on Ms. Bates's second postpartal day, the nurse should anticipate that the client will have a vaginal discharge called lochia
    a. Alba
    b. Rubra
    c. Serosa
    d. Serous
85. Rachel Barns is bottle-feeding her baby for the first time. In preparing her for this experience, the nurse's client teaching should include which of the following instructions?
    a. The best position for feeding is to have the baby lie flat in mother's arms

b. The collapsible, disposable bottles prevent swallowing of air while the infant is sucking
c. Milk should fill the entire nipple of the bottle when the baby is sucking
d. The infant should be bubbled at the end of each feeding

86. Barbara Tressler, g6p6, enters the obstetric recovery room. An hour ago she delivered a 9½ pound male infant. Low forceps were used after an 18-hour labor period. Which of the following complications is *most* likely?
    a. Placenta previa
    b. Postpartum hemorrhage
    c. Disseminated intravascular coagulopathy
    d. Retained secundines

87. Research has shown that maternal–child bonding most likely is set in motion when the mother first
    a. Hears her baby cry
    b. Breast-feeds her baby
    c. Has examined her baby for defects
    d. Has eye-to-eye contact with her baby

88. To promote the father's bonding, the nurse should
    a. Encourage him to touch the baby's skin
    b. Call the infant by its last name
    c. Discuss the newborn's characteristics
    d. Teach him to diaper his baby

89. Mary Jeffers has delivered a premature infant, at 26 weeks of gestation, weighing 3 pounds. The nurse expects Mary to
    a. Give the impression that this is no problem
    b. Seem depressed and withdrawn
    c. Show no interest in the baby
    d. All of the above

90. In the use of the rhythm method of birth control, it is important that the client know the time at which ovulation occurs. One indication that ovulation has just occurred is
    a. An abrupt rise in basal body temperature
    b. Absence of the fernlike pattern in the cervical mucus
    c. Decreased viscosity of the cervical mucus
    d. Tenderness and tingling of the breasts

91. A postpartum client asks, "When should a woman have the fit of her diaphragm checked?" The nurse's best response is
    a. "After a weight gain of 15 pounds but not after a weight loss."
    b. "Every 6 months."
    c. "After an abortion or a full-term pregnancy."
    d. "After the first pregnancy only."

92. Four days postpartum Ruth Johnson's physician diagnoses endometritis. Signs or symptoms of endometritis include
    a. Malaise, polydipsia
    b. Scant or profuse discharge of foul-smelling lochia
    c. Leg pains and edema
    d. All of the above

93. Lisa Bowman develops symptoms of mastitis. Which of the following statements about mastitis are true?
    a. Symptoms usually develop within 4 to 6 days after delivery
    b. The infection is most likely bilateral, due to the invasion of hemolytic *Streptococcus* organisms
    c. Localization of the infection with axillary adenopathy occurs rapidly after the initial infection
    d. Treatment will include sufficient support of the breasts, local application of heat, antibiotic and analgesic therapy

94. (Questions 94 and 95 refer to this situation) A 17-year-old client comes to the nurse and states "I think I'm pregnant. My period is late and I've been sick to my stomach. Is there a test that can tell me for sure?" The *most* helpful response for the nurse to make is
    a. "How late is your period?"
    b. "That's a scary situation, I know. Let's

talk more about why you think you're pregnant."
c. "You seem worried. Do you want to talk about it?"
d. "I know you're worried. Have you thought about the alternatives to pregnancy?"

95. In the previous situation, the nurse/client relationship will be enhanced if during the interview, the nurse
   a. Uses open-ended questions
   b. Promotes a comfortable climate
   c. Focuses on the client's intention
   d. Provides information that will solve the client's problem

96. Bill and Beth Weaver are a young couple, recently married, who are seeking family planning information. Beth says to the nurse, "We're really having problems. Bill's family keeps asking us when we're going to have a baby. Bill is one of seven children and I'm an only child. We don't want to start our family yet." The nurse's first response should be
   a. "You seem to be upset about your husband's relatives intruding on your privacy."
   b. "You're in an awkward situation and don't know how to handle it."
   c. "That's typical of some large families. They're making you feel guilty."
   d. "Are you upset at your relatives, or your husband?"

97. Select the underlying feeling *best* reflected in this statement: "Young people today really have a lot more sexual freedom than we did when I was growing up."
   a. Frustration
   b. Powerlessness
   c. Anger
   d. Confusion

98. (Questions 98–100 refer to this situation) In the newborn nursery, the nurse is plotting baby Timmy Jones' weight against gestational age on the intrauterine growth chart. His weight is above the 10th percentile and below the 90th percentile for any given gestational age and is therefore determined to be
   a. SGA
   b. AGA
   c. LGA
   d. Postterm

99. In caring for Timmy, which of the following preparations is inappropriate as a prophylactic agent for treating ophthalmia neonatorum?
   a. Nystatin liquid
   b. Penicillin drops
   c. Silver nitrate 1%
   d. Erythromycin (Ilotycin) ointment

100. The nurse assists in diagnosing an infection in Timmy by observing for the following symptom(s)
   a. Hyperthermia
   b. Lethargy and irritability
   c. Hyperactivity
   d. Daily weight loss of 1 ounce

101. In assessing the condition of a full-term, newborn girl, an abnormality might be present if the nurse observes
   a. That the infant regurgitates following nursing
   b. The presence of erythema toxicum
   c. Bloody discharge from the infant's vagina
   d. That the left arm is unflexed

102. A baby whose mother has diabetes is admitted to the nursery. The nurse should anticipate that the baby will need
   a. Phototherapy
   b. A RhoGam work-up
   c. Early glucose feedings
   d. Care for dry, cracking skin

103. Baby Cindy James's high-pitched, shrill cry should alert the nurse to observe for other signs of
   a. Caput succedaneum
   b. Cephalhematoma
   c. Intracranial pressure
   d. Erb–Duchenne paralysis

104. A mother who has a history of recurrent monilial infection should be alerted to report to her physician any signs of infection in her newborn. The sign, which will probably appear after the baby is discharged, and the appropriate treatment are
    a. Purulent eye drainage; penicillin drops
    b. Yellow discharge from the vagina; IV antibiotics
    c. Eruption of skin pustules; penicillin ointment
    d. White patches in the mouth; nystatin liquid or gentian violet
105. The nurse is assisting a mother as she bathes her 2-day-old infant, who weighs 5 pounds, 10 ounces. Which of the following comments would be *most* appropriate in regard to the infant's thermoregulation?
    a. "You can totally undress him, keep him covered with a light blanket, and quickly bathe him to keep him from getting cold."
    b. "Since your son is now past his first 24 hours, he can control his temperature quite well."
    c. "Uncover only the portion of the baby you are bathing at the time."
    d. "Since your baby is now eating well, this helps him control his temperature."
106. An infant is experiencing respiratory distress. Which one of the following observations relates to this condition?
    a. The chest and abdomen rise with inspiration
    b. There is a decrease in respiratory rate
    c. There is inspiratory grunting
    d. Intercostal muscles are indrawn
107. The nurse notices signs of jaundice in several newborns in the nursery. The newborn's immature liver is the major cause of physiologic jaundice, which occurs
    a. Within the first 24 hours of life
    b. When an infant receives phototherapy
    c. When the direct Coombs' test result is positive
    d. On the second or third day in the normal newborn
108. (Questions 108 and 109 refer to this situation) In caring for premature infant Matthew Brown, who is receiving phototherapy, the nurse should observe all of the following precautions *except*
    a. Temperature monitoring
    b. Applying eye patches
    c. Removing the infant from under the lights for 2-hour periods for stimulation
    d. Covering the genitalia
109. To determine whether or not premature Matthew might tolerate oral feedings, the nurse should look for
    a. The absence of respiratory distress and abdominal distention
    b. The presence of suck and swallow reflexes
    c. Gastric residuum of 1 mL or less before feeding
    d. All of the above
110. While caring for an infant born to a drug-addicted mother, the nurse should know that for withdrawal
    a. Symptoms may include tremors, shrill crying, and restlessness
    b. Symptoms are a result of narcosis
    c. Treatment includes hydration and administration of methadone
    d. The prognosis is good with or without treatment
111. A mother who is breast-feeding her infant for the first time says, "He's so fussy, I don't think he's getting enough." A facilitative response would be
    a. "Oh, newborns don't really need that much at first."
    b. "Maybe you're not holding him right. Let me prop you up more."
    c. "Why don't you try him on the glucose water this time?"
    d. "You're worried because you can't see how much he's getting."

Answer Sheet—Test 2

Answers and Rationales for Test 2

1. d. The client has had four pregnancies (gravida 4), of which two were carried to viability (para 2). A, H
2. c. Count back 3 months from the date of the client's last menstrual period (LMP), and add 7 days. A, H
3. d. The client should be aware of the possible teratogenic effects of drugs during pregnancy. I, D
4. b. A history of stillbirth is an indication of high risk. A, H
5. b. Kegel's exercise involves tightening and relaxing the muscles of the perineal floor. I, O
6. c. Gaining 22–32 pounds provides for growth of the fetus and strengthens supporting maternal tissues. I, O
7. a. Hemodilution occurs as blood volume increases and iron is stored in the fetal liver the last half of pregnancy; therefore, supplemental sources of iron are necessary for the mother and fetus. P, H
8. a. In a normal pregnancy, proteinuria should not be present. A, H
9. d. All these precautions are sound advice. I, O
10. d. Bladder irritability is present, causing urinary frequency, nocturia. A, H
11. c. Choices *a*, *b*, and *d* can be confused with other problems. A, H
12. a. Early acceptance of the pregnancy is essential. Choice *b* involves a second trimester focus; *c* is not a task, and *d* is a third trimester task. A, H
13. c. Stress is encountered by both partners. A couple's relationship is often strengthened by sharing this experience. A, H
14. c. Research studies show that the quality of care is enhanced through effective communication skills. A, C
15. d. The best way for him to cope is to accept his partner's physical and emotional concern for their unborn child. I, O
16. a. Cell differentiation occurs during the first trimester. A, H
17. c. Rubella vaccine is a live attenuated vaccine and could cause anomalies in embryo and fetus. I, O
18. d. Research studies indicate a relationship between these variables. E, C
19. b. Endocrine therapy may induce ovulation in anovulatory women. A, H
20. b. Women age 16 or under are at risk physically, emotionally, and socially. A, H
21. c. Vegetarian diets can be consistent with nutritional needs throughout pregnancy, if a variety of plant foods are eaten. I, N
22. b. Diets low in sodium place the normal mother and fetus at risk, especially for pregnancy-induced hypertension (PIH). I, N
23. c. Grains, meat, liver, eggs, nuts, dried fruits, and legumes are good sources of iron. I, N
24. c. Residue (fiber) in diet adds bulk and aids bowel evacuation. I, N
25. d. Rubella vaccine, being a live attenuated vaccine, would be given after delivery with instructions to avoid pregnancy for 2 to 3 months. The vaccine does not affect the breast-feeding infant. A titer of 1:8 or less indicates nonimmunity to rubella. P, D
26. c. A woman can be reinfected by her partner. I, O
27. b. This process is, to some extent, ongoing throughout pregnancy, but parents begin preparation in earnest in the last trimester. A, H
28. c. This exercise strengthens and relaxes back muscles and pelvis. I, O
29. b. Amniocentesis can provide prenatal diagnosis of genetic problems and an estimation of gestational age. A, H

30. d. A decreasing estriol level indicates a failing pregnancy. P, D
31. c. RhoGam is given in these situations if Coombs' test result is negative. Administration should take place within 72 hours after delivery to prevent isoimmunization. I, D
32. b. Management includes hospitalization with administration of parenteral fluids in the first 48 hours and cautious resumption of a diet, in 6 small feedings daily, with clear liquids given 1 hour after meals. I, O
33. c. These symptoms suggest hydatidiform mole. A, H
34. b. Excessive bleeding (hence risk of shock) occurs with ruptured tubal pregnancy; surgery should be performed as soon as possible. I, O
35. a. Choices b, c, and d are wrong: gestational diabetics tend to have large-for-gestational-age (LGA) babies; insulin requirements usually decrease during the first trimester; and infants need to be monitored for symptoms of hypoglycemia. A, H
36. a. Cardiac output increases rapidly as extravascular fluid returns to the vascular compartment and intraabdominal pressure is drastically reduced. A, H
37. b. Pregnancy-induced hypertension (PIH) develops after the 20th week of gestation, accompanied by a weight gain in excess of 4 to 4½ pounds per week with BP of 140/90 or more. A, H
38. d. Choices a, b, and c indicate toxic levels of $MgSO_4$. I, D
39. d. Magnesium sulfate has anticonvulsant properties. Protein and fluids should not be limited. There is always a threat of sudden advancement of pregnancy-induced hypertension (PIH) with convulsions occurring. I, D
40. c. Retroplacental bleeding may be present but not evident. A, H
41. d. Placenta previa presents with no pain and bright red bleeding in the third trimester. A, H
42. c. Indications of false labor include irregular contractions that can be relieved by walking. A, H
43. d. Psychologist Carl Rogers' theory cites these three elements. E, C
44. b. Identify the area of concern and ask an open-ended question. Don't probe unnecessarily or convey an assumption. I, C
45. c. Demonstrating understanding is essential. Seek more information from the client without using a judgmental tone. I, C
46. a. These events occur in the first stage of labor. The other choices are stage 2 events. A, H
47. b. The normal fetal heart rate (FHR) range is 120–160 beats/minute. I, O
48. d. The normal fetal heart rate (FHR) is between 120 and 160 beats/minute. E, H
49. b. Early deceleration patterns are related to head compression. Cord compression is related to variable decelerations; uteroplacental insufficiency and maternal hypotension are related to late decelerations. A, H
50. d. Latent phase is from 0 to 3 or 4-cm dilation. A, H
51. d. Dosage is increased gradually until an adequate pattern of uterine contractions is achieved. I, D
52. c. After rupturing, the uterus is no longer able to contract and the client will experience pain. A, D
53. d. Tranquilizers are antianxiety agents. P, D
54. b. How persons perceive and respond to pain varies cross-culturally. A, H
55. d. Do not administer analgesics if birth is expected within 2 hours. For nullipara, administer before full dilation. For multipara, administer before dilation

reaches 7 cm. Respiratory depression with deceleration of fetal heart rate and loss of short-term variability can occur. A, D

56. c. Danger of prolapsed umbilical cord increases with breech presentation, because the breech does not fill the pelvic cavity as completely as does the head. A, H

57. b. Pushing should not begin until the second stage of labor. Brisk blowing or panting will prevent her from pushing. I, O

58. b. The second stage of labor is the expulsive stage. Explicit directions from the nurse to the client are important to achieve efficient pushing. P, O

59. a. Vasodilation induces hypotension. A, D

60. d. Fetal depression and hypoxia are indicated by decreased fetal heart rate (FHR) baseline variability and late decelerations. Changing maternal position and administering oxygen should reverse the placental insufficiency. Fetal distress is a contraindication for oxytocin (Pitocin). The physician should be advised of the fetal distress. I, D

61. c. Secondary uterine inertia results when well-established, effective contractions become weak, brief, or cease altogether. Uterine inertia of the latent phase is primary inertia. R, H

62. c. The nurse should respond honestly and ask the client for more information in order to understand her real need. I, C

63. c. Cephalopelvic disproportion (CPD) is the most common indication for performing a cesarean section (CS). At least 30% of cesarean births performed each year in the United States are repeat cesarean sections. R, H

64. c. The occiput pulls the cervix posterior, and uterine contractions are not as effective. The back pain is a result of the occiput compressing the mother's sacral nerves. R, H

65. a. With occiput posterior position, there is accentuated backache. Applying counterpressure to the sacral area of the back is helpful. I, O

66. b. Early maternal contact with the infant is important in the bonding process. P, O

67. b. Prevention of fetal hypoxia due to compression of the cord is of utmost importance. Knee chest or Trendelenberg position and vaginal support of the presenting part away from the cord are continuously maintained until delivery is accomplished. P, O

68. a. Oxytocin stimulates the uterus to contract, thus decreasing bleeding from the placental site. I, D

69. b. Retention of fluid alters pulmonary function and interferes with oxygen exchange. The priority of newborn care is the establishment of respirations, which normally is accomplished within 1 minute of birth. I, O

70. d. Scores below 7 indicate an increasing degree of asphyxia and depression in the infant. Scores between 4 and 7 indicate that muscle tone is reduced and the infant is cyanotic. Scores below 4 indicate that the infant is severely depressed. A, H

71. a. The presence of intestinal flora is necessary for the synthesis of vitamin K. I, D

72. d. Complete assessment of the client's condition is important during the fourth stage, which is the most critical time for the mother in regard to hemorrhage. P, H

73. a. The nurse thinks the client is questioning the nurse's knowledge and responds accordingly. I, C

74. d. Empathy is a display of understanding of another's feelings and the reason for those feelings. E, C

75. c. Massage will stimulate the uterus to contract. P, O
76. c. Applying ice to the area decreases edema. I, O
77. c. A full bladder will displace the uterus to the right, and should be the first nursing assessment performed. A, H
78. c. The infant should be awakened. Nursing will stimulate milk production. I, O
79. b. Air-drying the breasts helps prevent nipple irritation. I, O
80. d. The baby's intake is sufficient if she sleeps for 2–4 hours between feedings. A lengthy feeding of 20–30 minutes on each breast is excessive, causing nipple irritation at this early stage. I, O
81. b. Increasing caloric intake by approximately 500 calories will provide adequate protein, carbohydrates, and fats for the infant's nourishment during lactation. I, O
82. d. Thromboembolic disease and other vascular problems are side-effects of oral contraceptives (OCs). I, O
83. d. Suckling stimulates the release of oxytocin, which causes contraction of smooth muscles. I, O
84. b. Lochia rubra is present for the first 2 to 3 days after delivery. A, H
85. c. This prevents the infant from swallowing air. I, O
86. b. Grand multiparity decreases uterine muscle tone; delivery of a large baby indicates an overdistended uterus; low-forceps delivery traumatizes the mother. All these factors predispose her to uterine atony and hemorrhage. A, H
87. d. Eye contact appears to have a strong effect on initiating and developing a trusting relationship. A, H
88. a. Touch enhances interaction and development of attachment. I, O
89. d. Anticipatory grief, denial, and depression are all common reactions of a mother following the birth of a premature infant. R, H
90. a. The basal body temperature (BBT) drops slightly before ovulation, then elevates slightly after ovulation. I, O
91. c. A diaphragm must be refitted after the loss or gain of 10 pounds or more, or after giving birth. I, O
92. b. This discharge is characteristic of endometritis. A, H
93. d. These are standard measures in treating mastitis. I, O
94. b. The nurse is communicating support and understanding, while at the same time, steering the interview toward obtaining more specific information. I, C
95. b. Promoting a comfortable climate in the initial interaction helps to establish a trusting nurse/client relationship. I, C
96. a. The nurse is able to clarify the underlying issue through active listening rather than by presuming to know what the problem is. I, C
97. c. Anger is often expressed as annoyance or irritation. It is sometimes a defense mechanism to mask fear. E, C
98. b. The infant's weight is appropriate for gestational age. A, H
99. a. Nystatin is the treatment of choice for thrush. I, D
100. b. Lethargy and irritability may be symptoms of infection. A, H
101. d. An unflexed left arm is a symptom of brachial paralysis. A, H
102. c. Babies of mothers with diabetes are likely to exhibit symptoms of hypoglycemia during the first few hours after delivery. P, O
103. c. A shrill, high-pitched cry is a symptom of intracranial pressure. A, H
104. d. Thrush can be relieved by administration of nystatin. A, H

105. c. Uncovering only a portion of the baby at a time helps to prevent hypothermia. I, O
106. d. Respiratory distress causes the intercostal muscles to become indrawn. Respiratory distress in infants causes respirations to increase, and expiratory grunting to occur. A, H
107. d. This may occur on the second or third day. Phototherapy is used to treat hyperbilirubinemia, and Coombs' test detects the presence of antibodies. A, H
108. c. Infants need stimulation, but for therapy to be of maximum benefit, they should be removed from under the light for feeding periods of no longer than 30 minutes. I, O
109. d. These are all indications of readiness for oral feeding, as is the presence of bowel sounds. A, H
110. a. These symptoms are a result of withdrawal; methadone is contraindicated because of possible addiction; at least a third of addicted infants will die if treatment is withheld. A, H
111. d. This statement shows that the nurse understands her feelings and the cause underlying her concern. I, C

DIAGNOSTIC GRID
Test 2

Directions: The diagnostic grid is used to reveal deficiencies in nursing content and nursing process knowledge. Determine which questions you answered incorrectly and circle the corresponding codes. Total each column and note the percentage of incorrect answers.

Nursing Process
A = Assessment
R = Analysis/nursing diagnosis
P = Planning
I = Implementation/intervention
E = Evaluation

Nursing Content
H = Health status
O = Nursing actions/interventions
D = Drugs/pharmacology
N = Nutrition
C = Communication skills

Question	A	R	P	I	E	H	O	D	N	C
1.	A					H				
2.	A					H				
3.				I				D		
4.	A					H				
5.				I			O			
6.				I			O			
7.			P			H				
8.	A					H				
9.				I			O			
10.	A					H				
11.	A					H				
12.	A					H				
13.	A					H				
14.	A									C
15.				I			O			

DIAGNOSTIC GRID (Continued)

Question	Nursing Process					Nursing Content				
	A	R	P	I	E	H	O	D	N	C
16.	A					H				
17.				I			O			
18.					E					C
19.	A					H				
20.	A					H				
21.				I					N	
22.				I					N	
23.				I					N	
24.				I					N	
25.			P					D		
26.				I			O			
27.	A					H				
28.				I			O			
29.	A					H				
30.			P					D		
31.				I				D		
32.				I			O			
33.	A					H				
34.				I			O			
35.	A					H				
36.	A					H				
37.	A					H				

DIAGNOSTIC GRID (Continued)

Question	Nursing Process					Nursing Content				
	A	R	P	I	E	H	O	D	N	C
38.				I				D		
39.				I				D		
40.	A					H				
41.	A					H				
42.	A					H				
43.					E					C
44.				I						C
45.				I						C
46.	A					H				
47.				I			O			
48.					E	H				
49.	A					H				
50.	A					H				
51.				I				D		
52.	A							D		
53.			P					D		
54.	A					H				
55.	A							D		
56.	A					H				
57.				I			O			
58.			P				O			
59.	A							D		

DIAGNOSTIC GRID (Continued)

Question	Nursing Process					Nursing Content				
	A	R	P	I	E	H	O	D	N	C
60.				I				D		
61.		R				H				
62.				I						C
63.		R				H				
64.		R				H				
65.				I			O			
66.			P				O			
67.			P				O			
68.				I				D		
69.				I			O			
70.	A					H				
71.				I				D		
72.			P			H				
73.				I						C
74.					E					C
75.			P				O			
76.				I			O			
77.	A					H				
78.				I			O			
79.				I			O			
80.				I			O			
81.				I			O			

DIAGNOSTIC GRID (Continued)

Question	Nursing Process					Nursing Content				
	A	R	P	I	E	H	O	D	N	C
82.				I			O			
83.				I			O			
84.	A					H				
85.				I			O			
86.	A					H				
87.	A					H				
88.				I			O			
89.		R				H				
90.				I			O			
91.				I			O			
92.	A					H				
93.				I			O			
94.				I						C
95.				I						C
96.				I						C
97.					E					C
98.	A					H				
99.				I				D		
100.	A					H				
101.	A					H				
102.			P				O			
103.	A					H				

DIAGNOSTIC GRID (Continued)

Question	Nursing Process					Nursing Content				
	A	R	P	I	E	H	O	D	N	C
104.	A					H				
105.				I			O			
106.	A					H				
107.	A					H				
108.				I			O			
109.	A					H				
110.	A					H				
111.				I						C
Total items this test	44	4	10	48	5	47	32	15	4	13
Your total										
Percent Incorrect										

Practice Test 3: Care of the Child

Read each question carefully and select the best answer from the choices presented. Mark your answers on the answer sheet on page 377.

1. (Questions 1–3 refer to this situation) Amy Brooks, an 8-month-old girl, comes to the clinic for a well child visit. She is sitting on her mother's lap resting quietly. She appears well nourished and clean. Her mother expresses concern about Amy's language development. Amy should be
   a. Saying "dada" and "mama" specifically ("dada" to father and "mama" to mother)
   b. Saying three other words besides "mama" and "dada"
   c. Saying "dada" and "mama" nonspecifically
   d. Turning when she hears a voice, but not imitating speech sounds
2. If Amy's gross motor skills are developing normally, the nurse will observe Amy
   a. Stand momentarily without holding onto furniture
   b. Stand alone well for long periods of time
   c. Pass cubes hand to hand
   d. Sit without support for long periods of time
3. Nutritional counseling for Ms. Brooks about Amy's diet should include which of the following points?
   a. Items from all four food groups should be introduced to Amy by the time she is 9 or 10 months old
   b. Solid foods should not be introduced until Amy is 10 months old
   c. Iron deficiency rarely develops before 8 or 9 months of age, so iron-fortified cereals should be introduced when she is 9 months old
   d. Amy's diet can be changed from formula to whole milk when she is 12 months old
4. To encourage 4-year-old Sarah's autonomy, her mother should
   a. Discourage her choice of clothing
   b. Button her coat and blouse for her
   c. Praise her attempts to dress herself
   d. Criticize her combination of clothes
5. Goals of developmental assessment include all of the following *except*
   a. Providing anticipatory guidance for parents
   b. Helping parents understand their child's behavior
   c. Identifying deviations from normal growth and development patterns
   d. Determining the child's future development

6. Two-year-old Jimmy tells his mother he is afraid to go to sleep because "the monsters will get him." Jimmy's mother is very concerned about his behavior. The nurse should tell his mother to
   a. Allow Jimmy to sleep with his parents in their bed whenever he is afraid
   b. Increase Jimmy's activity before he goes to bed, so he eventually falls asleep from being tired
   c. Read a story to Jimmy before bedtime and allow him to have a cuddly animal or a blanket
   d. Allow Jimmy to stay up an hour later with the family until he falls asleep

7. At which of the following ages does a child have a vocabulary of 300 words, combine 2 or 3 words in a phrase, and ask for objects by name?
   a. 12–15 months
   b. 36–39 months
   c. 24–27 months
   d. 18–21 months

8. When a child is able to grasp the idea that even though mommy placed the ball under the hat, the ball continues to exist, according to Piaget, the child is in which of the following stages in the development of logical thinking?
   a. Sensorimotor
   b. Preoperational
   c. Concrete operations
   d. Formal operations

9. At 10 months of age, Anna now looks for objects that have been removed from her view. This developmental principle illustrates that
   a. Her neuromuscular development enables her to reach out and grasp objects
   b. Her curiosity is increased
   c. She understands the permanence of objects even though she cannot see them
   d. She is able to transfer objects from hand to hand

10. Tommy called everyone "dada" before he began to associate the name only with his father. Which of the following principles describes this behavior?
    a. Development follows a proximal-distal pattern
    b. Development moves from general to specific
    c. Growth and development is a constant process
    d. Speech development occurs later than other skills

11. Toddlers establish ritualistic patterns to
    a. Establish a sense of identity
    b. Gain control over adults in their environment
    c. Establish sequenced patterns of learning behavior
    d. Establish a sense of security among inconsistencies they perceive in their environment

12. Four-year-old Anne Baker attends a nursery school that provides daycare while her parents work. Health screening required by the nursery school should include submission of Anne's immunization record and
    a. Physical exam, vision/hearing
    b. Tuberculin test, physical exam, rubella serology, blood pressure
    c. Tuberculin test, physical exam, blood pressure, vision/hearing
    d. Tuberculin test, physical exam, blood pressure, vision/hearing, hemoglobin, hematocrit

13. Ms. Smith brought her 2-year-old Lynne in for a well child visit. She was concerned about toilet training her daughter. Which of the following are not requirements for toilet training readiness?
    a. Adequate neuromuscular development for sphincter control
    b. Appropriate chronological age
    c. The child's ability to communicate the need to use the toilet
    d. The child's desire to please her parents

14. The anterior fontanelle is usually closed by age
    a. 18 months
    b. 2 months
    c. 7 months
    d. 24 months
15. Communicating with parents and children about health care has become increasingly significant because
    a. Consumers of health care are less knowledgeable about health
    b. Specialization has increased the complexity of managing health
    c. Nurse educators have recognized the value of communication
    d. Clients are more demanding that their rights be respected
16. Safety measures to prevent childhood accidents include all of the following *except*
    a. Placing guards in front of any heating appliance, fireplace, or furniture
    b. Placing a car seat in a front-seat, front-facing position
    c. Checking the safety of toys
    d. Placing toxic substances out of reach or in a locked cabinet
17. A mother of a toilet-trained 2½ year old expresses concern over her child's bed-wetting while hospitalized. The most appropriate response for the nurse to make is to tell the mother that
    a. "He was too immature to be toilet trained. In a few months he should be old enough."
    b. "Children are afraid in the hospital and frequently wet their bed."
    c. "Hospitalization is so frightening for a child that they often regress in development to feel in control and safe in their environment."
    d. "Don't worry about it, he probably received too much fluid the night before."
18. The most appropriate toys to give to a 5-month-old infant are
    a. Toy cars
    b. Games, puzzles
    c. Stuffed animals
    d. Soft washable toys
19. In nurse/client communication, the quality of the interaction
    a. Is the responsibility of the nurse
    b. Depends on the client's needs
    c. Reflects the knowledge base of the participants
    d. Improves as the nurse gains experience
20. Four-day-old Brian is admitted to the special care nursery for observation. His mother appears to remain distant from him when she visits him. A breakdown in the mother–infant relationship may have occurred because of
    a. The mother's feelings of inadequacy in her role
    b. The hostile hospital environment
    c. Maternal guilt
    d. All of the above
21. Cory Dean brings her 15-month-child in for a well baby visit. Immunizations that should be completed at 15 months of age include
    a. DTP 2, OPV 3, tuberculin skin test, measles, mumps, rubella
    b. DTP 3, OPV 2, tuberculin skin test, measles, mumps, rubella
    c. DPT 4, OPV 4, tuberculin test, measles, mumps, rubella
    d. DPT 2, OPV 2, tuberculin skin test, measles, mumps, rubella
22. Debbie Connors brings her 7-month-old infant into the well baby clinic for a checkup. She is concerned that the infant girl is overweight. She feeds the infant 20 calorie per ounce formula whenever she is hungry. The nurse's most appropriate response would be
    a. "It is okay to use the 2% milk formula, just add vitamins."
    b. "Skim milk is high in protein and lower in calories."
    c. "Decrease the amount of formula

feedings to 16 ounces daily, and supplement with juice and water."
d. "Continue with the formula, keep a 3-day record of your child's intake, and bring this back to the clinic for further evaluation."

23. Gina Meyers brings 15-month-old Michael to the well baby clinic. She states he has been taking approximately 18 to 20 ounces of whole milk per day from a bottle with meals and at bedtime. The nurse should suggest that she begin weaning Michael from the bottle to avoid risking
    a. Malnutrition
    b. Anemia
    c. Dental caries
    d. Malocclusion

24. When teaching parents about poisonous substances, the nurse should emphasize which of the following safety points?
    a. Children should be adequately supervised at all times
    b. All poisonous substances should be kept out of reach of children and stored in a locked cabinet if necessary
    c. The importance of the difference between pediatric and adult dosages of medicines and the potential harmful effects of adult dosages on children
    d. All of the above

25. Immediate care of the child who has ingested a poisonous substance includes all of the following actions *except*
    a. Inducing vomiting or neutralization
    b. Providing respiratory and cardiac support
    c. Offering reassurance to decrease anxiety
    d. Teaching parents home safety

26. Amoxicillin is prescribed for Jimmy's ear infection. While on this antibiotic Jimmy should not eat
    a. Whole grain breads and cereals
    b. Meats and eggs
    c. Dairy products
    d. Juice and carbohydrates

27. Two toddlers are arguing over a toy in the playroom. An appropriate nurse response is
    a. "If you can't play together, I'll have to put you back in your rooms."
    b. "Give the toy to me. Now neither of you will have it."
    c. "Guess what? I'll bet you can't get all those blocks in that box."
    d. "Oh, let me see if I can hold that."

28. (Questions 28 and 29 refer to this situation) Alice James, 9 months old, is hospitalized for respiratory complications of her cystic fibrosis. Her mother is very upset and the nurse finds her crying in the parents' lounge. This is the fifth admission for Alice this year. The nurse's most appropriate response to Ms. James is
    a. "This must be very difficult for you. Would you like to talk about how you are feeling?"
    b. "Ms. James, Alice will be fine, she's been through this before."
    c. "Ms. James, maybe you should go home so Alice doesn't see how upset you are."
    d. To allow Ms. James to cry alone and spend time with Alice while her mother is gone

29. Alice refuses to take her pancreatic enzyme supplement with her meals and snacks. Her mother does not like to force the child to take the supplement. The most appropriate way for the nurse to reason with Ms. James is to tell her
    a. "We will not give her the Pancrease with this small snack, but at meal time we must."
    b. "Alice needs these pancreatic enzymes to aid with absorption of fats and proteins. She needs this nutrition to grow stronger and fight infection."
    c. "If Alice doesn't take this, she will never leave the hospital."

d. "Please let me feed her, maybe she won't refuse me, I have a way with these children."

30. Steroid therapy is indicated in the management of nephrosis in children. The child must be monitored for drug side-effects, which include all of the following *except*
    a. Signs of edema, especially in the face
    b. Gastric and intestinal mucosal bleeding
    c. Increased susceptibility to infection
    d. Headaches and dizziness

31. Characteristics of a parent at risk for child abuse include all of the following *except*
    a. Low self-esteem
    b. History of substance abuse
    c. An inadequate knowledge of normal growth and development patterns
    d. A history of multiple births

32. Billy, who is 4 years old, continues to come to the nurses' station after being told children are not allowed there. Which of the following statements is confrontative in a constructive way?
    a. "Billy, remember I told you not to come to the nurses' station. I don't want to make you feel badly, but if you keep coming here, I'll have to make you stay in your room."
    b. "Billy, you know you're not supposed to be in here. You'll have to stay out or I'll get mad."
    c. "What do you want now, Billy? You know you're not allowed in here."
    d. "Billy, let's go back out and see if we can find the building blocks."

33. A small infant is brought to the emergency room vomiting and suffering diarrhea, which the mother states started 3 days ago. Clinical manifestations of dehydration include
    a. Decreased or absent tearing
    b. Dry mucous membranes
    c. Sunken fontanelles
    d. All of the above

34. Frank Simms, 2 years old, is brought into the well child clinic by his foster mother. She is concerned because Frank's right eye seems to turn in toward his nose when he is tired. The clinic nurse's *most* appropriate action would be to
    a. Assure the foster mother that this is a normal event when a child is tired
    b. Advise the foster mother to continue to watch his eyes closely, and if the problem persists to call the clinic
    c. Test the child with the cover/uncover test and refer mother and child immediately to an ophthalmologist
    d. Explain to the foster mother that the child will probably outgrow the weakness and she need not be concerned

35. Immediate nursing care of a child born with cleft lip and cleft palate includes
    a. Maintaining a clear and adequate airway
    b. Maintaining sufficient fluid and caloric intake
    c. Providing emotional support to the parents
    d. All of the above

36. Lisa Black called the well baby clinic to report that 9-month-old Melissa has had loose watery stools, with a bloody appearance for 5 days, and has been very irritable. Clinical manifestations in children infected with *Shigella* include all of the following except:
    a. Nausea and vomiting
    b. An afebrile condition
    c. Watery bloody stools
    d. Abdominal cramps

37. Three-year-old Tammy is brought into the ER in her mother's arms. The child's mouth is open and she is drooling, and is lethargic. Her mother states that she became ill rather suddenly within the past 1 or 2 hours. Immediate medical treatment

for children diagnosed with acute epiglottitis is to
a. Draw blood cultures and CBC
b. Start an intravenous line
c. Obtain a chest x-ray
d. Secure an airway by intubation or tracheostomy

38. A 2-year-old child returns to the clinic completing a 10-day course of amoxicillin prescribed to relieve an infection in his right ear. After completing the medication, the child has become fussy and has a low-grade fever. On physical examination, his right tympanic membrane is bulging and he is tugging at his ear. What should the nurse anticipate as his next course of treatment? The physician will
a. Prescribe a decongestant and tell the mother to call if the infection persists
b. Repeat the 10-day course of amoxicillin
c. Refer him to an ENT specialist for myringotomy tubes
d. Start him on another antibiotic for a 10-day course and have his ear re-checked after treatment

39. Jenny Carlson thinks her little boy has appendicitis. The nurse records a detailed history, knowing that appendicitis classically presents with
a. Periumbilical pain, anorexia, shift to RLQ pain, fever
b. Anorexia, RLQ pain, fever, shift to periumbilical pain
c. Fever, vomiting, sharp abdominal pain, shift to RLQ pain
d. RLQ pain, fever, vomiting, shift to periumbilical pain

40. Justin, a 10-month-old boy born with myelomeningocele and hydrocephalus with a ventricular shunt, is brought to the emergency room. His symptoms include vomiting, poor feeding, lethargy, and irritability. The admitting nurse should be suspicious of
a. Acute otitis media
b. Formula intolerance
c. Ventricular shunt malfunction
d. Colic

41. (Questions 41 and 42 refer to this situation)
Client: "My baby won't take her bottle. I don't think she likes the formula."
Nurse: "Babies require a lot of patience. Keep offering it to her. Every little bit helps."
In the above dialogue, the mother's perception can be expressed as follows:
a. "The baby needs to eat, so give her something she likes."
b. "Babies are fussy eaters."
c. "The baby's behavior is confusing."
d. "Babies are very frustrating."

42. The nurse's perception of the situation, reflected in her response, is that the mother
a. Needs to try harder to encourage the baby to take the formula
b. Is insecure, so teaching needs to be reinforced
c. Is typical of all new mothers
d. Will eventually adjust to the situation

43. Proper positioning of the infant with myelomeningocele is
a. Lying on the right side with a pad between the knees, in the high Trendelenburg position
b. Prone position, legs maintained in adduction with pad between knees and roll placed under ankle, in the low Trendelenburg position
c. Prone position with legs maintained in abduction with pad between knees and roll placed under ankle, in the low Trendelenburg position
d. Left side-lying position with pad between knees and roll placed under ankle, in the high Trendelenburg position

44. Prevention of urinary tract infections in a child with myelomeningocele is an im-

portant long-term goal. Interventions include all of the following *except*
   a. Meticulous skin care and using the Credé maneuver to empty the bladder
   b. Frequent emptying of the bladder
   c. Adequate fluid intake
   d. Tight-fitting diapers to prevent leakage
45. For a child admitted because of dehydration, accurate monitoring of fluid intake and output includes
   a. Weighing and recording the weight of the wet diaper
   b. Obtaining a urine specific gravity measure with every voiding
   c. Assessing and measuring of all intake, including IV fluids
   d. All of the above
46. Findings associated with sudden infant death syndrome include all of the following *except*
   a. Infants most at risk are between 10 and 18 months of age
   b. Bouts of apnea lasting 20 seconds or more are warning signs
   c. There is a higher incidence among siblings
   d. There may be a neurological cause for this syndrome
47. Postoperative nursing care of a 7-year-old child who has had a tonsillectomy includes frequent monitoring of the blood pressure. Proper cuff size is
   a. No less than half and no more than two thirds part of the extremity being measured
   b. No less than one third and no more than two thirds part of the extremity being measured
   c. 2.5 times the diameter of the extremity being measured
   d. (None of the above); the blood pressure should be obtained by an arterial line
48. Treatment of viral pharyngitis includes all of the following *except*
   a. Providing a cool mist vaporizer
   b. Providing a soft or liquid diet
   c. Administration of aspirin
   d. Administration of acetaminophen
49. The nurse notices that Lydia, a 2-day-old girl is having an increased number of drooling and choking episodes. Excessive amounts of mucous and cyanotic episodes may indicate
   a. Gastroesophageal reflex
   b. Tracheoesophageal fistula
   c. Bronchopulmonary dysplasia
   d. Hydrocephalus
50. The Ortolani manipulation is used to detect
   a. The startle reflex
   b. Head control
   c. Congenital hip dysplasia
   d. An abdominal mass
51. The squatting position is often assumed by a child with a cardiac defect because it
   a. Increases venous return
   b. Decreases venous return
   c. Relieves abdominal pressure
   d. Increases muscle tone
52. (Questions 52–54 refer to this situation) Christopher Smith, 18 months old, has been hospitalized and scheduled for open heart surgery for tetralogy of Fallot. The defects associated with tetralogy of Fallot are
   a. Left ventricular hypertrophy, overriding aorta
   b. Atrial septal defect, overriding aorta
   c. Right ventricular hypertrophy, overriding aorta, ventricular septal defect, pulmonic valve stenosis
   d. Left ventricular hypertrophy, atrial septal defect, pulmonic valve stenosis
53. Christopher will be discharged from the hospital today. He will be required to receive digoxin twice a day. The nurse should include which of the following points when teaching family members about the action and effects of digoxin?
   a. Digoxin enables the heart to pump

more effectively with a slower and more regular rhythm
b. Signs of toxicity include loss of appetite, vomiting, increased pulse, and visual disturbances
c. Digoxin is absorbed better if taken with meals
d. If the child vomits within 15 minutes of administration, the dosage should be repeated

54. Postoperative complications of cardiac surgery require close nursing observation. Clinical signs of low cardiac output include
a. Cool extremities, bounding pulses, cyanosis, altered levels of consciousness
b. Bounding pulses and cool extremities
c. Alterations in level of consciousness and warm extremities
d. Alterations in level of consciousness, cool extremities, cyanosis or mottled skin, thready pulse

55. Robin, a 12-month-old girl, has iron deficiency anemia. Parent education to prevent recurrence should include the following guidelines/information:
a. Administer iron supplements in combination with ascorbic acid; avoid contact with teeth; Robin's stools will be darker than normal
b. Administer iron supplements with meals; stools will be darker
c. Avoid contact with teeth; administer with meals; stools will be darker
d. Stools will become darker; avoid contact with teeth; administer with tea or milk products

56. A normal, healthy child of 9 or 10 years
a. Enjoys physical demonstrations of affection
b. Is selfish and insensitive to the welfare of others
c. Is uncooperative in play and in school
d. Has a strong sense of justice and fair play

57. (Questions 57–60 refer to this situation) Eleven-year-old Sarah is admitted for treatment of an asthma attack. Assessment of Sarah's condition on admission reveals
a. Thin, copious mucous secretions
b. That Sarah's cough is productive
c. Intercostal retractions
d. A respiratory rate of 16 breaths/min

58. On the third hospital day, Sarah is receiving IV hydrocortisone, ampicillin, and aminophylline. She vomits after breakfast and lunch, and is very irritable. Her heart rate is 120 beats per minute. From this data it appears Sarah is probably experiencing
a. Hypolcalemia
b. An allergic reaction to the hydrocortisone
c. Theophylline toxicity
d. Depression of the central nervous system

59. The nurse's first action should be to
a. Put Sarah on oxygen
b. Ask Sarah to stay in bed for the day
c. Stop the IV hydrocortisone
d. Notify the physician

60. Sarah wants to exercise. Which of the following activities should the nurse suggest to improve her breathing?
a. Board games
b. Swimming
c. Track
d. Gymnastics

61. When observing a child for seizures, the nurse should be aware that
a. Accurate reporting of the site of origin and spread of seizure activity may help in identifying the affected area of the brain
b. Restraining the extremities will decrease the risk of injury to the child
c. Accuracy in inserting the padded tongue blade during the seizure activity helps open the airway
d. Maintaining a prone position will en-

sure a patent airway and adequate ventilation

62. Which of the following should be part of the nurse's teaching plan for a child with epilepsy being discharged on a regimen of diphenylhydantoin (Dilantin)?
    a. To be sure the child drinks plenty of fluids
    b. To brush teeth daily
    c. Never leave the child alone
    d. Report any signs of infection

63. (Questions 63–67 refer to this situation) Becky, who is 15 years old, has been diagnosed with acute glomerulonephritis and has been in the hospital 1 day. When assessing her condition the next day, the nurse would most likely see
    a. A large amount of periorbital edema
    b. Urine specific gravity of 1.030
    c. Positive throat culture for streptococcus
    d. A normal serum sodium level

64. The nurse helps Becky fill out her menu. Which of the following meals would be *most* appropriate?
    a. Egg noodles, hamburger, canned peas, milk
    b. Baked ham, baked potato, pear, canned carrots, milk
    c. Baked chicken, rice, beans, orange, milk
    d. Hot dog on a bun, corn chips, pickle, cookie, milk

65. The nurse's plan for Becky's care includes
    a. Assessing her vital signs and providing a no-sodium diet
    b. Maintaining intake and output and isolation
    c. Forcing fluids and maintaining isolation
    d. Maintaining bedrest and monitoring intake and output

66. Becky is in the recreation room and complains of a headache and blurred vision. The nurse should immediately
    a. Put Becky to bed
    b. Obtain a blood pressure reading
    c. Notify the physician
    d. Administer acetaminophen (Tylenol)

67. Becky's IV of 1000 mL is to run over 20 hours. How many drops per minute would there be using a macrodrip with 10 gtt/mL?
    a. 6 gtt/min
    b. 8 gtt/min
    c. 16 gtt/min
    d. 32 gtt/min

68. (Questions 68 and 69 refer to this situation) James is 13 years old, and has been admitted with a diagnosis of rheumatic fever and is on bedrest. He complains of a sore throat with a temperature of 100.4°F, pulse 120, respirations 22, and BP 110/80. The nurse should inform the physician of
    a. Swollen and painful joints
    b. A red rash on his trunk
    c. Heart rate of 150 beats/min
    d. Twitching of his extremities

69. The nurse should plan to
    a. Stay with James for close observation
    b. Allow James to participate in activities that will not tire him, so he avoids becoming dependent
    c. Provide for long periods of rest between activities
    d. Encourage his family to be with him 24 hours a day

70. The nurse is to run 250 mL of Ringer's lactate and 150 mL of 0.9 NaCl over the next 6 hours. Using a microdrip set, how many gtt/min will be administered?
    a. 33 gtt/min
    b. 49 gtt/min
    c. 67 gtt/min
    d. 83 gtt/min

71. The nurse is to give meperidine hydrochloride (Demerol) 9 mg IM to a client. If 25 mg/mL is available, how much should the client receive?
    a. 0.18 mL
    b. 0.36 mL

    c. 1.5 mL
    d. 3.0 mL

72. The nurse received an order to administer atropine 0.1 mg. 0.4 mg/mL is available. How much will the client receive?
    a. 0.125 mL
    b. 0.25 mL
    c. 0.4 mL
    d. 0.5 mL

73. (Questions 73–75 refer to this situation) Molly is 10 years old, and thought to have a brain tumor. She has had a headache and has been vomiting in the morning. All of the following facts about brain tumors are true *except*
    a. Brain tumors are primarily growth of neurological tissue
    b. Growths in the cerebellum are classified as infratentorial
    c. Meningiomas are most prevalent in the childhood years
    d. Astrocytomas are slow growing and cystic, whereas medulloblastomas are rapid growing and tend to seed

74. In planning care for Molly the nurse should include
    a. Providing information to Molly and her parents about a low-sodium diet
    b. Teaching Molly about diagnostic procedures
    c. Making Molly npo after she vomits
    d. Encouraging Molly to engage in increased activity so she will sleep better

75. The nurse should make the following initial physical assessment of Molly
    a. Leg strength
    b. Level of consciousness
    c. Muscle size
    d. Liver span

76. The nurse plans to do some teaching with 17-year-old Mary, who has a severe gonorrheal infection. Which of the following is true?
    a. Once treated she will have immunity
    b. Her partner needs no treatment
    c. She will have no further problems once she learns to protect herself
    d. Scarring of her fallopian tubes may occur

77. (Questions 77–81 refer to this situation) Pam is 8 years old, a newly diagnosed diabetic, and is in the hospital for regulation and education about her diet. The nurse should instruct Pam that the ADA exchange method for dietary regulation includes
    a. Choosing what she wants from each exchange list
    b. Using a scale to weigh all food
    c. Selecting from lists that group food as to protein, fat, and carbohydrate content
    d. Substituting one food for another within the same list

78. Pam is placed on NPH and regular insulin before breakfast and before dinner. She will receive a snack of milk and cereal at bedtime. The snack will
    a. Help her to regain lost weight
    b. Provide carbohydrates for immediate use
    c. Prevent late night hypoglycemia
    d. Help Pam stay on her diet

79. Pam and her parents should be taught that when she is ill Pam will probably need
    a. More calories
    b. More insulin
    c. Less insulin
    d. Less protein and fats

80. If Pam were hyperglycemic, she would exhibit which of the following symptoms?
    a. Weakness and thirst
    b. Shakiness and hunger
    c. Headache and irritability
    d. Weakness and dizziness

81. Pam's mother tells the nurse she does not want the school to know about Pam's condition. The nurse should reply
    a. "I think that would be a good idea."

b. "This is your decision and I'll agree with what you decide."
c. "It is absolutely necessary that Pam's teacher know."
d. "It is not safe to keep her teacher uninformed."

82. (Questions 82 and 83 refer to this situation) Judy is 14 years old and is being screened for scoliosis. Which of the following statements about routine scoliosis screening is true?
    a. Teenagers, ages 14–16, should be screened yearly
    b. Routine gym shirt and shorts are worn for screening
    c. The student is assessed both standing and bending forward
    d. If findings are positive, the diagnosis of scoliosis is made

83. Judy has to wear a Milwaukee brace. The nurse's teaching plan should include which of the following instructions?
    a. The brace is only worn during waking hours
    b. Lotions and powders should be used generously to relieve skin irritations
    c. No clothing should be worn under the brace
    d. The skin under the brace should be bathed daily

84. A 9-year-old child is scheduled for an electromyelogram. How would the nurse *best* initiate teaching for the procedure?
    a. Wait until just before the test to tell the child what will be done
    b. Ask the child to draw a picture of the body structures involved
    c. Show the child the equipment that will be used in the test
    d. Verbally explain what will be done during the test

85. (Questions 85–89 refer to this situation) Renee is 15 years old and has been admitted to the hospital with the diagnosis of acute lymphocytic leukemia. The nurse would expect to see all of the following signs and symptoms except
    a. Fatigue and anorexia
    b. Fever and petechiae
    c. Edema and pallor
    d. Enlarged liver and spleen

86. One of the chemotherapeutic agents Renee will be taking is cyclophosphamide (Cytoxan). The nurse should assess for the side-effect of
    a. Photosensitivity
    b. Ataxia
    c. Cystitis
    d. Stomatitis

87. Renee will also be taking vincristine. Knowing the side-effects of vincristine, the nurse should encourage Renee to eat a diet that is
    a. High residue
    b. Low residue
    c. Low fat
    d. Regular

88. Renee is taking immunosuppressive drugs and should
    a. Continue with her immunizations
    b. Not receive any immunizations
    c. Receive vitamin and mineral supplements
    d. Stay away from her peers

89. Renee should be
    a. Excluded from school
    b. Restricted from participating in all athletic activities
    c. Treated as "special" because of her disease
    d. Treated as "normal" as much as possible

90. (Questions 90 and 91 refer to this situation) Bill has 5 pounds of Buck's traction on his left leg. The nurse should assess for all of the following *except*
    a. Dryness of the skin, by removing adhesive wraps
    b. Correct body alignment of shoulder, hips, knees

c. Frayed rope near pulleys
d. Correct amount of traction weight on fracture

91. Bill has just had a plaster cast placed on his lower left leg. Nursing care includes
   a. Petaling the cast as soon as it is put on
   b. Leaving bits of plaster inside the cast that can be reached
   c. Using only the palms of the hand when handling the cast
   d. Notifying the physician because Bill complains of the heat

92. (Questions 92–94 refer to this situation) Paul's diagnosis of cystic fibrosis was made 13 years ago, and he has since been hospitalized several times. Initial assessment during his hospitalization would include an assessment of which of the following systems?
   a. Respiratory
   b. Cardiac
   c. Neurologic
   d. Skin

93. The nurse encourages Paul to eat a diet high in all of the following *except*
   a. Protein
   b. Fats
   c. Carbohydrates
   d. Calories

94. Paul is taking numerous antibiotics for his respiratory infection, and one of his medications is tobramycin. Which of the following is a side-effect of tobramycin?
   a. Hearing loss
   b. Fluid retention
   c. Malaise
   d. Paresthesia

95. Billy, 10 years old, was playing in the kitchen and received a burn from a hot liquid. His mother should first
   a. Keep Billy warm
   b. Rub butter on the burned area
   c. Apply cool water to the burned area
   d. Call the emergency room

96. Nine-year-old Chris is admitted to the hospital because of vomiting, dehydration, and abdominal pain. The nurse is assessing Chris for pain, and he is crying. Chris probably
   a. Is not in pain if he can be distracted
   b. Is less tolerant of pain because he is upset
   c. Is irritable so he must be in pain
   d. Was medicated 4 hours ago, so he could not be in pain now

97. (Questions 97 and 98 refer to this situation) Kathy is a 14-year-old girl with sickle cell disease. This is her fourth hospitalization for sickle cell crisis. Next month Kathy and her family are going to the mountains for a ski vacation. The nurse should
   a. Encourage them to go
   b. Say nothing since this is a family trip
   c. Suggest the trip be postponed until next year
   d. Tell them the high altitude may cause a crisis

98. To help Kathy prevent another crisis, the nurse should teach her to
   a. Restrict her fluid intake to less than 1 quart per day
   b. Drink at least 2 quarts of fluids a day
   c. Stay away from other teenagers
   d. Increase her physical activity and ability

99. (Questions 99 and 100 refer to this situation) Twelve-year-old Kent was admitted with the probable diagnosis of acute rheumatic fever. Aspirin has been prescribed for Kent. The nurse should be alert to the implications of which of the following statements/questions?
   a. "Can you hear that ringing noise?"
   b. "Is it alright to put lotion on my itchy skin?"
   c. "My stomach hurts after I take those."
   d. "These pills make me cough."

100. Kent is on bedrest. Which of the following would be an appropriate diversional activity for the nurse to encourage?

a. Watching television with his roommate
  b. Coloring picture books with his brother
  c. Keeping up with his school work
  d. Making crafts for others

101. John, 17 years old, may have bone cancer. He has been admitted to the hospital for a biopsy to confirm the diagnosis. The nurse knows that the *most* common presenting symptom(s) of this disease is(are)
  a. Cough and dyspnea
  b. Pain and swelling
  c. Fever and anorexia
  d. Decreased range of motion

102. (Questions 102 and 103 refer to this situation) Seven-year-old Joe has been diagnosed as being mentally retarded. His parents have been told that retardation means
  a. Subaverage intelligence
  b. An IQ below 90
  c. Deficits in adaptive behavior
  d. Subaverage intellectual and behavioral functioning

103. The best indication of how Joe is progressing can be obtained by observing him
  a. At school with his teacher
  b. At home with his family
  c. In the clinic with his mother
  d. Playing soccer with his friends

104. (Questions 104 and 105 refer to this situation) A characteristic behavior of 7-year-old Mary is that she
  a. Likes to play only with other girls
  b. Prefers to play with her sister
  c. Prefers to play team games
  d. Likes to play alone

105. Mary has developed some new fears. She is probably afraid of
  a. Separation from parents
  b. Trying something new
  c. Injury and pain
  d. Opposite sex relationships

106. The growth spurt in adolescent boys, compared with the growth spurt of adolescent girls, usually occurs
  a. At the same time
  b. 2 years earlier
  c. 2 years later
  d. 3 years later

107. Gary is 15 years old, and his parents state that he is moody and rude. The nurse should advise his parents to
  a. Restrict his activities
  b. Discuss their feelings with Gary
  c. Obtain family counseling
  d. Talk to other parents of adolescents

108. Acne is a chronic skin disease caused by
  a. Not keeping the face clean
  b. Eating lots of junk food
  c. Picking lesions on the face
  d. Inflammation of the sebaceous glands

109. The admission interview of a parent and child is a means to
  a. Become aware of the client's personality and history
  b. Establish trust and collect data
  c. Collect data and engage in casual conversation
  d. Establish the boundaries for further interactions

110. (Questions 12 and 13 refer to this situation) A 12-year-old client says, "Gimme my pajamas. I'm not putting your silly gown on." An attentive response would be
  a. "I know they're funny but everyone here wears them."
  b. "You don't mean that, now. A big guy like you knows how hospitals are."
  c. "You're upset because you feel awkward and embarrassed in these gowns."
  d. "You're upset because you think we're unreasonable."

111. It is important to be especially sensitive to the above child because
  a. He is not going to comply with authority

    b. This initial interaction will establish the climate for the relationship
    c. The nurse's impression may distort his or her feelings about the child
    d. His needs are not being met
112. Tammy, an 11 year old, is recovering from an appendectomy performed 2 days ago. The nurse enters her room with a breakfast tray and Tammy says, "I told you I don't eat breakfast. When my mother comes she'll bring me a McDonald's." The nurse responds, "Tammy, this is the second day you have refused your meals. It upsets me when you don't try to eat some of your meal because I've explained to you the need to eat well in order to heal." This confrontative response serves to
    a. Satisfy the nurse's own needs
    b. Clear the air so the nurse can move on
    c. Redirect the child's aggressive behavior
    d. Show the child the nurse is in control
113. Six-year-old Jamie and his parents have come to the clinic for a weekly consultation regarding his sleeping problem. Jamie interrupts the nurse's conversation with his parents despite the nurse's repeated requests to let the parents talk. The nurse says, "Jamie, I need to talk to your parents. I know it's hard to wait so long. You can play with the top or you can go out and watch the fish tank." The nurse's response to the above situation is
    a. An assertive response
    b. An aggressive response
    c. An empathetic statement
    d. An ultimatum for a change in behavior
114. The nurse makes a home visit to assess an 8-year-old client's rehabilitation from a fractured leg. His father says, "Oh, I didn't expect you today." A facilitative response would be
    a. "Oh, I'm sorry. I have you on my schedule."
    b. "I apologize for the interruption, but Tommie needs to be evaluated today."
    c. "Well, if it's a problem I could come back tomorrow."
    d. "I don't know how we got mixed up, but I need to see Tommie."

Answer Sheet—Test 3

Answers and Rationales for Test 3

1. c. According to the Denver Developmental Screening Exam, at 8 months of age the child should say "mama" and "dada" nonspecifically and imitate speech sounds. A, H
2. d. According to the Denver Developmental Screening Exam, a child of 8 months should sit without support for long periods of time. A, H
3. d. Infants should be on formula until 1 year of age; if solids are adequate, until 6 months. Solids are started between 4 and 6 months. Iron deficiency rarely develops before 6 months of age because babies have iron stores. I, N
4. c. At age 4, the child should be learning to dress herself without supervision. A child will feel more autonomous if allowed to try things herself; this should be encouraged to increase self-esteem. I, O
5. d. Goals of developmental assessment include anticipatory guidance, identifying deviations from the norm, helping parents understand their child's behavior, and assessing parent–child interaction. P, O
6. c. Behavior problems related to sleep and rest frequently occur. Consistent rituals around bedtime help make the transition from waking to sleep easier. Children who are allowed to sleep with their parents frequently create more problems for the family and child. I, C
7. c. According to the Denver Developmental Screening Exam, a child of age 24–27 months should have a vocabulary of 300 words, be able to combine 2 or 3 words, and ask for what he wants by name. A, H
8. a. During the tertiary circular reaction stage of the sensorimotor stage (12–18 months of age), the infant comes to understand causality and object permanence, recognizing that objects placed out of sight continue to exist. R, H
9. c. Understanding object permanence means that the child is aware of the existence of objects that are covered or displaced. A, H
10. b. According to the Denver Developmental Screening Exam, development moves from general to specific. A child will initially say "dada" nonspecifically, then he will say "dada" specifically. A, H
11. d. Toddlers establish ritualistic patterns to feel secure despite inconsistencies in their environment. R, O
12. d. Health screening should provide an immunizations schedule; tuberculin titer (TB) test; physical exam; blood pressure, vision, and hearing testing; Hct; HGb; and anticipatory guidance. I, O
13. b. The nurse can introduce concepts of readiness and encourage parents to look for adaptive and psychomotor signs: ability to walk well, balance, climb, sit in a chair, dress oneself, please the parent and communicate awareness of the need to urinate or defecate. R, H
14. a. The anterior fontanelle is usually closed by 18 months. A, H
15. b. The health care network includes many specialized areas, such as respiratory therapy, medicine, laboratory, social services, and technical monitoring to name a few. E, C
16. b. For infants up to 20 pounds, recommended car seating is rear facing with shoulder restraints. The middle of the back seat is considered the safest area of the car. P, O
17. c. A child will regress to a behavior used in an earlier stage of development in

18. d. order to cope with a perceived threatening situation. I, C
18. d. Soft, washable toys are appropriate for infants, who tend to place everything in their mouths. These toys are not harmful. P, O
19. c. The literature supports this with studies done on outcome assessment of nursing care. E, C
20. d. A mother who is separated from her newborn because of illness may feel maternal guilt, feelings of inadequacy as a mother, and view the hospital environment as hostile. R, H
21. b. At 15 months, a normal healthy child should have received DPT 3 (diptheria-pertussis-tetanus), OPV (oral polio vaccine) 2, MMR (measles, mumps, rubella), and tuberculin skin test. A, H
22. d. A 3-day diet history is the best way to accurately assess the child's intake. I, N
23. c. Nursing bottle caries occur when a child is routinely given a bottle of milk or juice at nap or bedtime. Teeth become coated and bathed in sugar, which converts to acid, leading to decay. I, N
24. d. Safety measures for poisonous substances include close supervision of children, safely storing toxic substances, teaching proper dosages and differences between adult and child doses, and keeping all poisonous substances out of the reach of children. P, O
25. d. Immediate care of the child who has ingested a poisonous substance includes maintenance of respiratory and cardiac function, gastric decontamination either through vomiting, gastric lavage, neutralization, and decreasing anxiety. I, O
26. c. A child taking amoxicillin should be on a lactose-free diet to avoid the diarrhea caused by this antibiotic. P, D
27. c. The response avoids conflict by diverting their attention. A different interest is created and a cooperative idea is promoted. When children perceive themselves as being valued, they are more apt to comply. I, C
28. a. It is best to acknowledge Ms. James' feelings instead of ignoring them. This will allow her to open up and express her frustrations and concerns. This is important when caring for a child with a chronic illness. I, C
29. b. Alice *does* need the enzymes with meals and snacks. Parents should not be threatened or made to feel inadequate. If they understand the reason behind the treatment or medication, they are more likely to comply. I, D
30. d. Side-effects of steroid therapy include edema of the face and trunk, increased susceptibility to infection, and gastric and intestinal mucosal bleeding. P, D
31. d. From documented cases of child abuse, a profile has emerged of a high-risk parent as isolated, single, having low self-esteem, a history of substance abuse, lacking knowledge of normal growth and development, having been subject to multiple stressors in life, lacking patience, and impulsive. A, H
32. a. The nurse states the expectations and identifies the consequences for the child who is ignoring them. This statement, if spoken warmly, will recognize and convey respect for the child's feelings. I, C
33. d. Clinical manifestations of dehydration include sunken fontanelle, dry mucous membranes, decreased tearing, and behavioral changes. A, H
34. c. Strabismus is diagnosed through observation and use of the corneal light reflex test. The cover/uncover test will reveal movement of the affected eye

when the unaffected eye is covered, indicating abnormal fixation of the affected eye. The child should be referred to an ophthalmologist as soon as possible so that correct vision in the affected eye can be restored. I, O

35. d. All three measures are important, because of the infant's appearance and difficulty with sucking and swallowing. I, O

36. b. Clinical manifestations of *Shigella* are fever, nausea, and vomiting, some cramping, headache, seizures and rectal prolapse, loose watery stools containing pus, mucous, and blood. A, H

37. d. Securing an airway is the primary measure because the airway can be occluded at any time due to obstruction. An x-ray of the neck may also be obtained to view the obstruction. I, O

38. d. Treatment of otitis media involves antibiotic therapy for 10 days, with ears rechecked by the physician. If infection is not cleared, restart the client on another antibiotic. I, D

39. a. The child may originally complain of a generalized periumbilical pain, with this pain later localizing in the right lower quadrant (RLQ). Fever and vomiting are usually present, and the child may complain of diarrhea or constipation. A, H

40. c. Common shunt complications are obstruction, infection, and disconnection of the tubing. With obstruction, sudden or gradual symptoms of increased intracranial pressure (ICP) develop, including vomiting, poor feeding, lethargy, and irritability. A, H

41. a. One's perception is one's interpretation of reality. The mother thinks the baby does not like the taste. To her, when something does not taste good it is refused. R, C

42. b. The nurse's perception is that the mother is insecure. Her response, based on her perception of the situation, is to offer reassurance. I, C

43. c. The prone position allows optimal positioning of the legs. Hips should be maintained in abduction. A pad between the knees counteracts hip subluxation, while the roll placed under ankles maintains neutral foot position. I, O

44. d. Prevention of urinary tract infections includes adequate fluid intake, urine acidification, frequent emptying of the bladder, and using the Credé maneuver to empty the bladder. I, O

45. d. Accurate intake and output recording includes noting all intake, including IV fluids, weighing diapers, measuring urine specific gravity, monitoring serum electrolytes, and monitoring for signs of dehydration. I, O

46. a. Findings associated with sudden infant death syndrome (SIDS) include the following: apnea lasting 20 seconds or more is a warning sign; incidence is higher among siblings; peak incidence is 2 to 4 months; 90% occur by 6 months of age; and there may be a neurological cause. R, H

47. a. Proper blood pressure cuff size is important for accurate readings. It should be 1.5 times the diameter of the extremity being measured, or less than half and no more than two thirds part of the extremity being measured. I, O

48. c. Treatment of viral pharyngitis includes use of a cool mist vaporizor, feeding a soft or liquid diet, and administration of acetaminophen for comfort. I, O

49. b. Assessment of the infant with tracheoesophageal fistula (TEF) includes excessive salivation, choking, coughing, and sneezing at birth, and cyanosis from larynogospasm. A, H

50. c. Ortolani's sign is used to detect congenital hip dysplasia. The infant is supine and a click is heard when flexed

legs are abducted. This results from pressure causing the femoral head to slip out of the acetabulum. A, O

51. b. A child with a cardiac defect finds that squatting decreases venous return and workload to the heart, and increases comfort. R, H

52. c. The child with tetralogy of Fallot has a ventricular septal defect pulmonic valve stenosis, overriding aorta, right ventricular hypertrophy. A, H

53. a. Digoxin taken 1 hour before meals or 2 hours after meals results in better absorption of the drug. Signs of toxicity include decreased heart rate. If the child vomits within 15 minutes of administration, the dose should not be repeated. I, D

54. d. Clinical signs of low cardiac output and poor tissue perfusion include pale, cool extremities, cyanosis or mottled skin, delayed capillary refill, weak, thready pulses, oliguria, and alterations in level of consciousness. A, H

55. a. Parent teaching concerning a child with iron deficiency anemia should include directions to give iron combined with ascorbic acid, in divided doses between meals. It should not be given with milk, antacids, or tea. Contact with teeth should be avoided, and stools will become darker. I, D

56. d. School-age children are concerned about justice and fair play. They become upset when they think someone is not playing fair. They are concerned about others and are cooperative in play and school. A, H

57. c. During an asthma attack, secretions are thick, cough is tight, and respiration is difficult (shortness of breath may occur). A, H

58. c. Side-effects of theophylline include vomiting, irritability, and headache. R, O

59. d. The nurse should notify the physician when an asthmatic client taking theophylline has symptoms including vomiting, headache, and irritability. These are common signs of a high-theophylline blood level. I, O

60. b. Swimming is good "all-over" exercise. It also teaches controlled breathing. I, O

61. a. The nurse times the seizure and notes what area of the body the seizure starts in and where it spreads, in order to pinpoint the area of the brain involved. A, H

62. b. Diphenylhydantoin (Dilantin) can cause gingival hyperplasia. Children taking Dilantin should brush their teeth at least once daily. I, O

63. b. An adolescent with acute glomerulonephritis has a small amount of periorbital edema, a normal serum sodium level, and (usually) a negative throat culture. A, H

64. c. The best selection would include no added salt or salty food. I, N

65. d. Becky should be on bedrest and I and O (intake and output) monitoring because of her kidney disease. P, O

66. b. Hypertension occurs with acute glomerulonephritis (AGN). The symptoms of headache and blurred vision may indicate an elevated blood pressure. I, O

67. b. $$\text{gtt/min} = \frac{1000 \text{ mL} \times 10}{20 \times 60}$$
$$= \frac{10,000}{1,200} = 8 \quad \text{A, D}$$

68. c. James' heart rate of 150 beats/min is significantly above its rate at the time of his admission (120). The physician needs to be notified of the possible complication of carditis. I, H

69. c. The nurse should provide for long periods of rest to decrease James's cardiac workload. P, O

70. c. 400 mL of IV fluid will run over 6 hours. 400 divided by 6 = 66.67/hour. Using a microdrip set the mL/hour is the same at gtt/min. P, D

71. b.
$$\frac{25 \text{ mg}}{1 \text{ mL}} = \frac{9 \text{ mg}}{x}$$
$$25x = 9$$
$$x = 0.36 \text{ mL meperidine HCl}$$
(Demerol) P, D

72. b.
$$\frac{0.4 \text{ mg}}{1 \text{ mL}} = \frac{0.1 \text{ mg}}{x}$$
$$0.4 \text{ mg } x = 0.1 \text{ mg}$$
$$x = 0.25 \text{ mL atropine} \quad \text{P, D}$$

73. c. Astrocytomas are one of the most common brain tumors in children. A, H
74. b. Molly will be undergoing several diagnostic procedures and needs guidance in preparing for them. She will not be on a special diet, and she should be kept quiet so as not to increase intracranial pressure. P, O
75. b. Level of consciousness is the single best indicator of cerebral function. A, H
76. d. With a severe gonorrheal infection, scarring of the fallopian tubes may occur. A, H
77. d. The ADA exchange diet allows the substitution of one food for another on the same diet list. P, N
78. c. NPH insulin peaks in 6 to 8 hours, which would occur during sleep. A bedtime snack is needed to prevent late night hypoglycemia. A, N
79. b. Pam needs more insulin during an illness. I, O
80. a. Symptoms of hyperglycemia include weakness and increased thirst. The other symptoms are those of hypoglycemia. A, H
81. d. Pam may have a diabetic reaction at school. Her teacher needs to know about her diabetes to be able to help her. A, H
82. c. Screening is done with the child wearing minimal clothing, standing, and bending forward. A, H
83. d. The skin under the brace should be bathed daily to help prevent irritation from the brace. I, O
84. b. Before teaching a school-age child about a medical or nursing procedure, it is best to become familiar with the child's knowledge level. Begin with the body structure involved in the procedure. I, C
85. c. Fever, anorexia, pallor, petechiae, and hepatosplenomegaly are classic signs and symptoms of acute lymphocytic leukemia. A, H
86. c. Cystitis is a potential side-effect of cyclophosphamide (Cytoxan). A, D
87. a. Vincristine may cause constipation, so Rene should be encouraged to eat a high-residue (fiber) diet. A, D
88. b. Children who are immunosuppressed should not receive immunizations, because of their inability to develop antibodies. P, H
89. d. Any child with a chronic illness should be treated as normally as possible. P, H
90. a. Bill's adhesive wraps should *not* be removed unless there is a physician's order. A, O
91. c. The wet plaster cast should only be handled using the palms of the hands to prevent indentations of the cast surface. P, O
92. a. Any patient with a chronic respiratory illness should have an initial respiratory assessment to determine respiratory status. A, H
93. b. Fats are difficult to digest. P, N
94. a. Hearing loss may be a problem for a client taking aminoglycosides. A, D
95. c. To prevent further injury to the skin, cool water is applied to the burn site. A, O

96. b. Emotional or physical stress lowers a person's tolerance of pain. A, H
97. d. High altitude causes deoxygenation, which might precipitate a crisis. P, H
98. b. Increasing fluid intake and being well hydrated will help prevent stasis. P, H
99. a. Tinnitis is a side-effect of aspirin. A, D
100. c. Kent should be encouraged to keep up with his school work. A, H
101. b. Common symptoms of bone cancer are pain and swelling in the tumor area. A, H
102. d. The definition of mental retardation includes deficits in both intellectual functioning and behavior. A, H
103. a. Watching the child relate to his teacher and school work is the best indication of how he is progressing. A, H
104. a. Seven year olds like to play with friends of the same sex. A, H
105. b. Trying something new is usually frightening for a 7 year old. A, H
106. c. Research studies indicate that adolescent boys lag about 2 years behind adolescent girls in growth. A, H
107. b. Parents need to discuss with their adolescent how they perceive his behavior and how they feel about it. Moodiness is characteristic of adolescents. The adolescent may have a reason for feeling this way or not be aware he is acting like this. A, H
108. d. Acne is an inflammation of the sebaceous glands. A, H
109. b. This is a significant objective of the interview, which should involve more than just getting information needed for the chart. E, C
110. c. The nurse uses active listening, in which the client's feelings and the cause of those feelings are reflected back to him. I, C
111. b. First impressions set the stage for the development of a relationship. E, C
112. c. Confrontation points out aggressive behavior and promotes a working relationship. I, C
113. a. Assertiveness is stating your expectations without violating the other person's rights. E, C
114. b. The nurse acknowledges that he or she was not expected and indicates intention to see the client. E, C

DIAGNOSTIC GRID
Test 3

Directions: The diagnostic grid is used to reveal deficiencies in nursing content and nursing process knowledge. Determine which questions you answered incorrectly and circle the corresponding codes. Total each column and note the percentage of incorrect answers.

Nursing Process
A = Assessment
R = Analysis/nursing diagnosis
P = Planning
I = Implementation/intervention
E = Evaluation

Nursing Content
H = Health status
O = Nursing actions/interventions
D = Drugs/pharmacology
N = Nutrition
C = Communication skills

Question	Nursing Process					Nursing Content				
	A	R	P	I	E	H	O	D	N	C
1.	A					H				
2.	A					H				
3.				I					N	
4.				I			O			
5.			P				O			
6.				I						C
7.	A					H				
8.		R				H				
9.	A					H				
10.	A					H				
11.		R					O			
12.				I			O			
13.		R				H				
14.	A					H				
15.					E					C

DIAGNOSTIC GRID (Continued)

Question	Nursing Process					Nursing Content				
	A	R	P	I	E	H	O	D	N	C
16.			P				O			
17.				I						C
18.			P				O			
19.					E					C
20.		R				H				
21.	A					H				
22.				I					N	
23.				I					N	
24.			P				O			
25.				I			O			
26.			P					D		
27.				I						C
28.				I						C
29.				I				D		
30.			P					D		
31.	A					H				
32.				I						C
33.	A					H				
34.				I			O			
35.				I			O			
36.	A					H				
37.				I			O			

DIAGNOSTIC GRID (Continued)

Question	Nursing Process					Nursing Content				
	A	R	P	I	E	H	O	D	N	C
38.				I				D		
39.	A					H				
40.	A					H				
41.		R								C
42.				I						C
43.				I			O			
44.				I			O			
45.				I			O			
46.		R				H				
47.				I			O			
48.				I			O			
49.	A					H				
50.	A						O			
51.		R				H				
52.	A					H				
53.				I				D		
54.	A					H				
55.				I				D		
56.	A					H				
57.	A					H				
58.		R					O			
59.				I			O			

DIAGNOSTIC GRID (*Continued*)

Question	Nursing Process					Nursing Content				
	A	R	P	I	E	H	O	D	N	C
60.				I			O			
61.	A					H				
62.				I			O			
63.	A					H				
64.				I					N	
65.			P				O			
66.				I			O			
67.	A							D		
68.				I		H				
69.			P				O			
70.			P					D		
71.			P					D		
72.			P					D		
73.	A					H				
74.			P				O			
75.	A					H				
76.	A					H				
77.			P						N	
78.	A								N	
79.				I			O			
80.	A					H				
81.	A					H				

DIAGNOSTIC GRID (Continued)

Question	Nursing Process					Nursing Content				
	A	R	P	I	E	H	O	D	N	C
82.	A					H				
83.				I			O			
84.				I						C
85.	A					H				
86.	A							D		
87.	A							D		
88.			P			H				
89.			P			H				
90.	A						O			
91.			P				O			
92.	A					H				
93.			P						N	
94.	A							D		
95.	A						O			
96.	A					H				
97.			P			H				
98.			P			H				
99.	A							D		
100.	A					H				
101.	A					H				
102.	A					H				
103.	A					H				

DIAGNOSTIC GRID (Continued)

Question	Nursing Process					Nursing Content				
	A	R	P	I	E	H	O	D	N	C
104.	A					H				
105.	A					H				
106.	A					H				
107.	A					H				
108.	A					H				
109.					E					C
110.				I						C
111.					E					C
112.				I						C
113.					E					C
114.					E					C
Total items this test	46	8	19	35	6	47	30	14	7	16
Your total										
Percent Incorrect										

Practice Test 4: Care of the Client with a Mental Health Problem

Read each question carefully and select the best answer from the choices presented. Mark your answers on the answer sheet on page 405.

1. (Questions 1–6 refer to this situation) Jason Smith is a 42-year-old unemployed laborer who was arrested by the police for disturbing the peace and brought voluntarily to the hospital. His language is incoherent and he is hallucinating. He is admitted to the psychiatric unit with a diagnosis of chronic undifferentiated schizophrenia. During the admission interview, Mr. Smith cocks his head to one side and says, "Really? Oh yeah, I understand," and then begins laughing to himself. The nurse's *best* response is
   a. "Why are you laughing, Mr. Smith?"
   b. "Are you hearing voices, Mr. Smith?"
   c. "You are laughing, Mr. Smith. I wonder what's so funny."
   d. "I'm glad you find this hospital so amusing."
2. When Mr. Smith verbalizes thoughts related to his fantasy world, the nurse can *best* intervene by
   a. Quickly interrupting to change the subject
   b. Maintaining silence with him
   c. Talking to him about his past life
   d. Speaking in simple, concrete sentences about present happenings
3. During the early stages of a one-to-one relationship with a withdrawn client like Mr. Smith, the nurse should focus *most* of her attention on helping the client develop a sense of
   a. Trust
   b. Autonomy
   c. Independence
   d. Decisiveness
4. Mr. Smith attends a remotivational group session each day with three other clients who exhibit symptoms of withdrawal and regressive tendencies. The best topic for this group to discuss would be
   a. Concepts of love
   b. Marital relations
   c. Religious beliefs
   d. Types of occupations
5. An antipsychotic medication is prescribed for Mr. Smith, to be taken 4 times a day.

All of the following drugs are classified as antipsychotic agents *except*
   a. Haloperidol (Haldol)
   b. Trifluoperazine (Stelazine)
   c. Thioridazine hydrochloride (Mellaril)
   d. Meprobamate (Equanil)
6. The most accurate precautionary information to give Mr. Smith about phenothiazines is
   a. "You may experience increased libido."
   b. "Your blood pressure will increase."
   c. "You should not drive an automobile alone."
   d. "The drug you are taking is an experimental drug."
7. (Questions 7 and 8 refer to this situation) Stan Reed, age 36, glances disdainfully around the adult in-patient unit on his arrival at the hospital. He is neatly and attractively dressed and is tightly clutching a leather briefcase in his arms. Mr. Reed refuses to let the nurse touch his briefcase, or check it for valuables or contraband on admission. The *best* way for the nurse to determine the contents of the briefcase at this time is to
   a. Obtain help to take the briefcase from Mr. Reed
   b. Ask Mr. Reed to describe the items in the briefcase
   c. Inspect the briefcase when Mr. Reed is temporarily out of his room
   d. Tell Mr. Reed that it is necessary to observe hospital policy if he wants to receive care
8. Mr. Reed cannot find his slippers. During the community meeting, he accuses clients and staff of stealing them during the night. The *most* therapeutic nursing approach is to
   a. Listen without reinforcing his belief
   b. Logically point out to him that he is jumping to conclusions
   c. Inject humor to defuse his intensity
   d. Divert his attention
9. Which of the following statements about a client with catatonic schizophrenia is *incorrect*?
   a. The client may exhibit extreme negativism
   b. The client's posture frequently has symbolic meaning
   c. The client is unaware of his external surroundings
   d. The client may have hallucinations and delusions
10. (Questions 10–17 refer to this situation) Valerie Jones, 33 years old, has been admitted to a locked unit because she has been oblivious to her family's activities at home. Her husband states that she sat silently for long periods at a time and had become progressively unable to sleep, eat, talk, or perform any of her usual activities. Mrs. Jones had been treated for psychotic depressive reactions at age 24, following the birth of her second child, and again at age 31. She was given ECT therapy during her second admission. In addition to insomnia and anorexia, Mrs. Jones might also develop
    a. Menorrhagia
    b. Sordes
    c. Melena
    d. Constipation
11. Mr. Jones asks, "What made my wife sick this time?" The nurse's *best* response to Mr. Jones is
    a. "Your questions indicate an unreasonable feeling of guilt on your part."
    b. "No single person or event is responsible for your wife's health or illness."
    c. "I know you're worried about the cause of her illness."
    d. "The psychiatrist will be able to answer that question."
12. Mrs. Jones's depression is probably a manifestation of
    a. A paralyzing fear of something
    b. An inability to resolve conflicting responsibilities

c. A suspicion that others are trying to harm her in some way
d. Disillusionment with self

13. The feeling Mrs. Jones is *most* apt to demonstrate during her psychotic depression is
    a. Agitation
    b. Loneliness
    c. Suspicion of others
    d. Disillusionment with self

14. Mrs. Jones is at greatest risk of attempting suicide
    a. Immediately after her admission
    b. At the point of her deepest depression
    c. When her depression begins to abate
    d. Shortly before hospital discharge

15. In responding to Mrs. Jones's expressions of delusional thought the nurse should *not*
    a. Explore the delusional content
    b. Try to reason away the delusion
    c. Show disbelief in the delusion
    d. Convey the idea that delusions are temporary

16. Mrs. Jones is receiving imipramine hydrochloride (Tofranil). Side-effects that the nurse may observe are
    a. Hot flashes, flushing, fainting
    b. Hypertrophy and tenderness of lymph nodes
    c. Gingival hypertrophy and bleeding
    d. Dryness of the mouth, tachycardia, constipation

17. Mrs. Jones's physician prescribes a series of ECT. Immediately following treatment, Mrs. Jones is most likely to experience
    a. Dull pain
    b. Confusion
    c. Agitation
    d. Elation

18. Seventeen-year-old Alice Hart has a history of running away from home and "borrowing" other people's things without their permission. She denies that she steals and rationalizes that she thought "borrowing" was okay as long as no one was using the items. Alice arouses anxiety and frustration in the staff and tends to intimidate them by her manipulative patterns. One morning she shouts to the nurse, "Since you won't give me a pass, go away you fat pig or I'll hit you." The nurse's *most* effective response is to say
    a. "You are rude and I don't like it. It makes me not want to talk to you."
    b. "That kind of talk will keep you here longer."
    c. "What did I do wrong?"
    d. "I don't like to hear insults and threats. What is the matter?"

19. In establishing a therapeutic nursing approach with a client who is addicted to drugs, the nurse's primary goal is to
    a. Promote a permissive, accepting environment
    b. Use a straightforward and confrontative approach
    c. Meet the client's need for a chemical substitute for the drug
    d. Prevent the client from using the addictive drug.

20. Nina Sparks has refused to attend group therapy sessions at 9:00 a.m. because she says she has to wash her hands for at least 45 minutes from 9:00 a.m. to 9:45 a.m. To help reduce the client's stress and to help her find more adaptive means of handling anxiety, the nurse should
    a. Provide varied activities on the unit, because a change in daily routine can break a ritualistic activity
    b. Give her ward assignments that do not require her to achieve perfection
    c. Tell her of changes in routine at the last minute to avoid build-up of anxiety
    d. Provide an activity in which positive accomplishment can occur and she can gain recognition

21. (Questions 21–24 refer to this situation) Janet Carlson, a 28-year-old married woman, is admitted to the psychiatric service with the diagnosis of anxiety re-

action. The nurse and Mrs. Carlson walk to a quiet corner of the unit. Mrs. Carlson's anxiety mounts. She becomes increasingly restless, and shifts rapidly from one foot to the other and continuously wrings her hands. The nurse suddenly feels uncomfortable and wishes to leave the scene. The nurse's feeling is probably a reaction to
   a. The client's empathic communication of her anxiety
   b. The nurse's desire to go off duty after a busy day
   c. The nurse's inability to tolerate the client's bizarre behavior
   d. The nurse's fear of the client becoming assaultive

22. Mrs. Carlson cries and tells the nurse that she has never been in the hospital except to have her children. The nurse realizes that Mrs. Carlson's emotional stress can be reduced and her psychologic safety assured in an environment in which
   a. The client's needs are a primary concern
   b. All the client's needs are met
   c. Realistic limits and controls are set
   d. The physical environment is kept in order

23. Later in the day, Mrs. Carlson meets the nurse and says, "That was a terrible feeling I had this morning. I'm so afraid to talk about it." The *most* useful nursing response is
   a. "Okay, let's not talk about it."
   b. "It's best that you try to talk about it."
   c. "What were you doing this morning when you first noticed the feeling?"
   d. "Don't worry, it's not likely that that feeling will come back. It's in the past."

24. Mrs. Carlson cries bitterly after a conference with her psychiatrist. She pounds the bed in frustration and threatens to kill herself. The *most* helpful nursing intervention is to
   a. Pat her gently on the back and say, "I know it's hard to bear."
   b. Sit beside her and listen attentively if she wishes to talk about the situation
   c. Ask her to talk about her problems; reassure her that others also have problems
   d. Leave her alone for a short period until she regains control of herself

25. When talking to a psychiatric client for the first time, the nurse should remember that
   a. Hostile behavior from the client indicates that the nurse's initial approach has been inadequate
   b. A client's case history should be reviewed before interviewing him or her
   c. The client's physical appearance provides an accurate index as to whether he or she will be receptive to the nurse
   d. They (client and nurse) are strangers to each other

26. The *most* appropriate nursing response to a client's emphatic statement, "I hate them!" is
   a. "I will stay with you as long as you feel this way."
   b. "You hate them?"
   c. "I understand how you can feel this way."
   d. "What have they done to make you hate them?"

27. A client states, "That lady plans to murder me now." The *most* appropriate response from the nurse is
   a. "Have you talked to your doctor about this?"
   b. "If she starts toward you, let me know and I'll stop her."
   c. "I'll stay with you."
   d. "She cannot hurt you. She is a client here also."

28. Tony Day's frequent asthmatic attacks appear to be psychophysiologically based. One morning he has a severe attack and says, "I'm never going to get better;

I'm going to die." The nurse should respond by
   a. Telling him that we all have to die sometime
   b. Pointing out how much he really has to live for
   c. Sitting with him for awhile
   d. Telling him that he never has died from an attack yet

29. Barbara Fleming has been diagnosed as having a dysthymic disorder (depressive neurosis) following the death of her husband. Mrs. Fleming tells the nurse, "My husband hated me, and he had a reason to." The nurse should respond
   a. "Why do you think your husband hated you?"
   b. "Tell me about your husband."
   c. "Oh, I don't believe he really hated you."
   d. "Your husband hated you?"

30. Eleanor Jones is a young woman who exhibits the following behavior. Sometimes she sits alone, staring straight ahead. In the cafeteria, she snatches food from other people's trays. Other times she lies on the floor mute and uncommunicative. The nurse finds her staring into space, and sees that she has not dressed for the day. The nurse should say to her
   a. "Get your clothes out and dress carefully today."
   b. "Here are your clothes, now put them on."
   c. "Hurry up or you'll be late for breakfast."
   d. "Raise up your right foot, now put on your stocking."

31. A client experiencing paranoid delusions states, "They are conspiring against me; they pursue me night and day." A therapeutic nursing response is
   a. "They are out to get you; they are conspiring against you?"
   b. "I can understand how you feel, but it does not seem to me that this is being done."
   c. "Why do you feel they are pursuing you?"
   d. "You think this now because you are mentally ill. When you get well, you'll see it isn't so."

32. Paul Brown is in the manic stage of a bipolar disorder. He is using vulgar language on the unit. The nurse should intervene by saying
   a. "We don't like that kind of talk around here."
   b. "I thought that you were a gentleman."
   c. "You will not be allowed in the recreation room while you are talking that way."
   d. "I want you to help me straighten all of the chairs in the dining room, Mr. Brown."

33. The *most* appropriate comment to make to a client who is senile and exhibiting withdrawn and negativistic tendencies is
   a. "Would you like to go to your room where you can be alone?"
   b. "Your family will be terribly disappointed if you don't go to OT."
   c. "Your doctor wants you to participate in activities."
   d. "I need a partner to play checkers with me."

34. A client with sociopathic behavior makes advances toward the nurse. An appropriate comment is
   a. "You're making me uncomfortable; I'll have to leave if you continue."
   b. "Stop that immediately. What if your girlfriend knew how you were behaving?"
   c. "Don't do that or I'll tell your doctor."
   d. "If you continue, we will be forced to seclude you."

35. A symptom that characteristically differentiates an autistic child from one with Down's syndrome is

   a. Retardation of activity
   b. Short attention span
   c. Difficulty in responding to a nurturing relationship
   d. Poor academic performance
36. An important objective of nursing care for a client with chronic arteriosclerotic brain syndrome is to
   a. Minimize regression
   b. Correct memory loss
   c. Rehabilitate the client toward independent functioning
   d. Prevent further deterioration
37. The nursing role in group therapy may include serving as a
   a. Role model and catalyst
   b. Transference object and interpreter
   c. Participant, observer, and facilitator
   d. All of the above
38. Behavior modification treatment can *best* be described as
   a. Role repatterning
   b. Medical intervention
   c. Social learning
   d. Somatic conditioning
39. Key concepts in crisis counseling include all of the following *except*
   a. Immediate availability of services to the client
   b. Quick assessment of the emergency situation
   c. Providing purposeful, focused activity to guide the client toward adaptive coping
   d. Solving the client's problem for him or her
40. The activity therapy *best* suited for a manic depressive client is
   a. Reading
   b. Hammering on a metal in a jewelry OT project
   c. Playing chess
   d. Playing ping pong
41. (Questions 41–43 refer to this situation) Maureen Victor has cancer of the bowel. Surgery offers a reasonable chance of saving her life and does not have a high mortality risk. Mrs. Victor asks the nurse about the exact nature of the disease and the operation. The *most* therapeutic response from the nurse is to
   a. Give a direct, factual answer
   b. Give a brief, simple answer and let her know that you are interested in hearing more about her feelings
   c. Introduce her to another client who is recovering from a similar operation
   d. Offer to speak to her physician for her
42. Mrs. Victor tells the nurse about caring for her mother during a long, final illness following a stroke. The nurse should
   a. Reassure her that she must have given her mother the best possible care
   b. Ask her if this previous experience is making her anxious about the operation
   c. Nonverbally communicate attentive, gentle interest in hearing more about the matter
   d. Divert her from brooding on thoughts of death by changing the subject
43. Mrs. Victor tells the nurse that she has not told her husband or young daughter of the diagnosis of cancer. The nurse's *best* response is to
   a. Say a word or two about how difficult it is to express feelings
   b. Urge her to inform her family because her problem is more important than any they may have
   c. Agree that it is best to wait until more information is available
   d. Tell her that it is not fair to exclude her family from this critical period in her life
44. The *most* important task for a nurse in any health care setting is to develop skill as a(n)
   a. Advisor
   b. Observer
   c. Listener
   d. Conversationalist

45. All of the following may help a nurse understand the motives and behavior of self and others *except*
    a. Acquiring as much knowledge as possible about human behavior
    b. Interpreting behavior of others to them
    c. Making a conscious effort to be aware of his or her own behavior
    d. Discussing and exchanging observations with others skilled in the field of human relations
46. All of the following are useful to the nurse in establishing effective communication *except*
    a. Knowledge of world events, music, art, religion
    b. Personal experiences
    c. Knowledge of nursing, physical and behavioral sciences
    d. Concern with power, prestige, authority
47. Therapeutic interaction with clients primarily consists of
    a. Impressing upon clients the need for following exact, careful health care regimens
    b. Keeping the conversation focused on cheerful topics
    c. Discouraging expression (verbal and nonverbal) of negative feelings
    d. Assisting the client in accepting limitations imposed by their health status and making optimal use of existing capabilities
48. The purpose of a nurse/client relationship is to provide the client with a(n)
    a. Nonthreatening environment in which to interact with the nurse
    b. Understanding of past emotional responses
    c. Insights into present behavior
    d. Corrective emotional experience
49. A client usually drops out of group therapy when he or she
    a. Has accomplished his or her goal in joining
    b. Shares personal concerns with other group members
    c. Discovers that his or her feelings are shared by others in the group
    d. Experiences feelings of frustration in the group
50. The differentiating characteristic of a crisis state from other stressful situations is the feeling of
    a. Anxiety
    b. Immobility
    c. Hopelessness
    d. Confusion
51. When applying a systems approach to intervention in family therapy, the nurse can expect
    a. Restoration of equilibrium among other members when the deviant member is removed
    b. Blocking of mutual insights when the deviant member is exposed to the family's pathology
    c. Ineffective treatment of the deviant member if treated separate from the other members
    d. No family response to the support of the deviant member
52. (Questions 52–57 refer to this situation) Rosemary Moore, a 45-year-old mother of three daughters, has been referred to a crisis intervention center by her physician because she has severe bouts of anxiety and depression. At her last visit to the physician, she was told that she was entering early menopause. Her youngest daughter is to be married in a month; the two older ones are already married and living out of the state. An accurate assessment of Mrs. Moore's problem will require that the therapist
    a. Obtain a complete menstrual history
    b. Assess the circumstances directly relating to the immediate situation
    c. Use a slow-paced approach to gather all information
    d. Obtain a developmental history

53. Following an accurate assessment, the therapist plans a goal for intervention. The goal that is *most* compatible with crisis intervention theory in Mrs. Moore's case is that she will
    a. Demonstrate a major personality restructuring
    b. Return to a precrisis level of equilibrium
    c. Develop new coping skills to deal with future problems
    d. Gain insight into past behaviors
54. Which approach by the therapist will be *most* effective in Mrs. Moore's case?
    a. An exploratory one
    b. Passive observation
    c. Active participation
    d. Participant observation
55. The *most* therapeutic intervention for Mrs. Moore would be to
    a. Describe to her the relationship between her anxiety and the upcoming marriage of her youngest daughter
    b. Explain to her the advantages of hormonal therapy for early onset of menopause
    c. Encourage her to become more active in her community
    d. Discourage her from using past coping behaviors
56. Therapy has been successful if Mrs. Moore states
    a. "Getting old overnight doesn't seem so frightening."
    b. "I guess I'll learn to adjust without the children."
    c. "My energy level should return with more rest."
    d. "I know how important good looks are to my husband."
57. Mrs. Moore exhibited several behaviors associated with anxiety during her crisis intervention therapy. Which of the following behaviors is *not* evoked by anxiety?
    a. Anger
    b. Withdrawal
    c. Projection
    d. Crying
58. Severe anxiety involves
    a. A sense of being overpowered and that control is disintegrating
    b. A sense of becoming more alert
    c. A sense that experience is too difficult to bear
    d. A sense of narrowing of perception and selective inattention
59. Mary O'Sullivan, 27 years old, is extremely hyperactive. She has not slept for the past three nights, since her admission. She moves constantly. She talks loudly, rapidly, and often abusively to others. She is too busy to eat or drink. The nurse calls Ms. O'Sullivan for dinner. The client says she has too much to do to eat. The *best* nursing intervention is to
    a. Remind her that it is a hospital rule that all clients must come to the dining room for meals
    b. Return with a tray of food to the dayroom and sit close to the client to help her with the food
    c. Leave a tray of food in the dayroom within her reach, and sit apart from both her and the tray
    d. Ask the client if she would prefer to have a snack at bedtime, when she is not so busy
60. Ms. O'Sullivan is unable to sleep that night and has spread all of her belongings out on her bed when the nurse makes rounds. Her roommate is unable to sleep because of Mary's activity. The *most* effective nursing action is to
    a. Quietly and efficiently return the client's belongings to their original places
    b. Tell her that she has 15 minutes to put her things away or she will be secluded
    c. Suggest that she fold and arrange her belongings in the dayroom

d. Call the physician to obtain a sedative for Ms. O'Sullivan

61. A desirable outcome for nursing interventions for Ms. O'Sullivan's problem (not eating because of her distractibility) would be for Mary to
    a. Return to her previous eating patterns
    b. Become less distracted
    c. Take enough food and fluid to prevent malnutrition and dehydration
    d. Eat all meals in the dining room with the other clients

62. (Questions 62 and 63 refer to this situation) George Dobbins is a 55-year-old man who had to be assisted onto the unit. He stops at the door and the nurse must gently push him into his room, as he seems unable to walk in. The nurse asks Mr. Dobbins to place his things on the bed. Mr. Dobbins replies, "Is that a good bed? What about the other one?" When the nurse returns, he is moving his suitcase from one bed to the other. The nurse recognizes that Mr. Dobbins is so ambivalent that even when he appears to agree, he continues to be undecided. The nurse should
    a. Move the vacant bed into the hallway because there are no private rooms available
    b. Turn down the covers on one bed and place Mr. Dobbins' suitcase at the foot
    c. Give Mr. Dobbins the bed by the door so that he will not feel so confined
    d. Tell Mr. Dobbins that if he doesn't make up his mind he will have to sleep in the dayroom

63. When Mr. Dobbins has difficulty deciding which medicine to swallow first, the nurse should say
    a. "Follow my instructions. Put the pink pill in your mouth first."
    b. "I know that it is difficult for you to decide."
    c. "Would you prefer that I put your medicine in juice?"
    d. "The pills will help you. It is important to take them all."

64. The nurse approaches Sue Forbes, who is lying still and staring into space. The nurse recognizes that the client has withdrawn into her own world, and is out of touch with reality. The nurse should say
    a. "Are the voices bothering you again?"
    b. "Why are you looking so forlorn?"
    c. "I am here and touching you. You are real."
    d. "Don't be frightened. They can't hurt you."

65. (Questions 65–67 refer to this situation) John Dawson has been pacing all day. The nurse recognizes that Mr. Dawson is frightened by voices, and is also suffering from delusions. He believes that he is being stalked by members of organized crime. The nurse's *best* approach to Mr. Dawson is
    a. A decisive approach
    b. A cautious approach
    c. A minimally intrusive approach
    d. An eager approach

66. As Mr. Dawson's agitation increases, the nurse decides to lead him to the quiet room. The nurse should say to the client
    a. "You are out of control and you must go to the quiet room at once."
    b. "You need to be safe and I understand. Come walk with me to the quiet room."
    c. "You are upsetting everyone around you. It's time to go to the quiet room."
    d. "I will give you 15 minutes to quiet down and then I am going for help."

67. The nurse knows that Mr. Dawson is very frightened, and that his contact with reality is poor. The nurse's actions are based on which premise?
    a. It is important for the nurse to control the client's periods of seclusion
    b. Mr. Dawson must recognize the nurse's authority

    c. Physical force should always be employed to ensure client safety
    d. As long as clients have control, they should be allowed to use it

68. The physician has prescribed trifluoperazine hydrochloride (Stelazine), 10 mg bid for a client with schizophrenia who has been hospitalized for the third time in 2 years. What information from the client's drug history will be most important in determining the potential success of the choice of medicine?
    a. The psychiatrist's knowledge of the drug
    b. The client's knowledge of the drug
    c. The client's past experience with side-effects
    d. A family member's report of the client's response to this drug

69. The nurse administers chlorpromazine (Thorazine) 50 mg IM to counteract a client's extreme agitation. The client clutches his throat and rolls his eyes upward. The nurse recognizes this as an acute dystonic reaction. The nurse should
    a. Reassure the client that the symptoms are reversible and will diminish shortly
    b. Stay with the client and monitor vital signs every 15 minutes
    c. Instruct the client to remain supine for 30 minutes
    d. Administer benztropine 2 mg IM

70. Jessica Hughes, a 26-year-old cellist, applied for treatment after being dismissed from the community philharmonic orchestra. The orchestra's conductor stated that she was irritable, argumentative, and unable to concentrate. At practice, she would walk among the musicians, giving the members unsolicited advice. She would boast to them about what a great cello player she was. Ms. Hughes was started on lithium carbonate po 300 mg bid. The physician will probably
    a. Maintain this dose for the client for at least 1 week
    b. Increase the dose approximately every 3 days
    c. Decrease the dose after the second day
    d. Change the route of administration to IM if the client has difficulty swallowing tablets

71. Lithium has a significant number of side-effects that are not only troublesome, but potentially dangerous. The *most* effective way to assess for potential dangerous side-effects is
    a. Blood studies
    b. Vital sign monitoring
    c. Frequent observation
    d. Urinalysis

72. A client on lithium should be cautioned
    a. "Do not drive a car until you are sure that the medication does not make you dizzy."
    b. "If you skip a dose, double the dosage the next time."
    c. "When you start taking this medication, you may experience difficulty in urinating."
    d. "Be sure not to become dehydrated due to excessive heat or energy."

73. The drug of choice for treatment of a panic disorder, which involves extreme levels of anxiety, is
    a. Chlordiazepoxide
    b. Diazepam
    c. Imipramine
    d. Meprobamate

74. (Questions 74–76 refer to this situation) Michele Jones has been brought to the emergency room by her husband for examination after a fall at home. Her appearance is disheveled and her voice is loud and abusive. Mr. Jones states that his wife has a mild drinking problem. Her blood alcohol level is 0.11%. On admission to the hospital the physician's medication order includes chlordiazepoxide 100 mg po stat, to be followed after 4 hours by 100 mg po. The nurse should
    a. Withhold the medication

b. Call the physician to request an IM order
c. Administer the medication as ordered
d. Administer 50 mg and call the physician for further instructions

75. The nurse should expect the physician to discontinue the chlordiazepoxide
    a. In stepwise reductions over a 1 to 2 week period
    b. Within 72 hours of the client's admission
    c. When Mrs. Jones has ceased to be verbally or physically abusive
    d. When Mrs. Jones becomes sedated

76. The principal rationale for administering chlordiazepoxide is to
    a. Protect Mrs. Jones from injuring herself while intoxicated
    b. Reduce Mrs. Jones's anxiety during detoxification
    c. Prevent acute withdrawal symptoms
    d. Ensure that Mrs. Jones has adequate rest

77. Steve Danvers has been observed to walk with a shuffling gait during the second week of his admission. His posture appears more rigid and his voluntary movements have slowed down. He is taking perphenazine (Trilafon) 8 mg po, tid. After reporting these symptoms to the physician, the nurse might anticipate an order to
    a. Lower the dosage of the antipsychotic
    b. Discontinue the present antipsychotic
    c. Begin oral administration of trihexyphenidyl hydrochloride (Artane)
    d. Increase the dosage of the antipsychotic

78. (Questions 78–85 refer to this situation) Monica Woods, 22, a college student, is admitted to the unit. In the hospital, she speaks to no one, does not appear to be aware of what is going on about her, resists all nursing overtures, and assumes and holds unusual body positions. She has not left her room and spends hours sitting and staring into space. Her personal hygiene is neglected. Schizophrenia may be regarded as an individual's maladjustment to life's problems. This unhealthy adjustment is accomplished through
    a. Flight into fantasy
    b. Attempting to dominate reality through aggressiveness
    c. Regressing to a more satisfying period of development
    d. Withdrawing from social activities

79. In working with clients with a diagnosis of schizophrenia, the nurse should
    a. Recognize reality as it is, and expect the client to adapt
    b. Understand that no matter how inappropriate or bizarre the client's behavior may be, it does have real meaning to the person
    c. Accept the fact that the meaning of verbal and nonverbal communication rarely is obvious and should not be explored
    d. Support the client's perception of reality

80. Ms. Woods is occasionally incontinent on the floor. The *best* intervention is
    a. Restrict her intake of fluids
    b. Provide more frequent toileting
    c. Ration her intake of coffee and use of cigarettes
    d. Accept the behavior as being beyond the client's control

81. Ms. Woods cannot make decisions for herself. The nurse should respond
    a. "Let's take our bath now, Ms. Woods."
    b. "It's time for your bath, go get it done."
    c. "When you are ready to take your bath let me know."
    d. "Take your bath, Ms. Woods. I will be here to help."

82. Ms. Woods turns her head and gives an affirmative nod. To assess if she is hallucinating, the nurse should say
    a. "Is that your father speaking to you?"
    b. "What is it that you're hearing?"

    c. "You are distracted: are you hearing something?"
    d. "Tell me what the voices are saying."
83. The *most* effective nursing intervention to minimize the disruption in Ms. Woods' socialization skills is to
    a. Let her know that the nurse is available at anytime she chooses
    b. Tell her what the nurse expects when in her presence and how long the nurse will stay
    c. Sit in proximity and allow her to initiate conversation
    d. Maintain eye contact with her throughout the time spent together
84. The *most* important factor to consider in setting therapeutic goals for Ms. Woods is her
    a. Behavior
    b. Diagnosis
    c. Past history
    d. Age
85. An initial recreational goal for Ms. Woods while she remains withdrawn is to
    a. Attend the client dances
    b. Join in a game of euchre
    c. Model clay
    d. Participate in an off-unit nature walk

Each of the following situations illustrates maladaptive psychological responses to anxiety. Assess the situation and identify the maladaptive response.

86. Kim Norris complains of a stomachache and asks to stay home from school on the day of her chemistry test. Her behavior is an example of
    a. Conversion
    b. Hypochondriasis
    c. Malingering
    d. Somatization
87. Jane Taylor informs the nurse that her migraine headaches occur most frequently when she is under pressure to meet deadlines at work. She is experiencing
    a. Conversion
    b. Hypochondriasis
    c. Malingering
    d. Somatization
88. Within the last year, Gordon Duncan has had three colon examinations that revealed no symptoms, but he is still seeking a new physician to assure him that he does not have rectal cancer. This behavior is an example of
    a. Conversion
    b. Hypochondriasis
    c. Malingering
    d. Somatization
89. Jack Simpson feigned symptoms of whiplash following a rear-end car collision, and is applying for disability insurance. His behavior reflects
    a. Conversion
    b. Hypochondriasis
    c. Malingering
    d. Somatization
90. Betty Casey has been unable to lift her right arm since she slapped her daughter in anger following an argument. This problem reflects
    a. Conversion
    b. Hypochondriasis
    c. Malingering
    d. Somatization
91. Lester Jeffers, a college professor, keeps a supply of antacids in his office for temporary relief of heartburn before he lectures. He experiences
    a. Conversion
    b. Hypochondriasis
    c. Malingering
    d. Somatization
92. After her mother died from cardiovascular disease, Ruth Nichols purchased a blood pressure monitoring device, and checks her blood pressure after any physical activity (three or four times daily). This behavior is
    a. Conversion
    b. Hypochondriasis

c. Malingering
d. Somatization

93. Don Evans is uncomfortable around dogs and develops symptoms of upper respiratory distress whenever he comes in close contact with them. He is experiencing
    a. Conversion
    b. Hypochondriasis
    c. Malingering
    d. Somatization

94. The prototype of later anxiety is thought to be established
    a. During prenatal development
    b. At birth
    c. At birth and during the first days of extrauterine life
    d. During the second year of life

95. (Questions 95–100 refer to this situation. Select the phase of the nursing process that is reflected in the questions the nurse asks himself or herself about this situation) Barbara Carlyle has been admitted to the hospital directly from the offices of the publishing company where she is the fashion editor of a women's magazine. Her manner is very dignified, reserved, and haughty. She says, "I am here for a much needed rest." The nurse thinks, "What do I know about Ms. Carlyle?"
    a. Assessment
    b. Analysis/diagnosis
    c. Planning
    d. Evaluation

96. "What additional information do I need to understand as I work with her?"
    a. Assessment
    b. Analysis/diagnosis
    c. Planning
    d. Evaluation

97. "What do my observations about this woman mean?"
    a. Assessment
    b. Analysis/diagnosis
    c. Planning
    d. Evaluation

98. "Why is she here for help?"
    a. Assessment
    b. Analysis/diagnosis
    c. Planning
    d. Evaluation

99. "What are my nursing goals for Ms. Carlyle? How can these be met with maximum benefit for her?"
    a. Assessment
    b. Analysis/diagnosis
    c. Planning
    d. Evaluation

100. "What factors seemed to change Ms. Carlyle's behavior?"
    a. Assessment
    b. Analysis/diagnosis
    c. Planning
    d. Evaluation

101. (Questions 101–105 refer to this situation) Establishing a therapeutic relationship will facilitate operationalizing the nursing process with Ms. Carlyle. A one-to-one relationship can be established only if the nurse
    a. Has a sincere interest in helping her
    b. Can understand his or her own feelings about Ms. Carlyle
    c. Approaches her at the level at which she is currently functioning
    d. Accepts the role of becoming Ms. Carlyle's friend

102. The nurse's therapeutic relationship with Ms. Carlyle will be enhanced if the nurse uses verbal and nonverbal methods to communicate
    a. Acceptance of Ms. Carlyle as a person
    b. Recognition of her needs for attention
    c. Disappointment when Ms. Carlyle's condition does not improve
    d. Understanding of her problems

103. A therapeutic nurse/client relationship can be described as
    a. An automatic process based on established protocol
    b. Occurring exclusively in psychiatric settings

c. An interactional process between two people, involving a series of purposeful activities
d. Insightful, from the perspective of nursing

104. All of the following techniques are used in a therapeutic relationship *except*
    a. Offering self
    b. Using silence
    c. Voicing personal opinions
    d. Helping to identify feelings

105. The nurse suggests to Ms. Carlyle that perhaps the two of them can discuss and discover what produces Ms. Carlyle's anxiety. The nurse is using the technique of
    a. Exploring
    b. Reassuring
    c. Offering self
    d. Suggesting collaboration

106. (Questions 106–113 refer to this situation) Substance abuse is a growing problem in our society and one that crosses all socioeconomic boundaries. The indiscriminate use of drugs has been described as a behavior pattern by which individuals cope with the stress of overwhelming and perceived uncontrollable changes or disruptions in their lives. Whatever agent is abused, all but one of the following statements apply. Select the response that is *not* true. Effects can broadly be described as
    a. Contentment-inducing
    b. Predictable
    c. Hallucinogenic
    d. Tension-reducing

107. Nurses are susceptible to drug dependency in part because of their easy access to drugs, and because of the role strain many are under. Which additional statement below *best* supports the premise of susceptibility?
    a. Nurses are unaccountable for drug distribution
    b. Nursing practice promotes alienation because of its increasingly mechanized nature
    c. Nurses may have tolerant or even omnipotent attitudes toward drugs
    d. Nursing is a woman's profession and middle-aged women are most at risk

108. Some theorists believe that drug-dependent persons as a group do not know how to indulge in pleasurable activities (at least not without their drug). They suggest that treatment should be directed toward helping abusers become agents of their own pleasure. Which treatment modality would *not* be appropriate?
    a. Body/sensory awareness
    b. Meditation
    c. Art therapy
    d. Behavior modification

109. Drugs that are most commonly abused are divided into four major groups: CNS depressants, stimulants, narcotics, and hallucinogens. Which of the drugs listed below makes up the fifth category (less commonly abused)?
    a. Mescaline
    b. Marihuana
    c. Cocaine
    d. Librium

110. Which of the following drugs initially may improve the ability to think quickly and to concentrate?
    a. Cocaine
    b. Chloral hydrate
    c. Propoxyphene hydrochloride (Darvon)
    d. Chlordiazepoxide hydrochloride (Librium)

111. Flashbacks—a sudden recrudescence of symptoms, days, weeks, or months after ingestion—are most common with
    a. Alcohol
    b. Cocaine
    c. Marihuana
    d. LSD

112. All of the drug groups below necessitate withdrawal *except*
    a. Stimulants
    b. Depressants
    c. Hallucinogens
    d. Opiates

113. Withdrawal must be controlled over a specified period with decreasing dosage for which of the following drugs?
    a. Heroin
    b. Morphine
    c. Barbiturates
    d. Amphetamines

114. Dean Jones is admitted to the detoxification unit for withdrawal from an overdose of secobarbital (Seconal). A necessary piece of equipment at the bedside is a
    a. Catheterization tray
    b. Tracheostomy tray
    c. Cut-down tray
    d. Padded tongue blade

115. (Questions 115–118 refer to this situation) Greg Smith is brought to the emergency room by his fraternity brothers on a bad "trip" with LSD. The nurse is aware that he may be placed in life-threatening circumstances because of
    a. His maladaptive behavior
    b. The possibility of respiratory collapse
    c. His distorted perception
    d. The possibility of circulatory collapse

116. After detoxification, Greg is placed in a drug treatment in-patient program. Programs vary in philosophy and treatment modality with the exception of
    a. Therapeutic milieu
    b. Length of treatment
    c. Cost
    d. Psychotherapeutic techniques

117. Greg's friends visit on a regular basis. At each visit, they are asked to leave all packages at the nurses' station. This is necessary because
    a. They may forget them when leaving
    b. Greg is not to receive any packages from outside
    c. Greg's visitors are quite likely to be substance abusers themselves
    d. The other clients might take them

118. Greg is complaining of numerous physical ailments. The nurse recognizes that drug abusers often have hypochondriacal complaints. The *most* appropriate intervention is to
    a. Ignore his physical complaints and encourage Greg to rechannel his energy
    b. Carefully monitor vital signs and BP, and watch for symptoms
    c. Tell Greg that he is imagining the physical problems and that they will go away over time
    d. Offer Greg pain medication for severe complaints

119. In general, when medication is ordered for the drug abuser, it should be administered
    a. As seldom as possible
    b. In reduced dosage
    c. Only on a prn basis
    d. Orally if possible

120. School nurses are likely to encounter drug abuse in the adolescent community. The nurse who will be *most* helpful in the school environment should
    a. Be prepared to tell the students about the dangers of drugs
    b. Monitor restrooms, locker rooms, and the cafeteria carefully for signs of drug trafficking
    c. Work to gain a reputation of being understanding and "with it"
    d. Maintain contact with parents to be able to report their childrens' activities

Answer Sheet—Test 4

Answers and Rationales for Test 4

1. c. This response shares the nurse's observation and focuses on the client. Questions including "why" intimidate. Questions that can be answered "yes" or "no" elicit little information. Sarcasm should never be used. I, C
2. d. Gain the client's attention with simple statements; interrupting may antagonize or startle him. I, C
3. a. A person must feel safe with a therapist before he or she will discuss symptoms or become more self-sufficient. P, H
4. d. Simple, concrete subjects are best. P, O
5. d. Meprobamate (Equanil) is classified as an antianxiety medication. P, D
6. c. A major side-effect of antipsychotic drugs is drowsiness. I, D
7. b. This poses the least threat to the client. The other choices involve secrecy, dishonesty, and threats, which are less desirable. A, O
8. a. A key consideration in interactions with paranoid clients is to avoid the use of logic and argument. Humor intensifies anger and suspiciousness. Changing the topic may reinforce his belief about the others' guilt. I, O
9. c. It is generally accepted that catatonic clients are in contact with, and aware of, their environment. A, H
10. d. Depression causes a decrease or slowing down in all physiological system functions including that of the gastrointestinal (GI) tract. A, H
11. b. An honest response focuses on the husband's concerns. I, C
12. d. Depression is a response to a real or imagined loss. Loss results in anger, and anger is turned upon the self. A, H
13. d. Agitation refers to a psychomotor activity. Delusions of unworthiness (self-reproach) are common psychotic symptoms. A, H
14. c. When depression abates, the client has more energy and is better able to formulate self-destructive plans. A, H
15. b. A delusion is a belief which is not true to fact and cannot be corrected by an appeal to the reason of the person entertaining it. I, O
16. d. These are side-effects of anticholinergics. A, D
17. b. After five or six treatments, frequent complaints of confusion and loss of memory of recent events are common. A, H
18. d. Let the client know without anger how you feel, show that you are not intimidated, and help her examine what she is doing and why. I, C
19. b. It is important to provide external support to help develop the superego and to lessen the client's manipulative behavior. P, O
20. d. The first three choices produce the opposite of the desired result. Clients like Ms. Sparks do best when provided routine activities to follow. Changes produce anxiety. Activities at which the client can succeed bring satisfaction. Changes in routine need to be announced ahead of time. I, O
21. a. Anxiety is an interpersonal experience, which is easily communicated and contagious. A, O
22. c. Personnel should demonstrate acceptance of the client, but set limits on her behavior. P, H
23. c. It is useful to help the client focus on situations that precipitate feelings. I, C
24. b. Sitting with her indicates acceptance and demonstrates that the nurse feels she is worthy of spending time with. I, O
25. d. In therapeutic alliances, psychiatric nurses present themselves as real per-

sons working toward forming a mature alliance with the client. E, H
26. b. In reflecting the content of a message, the client has the opportunity to hear and mull over what he or she has said. I, C
27. d. The nurse recognizes that the client is frightened and in poor contact with reality, and provides assurance that he or she will be safe. I, C
28. c. In anxiety intervention, the nurse remains calm and stays with the client to help reduce feelings of panic. I, O
29. d. See answer 26. A, H
30. d. In withdrawn, regressed behaviors, interventions are concrete, simple, and directive. I, C
31. b. Don't argue or disagree with delusions. Let the client know you know it seems real to them, but it does not seem real to you. I, C
32. d. The use of profanity may increase in the manic stage. The best intervention is to create a diversionary activity. I, C
33. d. Interventions should be concrete and reality based. I, C
34. a. Confrontation of behavior should not incorporate threats or consequences that one cannot carry through. Avoid escalation. I, C
35. c. Most children with Down's syndrome are affectionate and enjoy being held and cuddled. A, H
36. a. Memory loss is usually permanent; however, disorientation resulting from memory loss can be minimized. Clients usually become more dependent in the course of illness and deteriorate progressively. Use of regression as a coping response can be minimized. P, O
37. d. All of the choices are correct. They are roles assumed in therapeutic relationships. I, O
38. c. Medical intervention is psychopharmacology. Somatic conditioning is biofeedback. Social learning implies accepting and adapting to rules, regulations, and norms to more effectively adjust to living. A, O
39. d. This is not a therapeutic goal for any modality. E, O
40. b. Manic depressive clients are unable to sit still for sedentary activities. Ping pong introduces a competitive factor that the client may not be able to tolerate. P, O
41. b. A therapeutic relationship encourages the client to share her feelings. I, O
42. c. The nurse implies empathy, honesty, and genuineness in a one-to-one relationship. I, O
43. a. This may encourage the client to provide more information about her reasons for withholding this from her family. Feelings are more important than facts. Avoid giving advice. I, C
44. c. Listening for three levels is considered crucial to therapeutic communication. E, O
45. b. The client must understand his or her own behavior. It cannot be interpreted by others. A, O
46. d. These concerns are nonproductive for establishing a one-to-one relationship. P, C
47. d. The first three choices are not therapeutic. The fourth choice will help the client adjust to the situation. E, O
48. d. This is the primary goal of a therapeutic relationship. P, O
49. d. The first three choices are positive gains of group therapy. Dropping out is a negative response. E, H
50. d. Normal coping strategies disintegrate, causing confusion. E, H
51. c. Systems theory evaluates each member within the family setting. E, O
52. b. Crisis intervention focuses on the present, nonfunctioning behavior. A, H

53. b. This is the main purpose of crisis intervention. P, O
54. c. The therapist must structure the setting to ensure the greatest return in the shortest time. I, O
55. a. The therapist first focuses on identifying the problem. I, H
56. a. Mrs. Moore has identified her problem. E, O
57. b. Withdrawal is a behavior associated with schizophrenia, a major psychosis. A, H
58. d. This represents 4+ anxiety. A, H
59. c. Bring the food to Mary. Sitting close may agitate the client. I, O
60. c. Mary cannot control her hyperactivity. The nurse helps her to channel her energy in a safe manner to avoid disturbing the roommate. I, O
61. c. Malnutrition and dehydration are serious complications for manic clients. P, O
62. a. Removing all choices for George allows for closer observation. I, O
63. a. Give direct, concrete instructions to an indecisive client. I, O
64. c. Orient the client toward reality. I, O
65. c. Recognizing the concept of territoriality is important. I, O
66. b. Offering reassurance and giving concrete guidance will lessen anxiety. I, C
67. d. This poses the least threat and gives the client control. E, O
68. c. Noncompliance with a medication regimen is the primary reason for exacerbation of schizophrenic symptoms. The client's recall of side-effects will influence compliance. E, D
69. d. Cogentin (benztropine) is the drug of choice to counteract an EPS (exophthalmos-producing substance) reaction. E, D
70. b. Lithium is increased and blood studies monitored until therapeutic blood levels are reached. P, D
71. a. Lithium is the only antipsychotic medicine that can be measured by blood level studies. A, D
72. d. Lithium is a natural salt that replaces sodium. I, D
73. c. Imiprimine (Tofranil) is an antidepressant used to treat panic attacks. P, D
74. c. The medication prevents the occurrence of delirium tremors (DTs). I, D
75. a. Stepwise reduction of dosage is the treatment of choice for DTs. E, D
76. c. Chlordiazepoxide is the drug of choice for acute withdrawal. E, O
77. c. Trihexyphenidyl (Artane) is an antiparkinsonian drug that controls extrapyramidical symptoms. A, D
78. c. Regression is a common schizophrenic behavior. A, H
79. b. The nurse must accept this principle to effectively use reality testing. E, O
80. b. The nurse must assist clients with acute symptoms of schizophrenia to perform activities of daily living (ADLs). I, O
81. d. Give direct, concrete instruction and provide supervision. I, C
82. c. The nurse should acknowledge the client's behavior and ask the client to validate the nurse's perception. A, O
83. b. This firmly establishes a contract for the one-to-one interaction between nurse and client. I, O
84. a. The nurse accepts the here and now and is concerned with the client's behavior. P, O
85. c. Modeling clay is a nonthreatening therapeutic activity. P, H
86. d. Somatization is a process in which anxiety is expressed through physical changes that have an organic basis. A, H
87. d. See answer 86. A, H
88. b. Hypochondriasis involves the expres-

sion of anxiety through physical symptoms that have no organic basis. A, H
89. c. Malingering is a purposeful, conscious feigning of illness and physical symptoms that have no organic basis. A, H
90. a. Conversion expresses anxiety through physical changes that have no organic basis. A, H
91. d. See answer 86. A, H
92. b. See answer 88. A, H
93. d. See answer 86. A, H
94. c. This is when bonding occurs. If successful, a sense of trust and security is established. A, H
95. a. Assessment involves gathering information. A, H
96. b. Analysis involves grouping and validating information. R, H
97. b. Analysis involves grouping and validating information. R, H
98. a. Assessment involves gathering information. A, H
99. c. Goals always are established with the client. P, H
100. d. Evaluation involves asking, "Did the interventions work?" E, H
101. b. The nurse must first recognize his or her own feelings if a therapeutic one-to-one relationship is to be successful. I, O
102. a. A one-to-one relationship requires acceptance of the client. E, C
103. c. A therapeutic relationship is a goal-directed, purposeful contract between the nurse and client. A, C
104. c. Voicing personal opinions inhibits full self-disclosure on the client's part and puts the nurse "in charge." I, C
105. d. Collaboration between the nurse and client is a key component in a therapeutic relationship. I, C
106. b. Effects of drugs vary enormously among users and are never predictable. A, D
107. c. Because of their familiarity with the analgesic properties, many nurses feel that they can control their drug use. R, H
108. d. Behavior modification emphasizes good behavior and deemphasizes the importance of pleasurable feelings. I, O
109. b. Marihuana is the fifth category and falls under cannabinols. A, D
110. a. Cocaine is a stimulant. Users describe an initial feeling of increased alertness and ability to concentrate. R, D
111. d. Lysergic acid diethylamine tartrate 25 (LSD) is a hallucinogen. Flashbacks occur with this drug category. R, D
112. c. Hallucinogens are not addictive. R, D
113. c. The correct answer is barbiturates, because of the life-threatening syndrome, including grand mal seizures, which accompanies withdrawal. Withdrawal from amphetamine addiction can be abrupt or gradual because there is no physiological, life-threatening abstinence syndrome. Heroin and morphine are similar and withdrawal can be "cold turkey." I, D
114. b. The first priority in the treatment of barbiturate overdose is maintaining respiration, which requires an open airway. I, O
115. c. Hallucinogens have no real overdose limit resulting in physiologic emergency. Distorted perceptions induced by them, however, lead people to believe that they are superhuman and to attempt suicidal activities. A, H
116. a. This is a secure, predictable, limit-setting environment in which Greg can learn new coping behaviors, acquire a sense of responsibility, and regain his self-esteem. P, O

117. c. In a residential treatment program, it is very important to block all attempts by the abuser to obtain drugs. It is very likely that Greg's friends would be his best source. I, O
118. b. Drug abusers are particularly vulnerable to illness, so the nurse must continuously assess the validity of the client's physical complaints, to separate valid complaints from manipulative hypochondria. I, O
119. d. To continue to inject the abuser is to reinforce his or her former life-style. I, D
120. c. Being an understanding listener is a prerequisite to helping adolescents with their problems. No progress can be made helping an abuser until the adolescent feels close enough to the nurse to discuss with him or her the consequences of taking drugs. P, O

DIAGNOSTIC GRID
Test 4

Directions: The diagnostic grid is used to reveal deficiencies in nursing content and nursing process knowledge. Determine which questions you answered incorrectly and circle the corresponding codes. Total each column and note the percentage of incorrect answers.

Nursing Process
A = Assessment
R = Analysis/nursing diagnosis
P = Planning
I = Implementation/intervention
E = Evaluation

Nursing Content
H = Health status
O = Nursing actions/interventions
D = Drugs/pharmacology
N = Nutrition
C = Communication skills

Question	Nursing Process					Nursing Content				
	A	R	P	I	E	H	O	D	N	C
1.				I						C
2.				I						C
3.			P			H				
4.			P				O			
5.			P					D		
6.				I				D		
7.	A						O			
8.				I			O			
9.	A					H				
10.	A					H				
11.				I						C
12.	A					H				
13.	A					H				
14.	A					H				
15.				I			O			

411

DIAGNOSTIC GRID (Continued)

Question	Nursing Process					Nursing Content				
	A	R	P	I	E	H	O	D	N	C
16.	A							D		
17.	A					H				
18.				I						C
19.			P				O			
20.				I			O			
21.	A						O			
22.			P			H				
23.				I						C
24.				I			O			
25.					E	H				
26.				I						C
27.				I						C
28.				I			O			
29.	A					H				
30.				I						C
31.				I						C
32.				I						C
33.				I						C
34.				I						C
35.	A					H				
36.			P				O			
37.				I			O			

DIAGNOSTIC GRID (Continued)

Question	Nursing Process					Nursing Content				
	A	R	P	I	E	H	O	D	N	C
38.	A						O			
39.					E		O			
40.			P				O			
41.				I			O			
42.				I			O			
43.				I						C
44.					E		O			
45.	A						O			
46.			P							C
47.					E		O			
48.			P				O			
49.					E	H				
50.					E	H				
51.					E		O			
52.	A					H				
53.			P				O			
54.				I			O			
55.				I		H				
56.					E		O			
57.	A					H				
58.	A					H				
59.				I			O			

DIAGNOSTIC GRID (Continued)

Question	Nursing Process						Nursing Content				
	A	R	P	I	E		H	O	D	N	C
60.				I				O			
61.			P					O			
62.				I				O			
63.				I				O			
64.				I				O			
65.				I				O			
66.				I							C
67.					E			O			
68.					E				D		
69.					E				D		
70.			P						D		
71.	A								D		
72.				I					D		
73.			P						D		
74.				I					D		
75.					E				D		
76.					E			O			
77.	A								D		
78.	A						H				
79.					E			O			
80.				I				O			
81.				I							C

414

DIAGNOSTIC GRID (Continued)

Question	Nursing Process					Nursing Content				
	A	R	P	I	E	H	O	D	N	C
82.	A						O			
83.				I			O			
84.			P				O			
85.			P			H				
86.	A					H				
87.	A					H				
88.	A					H				
89.	A					H				
90.	A					H				
91.	A					H				
92.	A					H				
93.	A					H				
94.	A					H				
95.	A					H				
96.		R				H				
97.		R				H				
98.	A					H				
99.			P			H				
100.					E	H				
101.				I			O			
102.					E					C
103.	A									C

DIAGNOSTIC GRID (*Continued*)

Question	Nursing Process					Nursing Content				
	A	R	P	I	E	H	O	D	N	C
104.				I						C
105.				I						C
106.	A							D		
107.		R				H				
108.				I			O			
109.	A							D		
110.		R						D		
111.		R						D		
112.		R						D		
113.				I				D		
114.				I			O			
115.	A					H				
116.			P				O			
117.				I			O			
118.				I			O			
119.				I				D		
120.			P				O			
Total items this test	35	6	18	45	16	36	45	19		20
Your total										
Percent Incorrect										

PRACTICE TEST SUMMARY

Directions: Use this sheet to summarize results from all four practice tests. Enter your score from each practice test and the item code summary from each diagnostic grid.

	Test 1	Test 2	Test 3	Test 4
Test Score	___	___	___	___
Nursing Process				
Assessment	___	___	___	___
Analysis	___	___	___	___
Planning	___	___	___	___
Implementation	___	___	___	___
Evaluation	___	___	___	___
Nursing Content				
Health Status	___	___	___	___
Nursing Actions	___	___	___	___
Drugs	___	___	___	___
Nutrition	___	___	___	___
Communication	___	___	___	___

Index

Page numbers followed by *f*, *t*, and *n* indicate figures, tables, and notes, respectively.

abortion, 171, 183
   practice test for, 338
abruptio placenta, 171
   practice test for, 343
abscess, anal, 85–86
accidents
   adolescent and, 235
   practice test for, 365
   preschooler and, 220
   school-age child and, 223
acetylsalicylic acid
   for myocardial infarction, 42
   practice test for, 301
   diabetes and, 94*t*

   drome, 149–152

acne, 239, 375
bone tumors, 236, 375
convulsive disorders, 237, 303–304
drug abuse, 238, 392, 403–404
obesity, 235–236
scoliosis, 236–237, 373
suicide, 238–239, 391–392
venereal diseases, 237–238. *See also* sexually transmitted diseases
hospitalization and, 235
leisure activities for, 235
nutritional requirements for, 234
sexuality and, 235
sleep and rest for, 234
adrenocorticotropic hormone, for multiple sclerosis, 114
adult respiratory distress syndrome, 71–73
affect, schizophrenia and, 268
AGA infant. *See* appropriate-for-gestational-age infant
agoraphobia, 271
AIDS. *See* acquired immunodeficiency syndrome
   related complex, 149
   ol amnestic disorder, 259
   hol coma, 261
   ohol hallucinosis, 259
   coholic dementia, 259, 260
   lcohol intake
      cirrhosis and, 88
      detoxification from, 259
      general considerations for, 260
      laryngeal tumors and, 118
      medical conditions associated with, 261
      mental disorders and, 259–262
      practice test for, 404
allergies
   contact dermatitis and, 105–106
   infant and, 207–208

allopurinol
  for leukemia, 103
  for renal calculi, 154
alprazolam (Xanax), 252t. *See also* benzodiazepines
Alzheimer dementia, 257–259
American College Testing Program's Proficiency Examination Program, 3–4
American Diabetic Association exchange diet, 95–96, 231
  practice test for, 372
amitriptyline hydrochloride (Elavil), 248t. *See also* antidepressant agents
amniocentesis, 168
  practice test for, 341
amniotic fluid, meconium stained, 175
amobarbital (Amytal), 252t. *See also* barbiturates
amoxapine (Asendin), 248t
amoxicillin, for otitis media, 215. *See also* ampicillin
  practice test for, 366, 368
amphetamine abuse, 264–265. *See also* drug abuse
ampicillin, for otitis media, 214. *See also* amoxicillin
amputations, 59, 128–129, 236
Amytal (amobarbital), 252t
anal abscess, 85–86
anal fistula, 86
analgesics
  for detached retina, 124
  for diverticulitis, 88
  for gout, 131
  for herpes zoster, 105
  for labor, 175
    practice test for, 344
  for osteoarthritis, 130
  for ovarian cancer, 138
  for rheumatoid arthritis, 132
anemia
  iron deficiency, 100–101, 170, 205–206, 370
  nutritional, 100–101, 297
  pernicious, 99–100
  sickle cell, 101–102, 230, 299, 374
anesthesia, for labor and delivery, 175–176
aneurysm, 51–53
angina pectoris, 37–39
  practice test for, 287
anorexia nervosa, 275
Antabuse (disulfram), for alcohol intoxication, 261–262
antacids
  for Addison's disease, 99
  for hiatal hernia, 76
  for peptic ulcer, 77–78
antianxiety agents, 250–251, 252t, 253t. *See also names of specific antianxiety agents*
antibiotic agents. *See also names of specific antibiotic agents*
  for burns, 107
  for cataracts, 123
  for contact dermatitis, 106
  for detached retina, 124
  for diverticulitis, 88
  for gallbladder disease, 80
  for gonorrhea, 147
  for leukemia, 103
  for meningitis, 113
  for mitral stenosis, 48
  for ovarian cancer, 138
  for pelvic inflammatory disease, 136
  for regional enteritis, 81
  for rheumatic heart disease, 46
  for spinal cord injuries, 128
  for syphilis, 146
anticholinergic agents. *See also names of specific antibiotic agents*
  for asthma, 70
  for chronic obstructive pulmonary disease, 65
  for Meniere's sundrome, 121
  for Parkinson's disease, 117
anticholinesterase agents, for myasthenia gravis, 116
anticoagulant agents. *See also names of specific anticoagulant agents*
  for cerebrovascular accident, 57
  for mitral stenosis, 48
  for thrombophlebitis, 54
anticonvulsant agents. *See also names of specific anticonvulsant agents*
  for head injury, 109
  for seizures, 237
antidepressant agents, 246, 248, 248t. *See also names of specific antidepressant agents*
antidiarrheal agents, for ulcerative colitis, 82
antiflatulent agents, for ovarian cancer, 138
antigonadotropin, for endometriosis, 137
antihistamine agents, 251, 253
  for hepatitis, 92
antimania agents, 248–250, 251t
antiparkinsonian agents, 251, 253
antipsychotic/neuroleptic agents, 245–246, 246t
  practice test for, 390–391, 400
antispasmodic agents, for diverticulitis, 88
antitubercular agents, 68–69
  practice test for, 289
antivertiginous agents
  for Meniere's sundrome, 121
  for otosclerosis, 120
anxiety management strategies
Apgar scoring, 176
  practice test for, 346
appendicitis and appende
  practice test for, 368,
appropriate-for-gestat
ARC. *See* AIDS-rela

ARDS. *See* adult respiratory distress syndrome
arteriosclerosis, 61–62
　aneurysm and, 52
Asendin (amoxapine), 248t
aspirin. *See* acetylsalicylic acid
assessment, definition of, 13, 14t, 15
asthma, 69–70, 226–227
　practice test for, 370, 393–394
atherosclerosis, 37–39, 40
Ativan (lorazepam), 250, 252t
Atromid-S (clofibrate), for arteriosclerosis, 62
atropine
　for chronic obstructive pulmonary disease, 65
　practice test for, 372
attachment, parental, 181. *See also* bonding, parent-child autonomy
　in nurse-client relationship, 22–23
　practice test for, 363
Aventyl (nortriptyline hydrochloride), 248t

baccalaureate degree in nursing, enrollment data on, 3
Bacillus Calmette-Guerin, 69
barbiturates, 250–251, 252t, 253t
　abuse of, 262–263
BCG. *See* Bacillus Calmette-Guerin
behavioral objective, definition of, 17
behavior change, interpersonal skills and, 31–32
behavior therapy, 254
　practice test for, 395
Benemid (probenecid), 131, 136
benign prostatic hypertrophy, 141–142
　practice test for, 310–311
benzodiazepines, 250–251, 252t, 253t. *See also names of specific benzodiazepines*
Berne, E., 24–28, 27f
beta-adrenergic blocking agents
　for angina pectoris, 39
　for glaucoma, 122
　for hypertension, 63
　for myocardial infarction, 42
bilateral salpingo-oophorectomy, 137
　practice test for, 312
biopsy, liver. *See* liver biopsy
bipolar disorders, 269–270
　practice test for, 394
birth control methods, 183
　practice test for, 346–348
bladder infection, 159
bladder tumors and neoplasms, 160–161
　practice test for, 308
blindness. *See* eye impairment
blood abnormalities, 99–105. *See also names of specific blood abnormalities*
blood and body fluid precautions, 150t

chemotherapeutic agents and, 102
　practice test for, 295
blood transfusion, 137
bloody show, pregnancy and, 169
bonding, parent-child, 176–177, 181, 193
　practice test for, 348
bone tumors
　adolescent and, 236
　practice test for, 375
Boniface, W. J., 23–24
bottle-feeding, 182
　practice test for, 347–348
botulism, 74–75
BPH. *See* benign prostatic hypertrophy
brain tumors, 109–111, 225–226
　practice test for, 303, 372
Braxton-Hicks contractions, 166
breast cancer, 139–140
　practice test for, 312–313
breast-feeding, 179, 180–181
　practice test for, 341, 347, 350
breathing exercises
　during labor, 175
　for test-taking, 11
bronchitis, chronic, 64–66
bronchodilators
　for asthma, 70
　for chronic obstructive pulmonary disease, 65
bronchogenic cancer of lung, 66–68
　practice test for, 286
BSN. *See* baccalaureate degree in nursing
Buerger's disease, 59–60
bulimia, 275–276
burns, 106–107
　practice test for, 297–298, 374
butabarbital (Butisol), 252t. *See also* barbiturates
Butisol (butabarbital), 252t
butyrophenones, 246t. *See also* antipsychotic/neuroleptic agents

CABG. *See* coronary artery bypass graft
CAD. *See* coronary artery disease
calcium channel blocking agents, for angina pectoris, 39
cancer
　bone, 236, 375
　breast, 139–140
　cervical, 140–141, 148
　colon, 82–83, 84t, 85t, 295
　liver, 91
　lung, 66–68
　ovarian, 138–139
　practice test for, 286, 309–313, 375, 395
　prostatic, 143–144

cancer (*continued*)
    renal, 154–155
    testicular, 144–145
    uterine, 140–141
carafate (Sucralfate), for peptic ulcer, 77–78
carbamazepine (Tegretol), for epilepsy and seizures, 112
cardiac catheterization, 38*t*
cardiac dysfunction, 37–51
    angina pectoris as, 37–39, 287
    congestive heart failure as, 43–45, 289–290
    heart block as, 49–51, 290–291
    mitral stenosis as, 47–49
    myocardial infarction as, 40, 41*t*, 42
    rheumatic heart disease as, 45–47, 342, 371, 374–375
cardiac enzyme level
    after acute myocardial infarction, 40, 41*t*
    practice test for, 286–287
cardiac surgery, 39, 46, 47
    practice test for, 370
cardiogenic shock syndrome, 40, 41*t*
cardiovascular dysfunction, pregnancy and, 170
cataracts, 122–123
    practice test for, 306
celiac disease, 217
Centers for Disease Control blood and body fluid precautions, 150*t*
central nervous system impairment, 108–111
cerebrovascular accident, 56–58
    practice test for, 292
cervical cancer, 140–141
    genital herpes and, 148
cervix, dilation of, 169
cesarean birth, 176
    neonate and, 189
    postpartal care and, 180
Chadwick's sign, pregnancy and, 166
chemotherapy
    for acute lymphocytic leukemia, 225
    for bladder tumors and neoplasms, 160
    blood and body fluid precautions and, 102
    for breast cancer, 140
    for cancer of testes, 144–145
    for Hodgkin's disease, 104
    for leukemia, 102–103
chest pain, 37, 40
    practice test for, 287
CHF. *See* congestive heart failure
child abuse and neglect, 208–209
    practice test for, 367
childbearing. *See* delivery; labor; pregnancy
childbirth education, 168
children, care of, 193–233. *See also* adolescent; infant; neonate; preschooler; school-age child
    practice test for, 363–376

chlamydia, 148–149
    adolescent and, 238
    pregnancy and, 172
chloral hydrate (Noctec Somnos), 252*t*. *See also* antianxiety agents
chlorazepate dipotassium (Traxene), 250, 252*t*. *See also* benzodiazepines
chlordiazepoxide (Librium), 250, 252*t*. *See also* benzodiazepines
    for alcohol intoxication, 261
    practice test for, 399–400
chlorpromazine (Thorazine), 246*t*. *See also* antipsychotic/neuroleptic agents
    practice test for, 399
chlorprothixene (Taractan), 246*t*. *See also* antipsychotic/neuroleptic agents
cholecystectomy, 79
cholecystitis, 78–80
cholecystogram, 79, 79*t*
    practice test for, 294
cholelithiasis, 78–80
cholestyramine (Questran)
    for arteriosclerosis, 62
    practice test for, 295
Christmas disease, 219
chronic obstructive pulmonary disease, 64–66
    practice test for, 288–289
chronic renal failure, 157–158
cigarette smoking, 64
    ear impairment and, 119–121
    laryngeal tumors and, 118
    lung cancer and, 66
    pregnancy and, 167
cimetidine
    for pancreatitis, 93
    for peptic ulcer, 77
    practice test for, 294
circumcision, infant care and, 181
cirrhosis, 88–91
    practice test for, 295–296
cleft lip and cleft palate, 198–199
    practice test for, 367
cloasma, pregnancy and, 166
Cloestid (colestipol hydrochloride), for arteriosclerosis, 62
clofibrate (Atromid-S), for arteriosclerosis, 62
closed questions, definition of, 32
cocaine abuse, 265–266. *See also* drug abuse
colestipol hydrochloride (Cloestid), for arteriosclerosis, 62
colon cancer, 82–83, 84*t*, 85*t*
    practice test for, 295
colon surgery, 84*t*, 85*t*
colostomy, 83
    practice test for, 299

coma
  alcohol-induced, 261
  diabetes and, 94t
  hepatic, 89
commissurotomy, for mitral stenosis, 47
communication, nurse-client, 21–23, 243–244
  autonomy and, 22–23
  behavior change and, 31–32
  conflict resolution skills and, 30–31
  congruence and, 24, 34
  decoding in, 23
  ego and, 24–28, 27f
  empathy and, 24, 27
  encoding in, 23
  facilitation skills for, 27–28
  general considerations for, 21–22
  importance of, 22–23
  interviewing skills and, 28–30
  key terms in, 32–33
  listening skills and, 27–28
  models for, 23–28, 24
    Gerrard, Boniface, and Love's communication model, 23–24
    King's interaction model, 24
    Rogerian model, 24
    Transactional model, 24–28, 27f
  positive regard and, 24
  practice test for, 293–294, 339–340, 365, 396
  trust and, 33
  value systems and, 21–23
complementary transactions, definition of, 32
concussion, 108–109
condom, for birth control, 182
conflict, definition of, 32
conflict resolution skills, 30–31
confrontation, definition of, 32
confrontation skills, 30–31, 32
  practice test for, 294, 367
congenital aganglionic megacolon, 206–207
congenital anomalies, 187. See also names of specific congenital anomalies
congenital heart disease, 200–201
congenital hip dysplasia, 199–200
congestive heart failure, 43–45
  practice test for, 289–290
congruence, definition of, 24, 32
constipation, pregnancy and, 166
contact dermatitis, 105–106
contracoup, 108–109
contusion, 108–109
conversion disorder, 272, 273
convulsive disorder(s), 111–118
  adolescent and, 237
  epilepsy and seizures as. See epilepsy and seizures
  meningitis as, 112–113

  multiple sclerosis as, 113–114
  Parkinson's disease as, 116–118
  practice test for, 303–304
COPD. See chronic obstructive pulmonary disease
cord, infant, care of, 181
coronary artery bypass graft, 39
coronary artery disease, 37–39
corticosteroids. See also names of specific corticosteroids
  for asthma, 70
  for cerebrovascular accident, 57
  for chronic obstructive pulmonary disease, 65
  for contact dermatitis, 106
  for head injury, 109
  for myasthenia gravis, 116
  for nephrosis, 219
  for renal transplantation, 158
  for rheumatic heart disease, 46
  for spinal cord injuries, 128
cortisone. See also steroid therapy
  for Addison's disease, 99
coughing technique, 65, 66
  practice test for, 288
Coumadin (warfarin sodium crystalline), 54, 55, 293
coup, 108–109
cretinism, 97–99
crisis intervention, 254–255
  for adjustment disorder, 278, 279
  practice test for, 395, 396–397
Crohn's disease, 80–81
  practice test for, 299
cromones, for chronic obstructive pulmonary disease, 65
crossed transactions, definition of, 32
CVA. See cerebrovascular accident
cyanotic heart disease, 200–201
cyclophosphamide (Cytoxan), 225
  practice test for, 373
cycloplegics, for detached retina, 124
cystic fibrosis, 215–216, 227–228
  practice test for, 374
cystitis, 159
cytomegalovirus, pregnancy and, 172
Cytoxan (cyclophosphamide), 225, 373

Dalmane (flurazepam), 252t
Decadron (dexamethasone), 109, 301
decoding, 23
deep vein thrombosis, 53–55
  practice test for, 293
degenerative joint disease, 129–130
dehydration, diarrhea and, 204–205
  practice test for, 367, 369
delirium, 256–257
  amphetamine abuse and, 264–265

delirium tremens, 259
delivery, 175–178. *See also* labor; neonate
　anesthesia during, 175–176
　complications of, 177–178
　emergency, 178
　forceps, 178
　maternal physiological assessment during fourth stage of, 177
　practice test for, 345–347
delusional thought, 267–268
　practice test for, 391–392, 394, 398
dementia(s), 257–259, 260
　alcohol-induced, 259–260
Demerol (meperidine hydrochloride), 93, 371–372
dental health
　adolescent and, 235
　hydrogen peroxide mouthwash for, 118
　preschooler and, 212
　school-age child and, 222
dependent nursing interventions, definition of, 14t, 18
depressive disorders, 270–271
　practice test for, 391–392, 394
dermatitis, contact, 105–106
desipramine hydrochloride (Norpramin, Pertofrane), 248t. *See also* antidepressant agents
Desyrel (trazadone), 248t
detached retina, 123–124
　practice test for, 306–307
detoxification, for alcoholic, 259
　practice test for, 404
deviated septum, 124–125
dexamethasone (Decadron), 109
　practice test for, 301
diabetes, 93, 94t, 95–96
　diet and, 95–96, 231
　metabolic acidosis and, 94t
　neonate and, 188–189
　practice test for, 296–297, 342, 349
　pregnancy and, 169–170
diabetic acidosis, diabetes and, 94t
Diagnostic and Statistical Manual of Mental Disorders, 267n
　adjustment disorders and, 277
　agoraphobia and, 271n
　bipolar disorders and, 269
　schizophrenia and, 267
dialysis, peritoneal, 158. *See also* hemodialysis
diaphragm, for birth control, 182
diarrhea, dehydration and, 204–205
　practice test for, 367, 369
diazepam (Valium), 250, 252t. *See also* benzodiazepines
　for alcohol intoxication, 261
　for epilepsy and seizures, 112
　for myocardial infarction, 42
dibenzoxazepines, 246t. *See also* antipsychotic/neuroleptic agents

digitalis (Lanoxin)
　for congenital heart disease, 201
　for congestive heart failure, 44
　for mitral stenosis, 47
　practice test for, 289, 290, 369–370
　for pulmonary embolism, 56
digoxin. *See* digitalis
dihydroindolones, 246t. *See also* antipsychotic/neuroleptic agents
Dilantin, for epilepsy and seizures, 112, 237
dilation, labor and, 174
discipline, preschooler and, 212
disulfram (Antabuse), for alcohol intoxication, 261–262
diuretics
　for cerebrovascular accident, 57
　for cirrhosis of liver, 90
　for congestive heart failure, 44
　for head injury, 109
　for hypertension, 63
　for Meniere's syndrome, 121
　for mitral stenosis, 47
diverticulitis, 87–88
　practice test for, 299
DJD. *See* degenerative joint disease
docusate sodium (Colace), for myocardial infarction, 42
Doppler study, for thrombophlebitis, 53
doxepin hydrochloride (Adapin, Sinequan), 248t. *See also* antidepressant agents
D-penicillamine, for rheumatoid arthritis, 132
drug abuse
　adolescents and, 238
　alcohol intoxication as, 259–262
　amphetamine and sympathomimetic organic mental disorders and, 264–265
　barbiturate and sedative/hypnotic mental disorders and, 262–263
　cocaine organic mental disorders and, 265–266
　opioid organic mental disorders and, 263–264
　practice test for, 392, 403–404
DSM. *See Diagnostic and Statistical Manual of Mental Disorders*
dysmorphic disorder, 272–273
dystocia, 177

ear
　impairment of, 119–121
　inflammation of, 214–215
eating disorders, 275–276
eclampsia, 170
ECT. *See* electroconvulsive therapy
ectopic pregnancy, 171, 183
EDC. *See* expected date of confinement
ego, in Transactional Analysis model, 24–28, 27f
Elavil (amitriptyline hydrochloride), 248t

electrocardiographic abnormalities
   in angina pectoris, 37
   in heart block, 50–51, 47, 48–49f
   in mitral stenosis, 47
   in myocardial infarction, 40
   practice test for, 286
   in rheumatic heart disease, 45
electroconvulsive therapy, 253–254
   practice test for, 392
electrolyte replacement, for mitral stenosis, 47
embolectomy, for pulmonary embolism, 55
embryo, definition of, 165
emotional tone, definition of, 32
empathy, 24, 27, 32
encoding, 23
endometriosis, 136–138, 183
   practice test for, 312, 348
enema
   for hepatic coma, 89
   practice test for, 295, 307
epiglottitis, acute, 202–203
   practice test for, 367–368
epilepsy and seizures, 111–112. *See also* seizures
   adolescent and, 237
   practice test for, 371
episiotomy, 178, 179
   infection and, 183
Equanil (meprobamate), 252t
Escherichia coli, 204
esotropiamyringotomy tube insertion, 200
estriol test
   for fetal well-being, 167–168
   practice test for, 341
estrogen therapy, for prostatic cancer, 144
ethchlorvynol (Placidyl), 252t. *See also* antianxiety agents
ethosuximide (Zarontin), for seizures, 237
evaluation, in nursing process, 14t, 18, 20
exhibitionism, 274
exotropia, 200
expected date of confinement, 166
   practice test for, 338
eye impairment, 121–124
   cataracts as, 122–123
   detached retina as, 123–124
   glaucoma as, 121–122
eye surgery, postoperative care for, 123, 124

facilitation skills, definition of, 32
failure to thrive, 210–211
family planning, 182
family relationships
   adolescent and, 235
   preschooler and, 212–213
   school-age child and, 222
family therapy, 254
   practice test for, 396
feeding problems, neonatal, 187
ferrous gluconate, for ulcerative colitis, 82
fetal assessment, 167–168
fetal development, 165
fetal heart rate, 175t, 175–176
   practice test for, 343, 345
fetal loss, 183
fetal response to labor, 174–175, 175t
fetishism, 274
fever
   acute respiratory infections and, 203
   hepatitis and, 91
   Hodgkin's disease and, 103–104
   myocardial infarction and, 40
   pancreatitis and, 93
   pelvic inflammatory disease and, 135
   rheumatic heart disease and, 45
fibroids, uterine, 133–134
fistula
   anal, 86
   tracheoesophageal, 201–202
fluphenazine decanoate (Prolixin Decanoate), 246t. *See also* antipsychotic/neuroleptic agents
fluphenazine hydrochloride (Prolixin), 246t. *See also* antipsychotic/neuroleptic agents
flurazepam (Dalmane), 252t. *See also* benzodiazepines
folic acid
   for mitral stenosis, 47
   for sickle cell anemia, 101
food poisoning, 74–75
forceps delivery, 178
fractures, 125–127. *See also* hip fracture
   children and, 232–233
fundus, postpartal, 179
   practice test for, 347
furosemide (Lasix), for congenital heart disease, 201

gallbladder disease, 78–80
Games People Play, 24–28, 27f
gamma globulin therapy, for AIDS, 151
gastrectomy
   for peptic ulcer, 77
   practice test for, 294
gastrointestinal dysfunction
   bleeding and, 89–80
   large bowel, 81–88
      anal abscess as, 85–86
      anal fistula as, 86
      appendicitis as, 86–87
      colon cancer as, 82–83, 84t, 85t
      diverticulitis as, 87–88

gastrointestinal dysfunction, large bowel (*continued*)
    hemorrhoids as, 83–85
    pilonidal cyst as, 86
    ulcerative colitis as, 81–82
  upper, 72–81
    food poisoning as, 74–75
    gallbladder disease as, 78–80
    hiatal hernia as, 75–76
    peptic ulcer as, 76–78
    regional enteritis as, 80–81
gavage, for neonate, 187
general anxiety disorder, 271–272
genital herpes. *See* herpes II
genitourinary and reproductive problems. *See* renal dysfunction; reproductive problems; sexually transmitted diseases
Gerrard, B. A., 23–24
glaucoma, 121–122
  practice test for, 300
glomerulonephritis, 152–153
  acute, 226
    practice test for, 371
glucose, for alcohol intoxication, 261
gold salts, for rheumatoid arthritis, 132
gonorrhea, 146–147
  adolescent and, 238
  practice test for, 308–309, 372
  pregnancy and, 172
gout, 130–131
  practice test for, 302
grandparents, 181
gravida, definition of, 166
group therapy, 254
guanethidine (Ismelin), for hypertension, 63

Haldol (haloperidol), 246t
hallucinations, 267
  alcohol-induced, 259
  practice test for, 400
haloperidol (Haldol), 246t. *See also* antipsychotic/neuroleptic agents
  for adjustment disorder, 279
  for delirium, 257
head injury, 108–109
  practice test for, 300
hearing loss, 119–121
heart block, 49–51
  practice test for, 290–291
heartburn, 166
  practice test for, 294
heart disease. *See also* cardiac dysfunction
  congenital, 200–201
heavy metal antagonist, for rheumatoid arthritis, 132
helminthic infections, 223–224

hemodialysis, 158
  for hepatic coma, 89
hemophilia, 219–220
hemorrhage
  postpartal, 182–183
  pregnancy and, 171
  ruptured spleen and, 104
hemorrhoidectomy, 84–85
  practice test for, 295
hemorrhoids, 83–85
  postpartal, 180
  pregnancy and, 167
heparin therapy
  practice test for, 291, 292
  for pulmonary embolism, 55
  for thrombophlebitis, 54
hepatic coma, 89
hepatitis, 91–92
  practice test for, 295
hernia
  hiatal, 75–76, 294
  inguinal, 228, 340
heroin addiction, 264. *See also* drug abuse
herpes II, 147–148
  practice test for, 309
  pregnancy and, 172
  transplacental infection and, 189
herpes zoster, 105
hiatal hernia, 75–76
  practice test for, 294
hip, congenital dysplasia of, 199–200
hip fracture, 125–127
  practice test for, 305–306
hip replacement, 126–127
Hirschsprung's disease, 206–207
Hodgkin's disease, 103–104
  practice test for, 299
Holmes and Rahe scale, 278
Homan's sign, for thrombophlebitis, 53
hormone replacement, for hyperthyroidism, 97
hospitalization
  adolescent and, 235
  infant and, 196
  practice test for, 365, 375–376
  preschooler and, 213
  school-age child and, 222–223
H_2-receptor antagonists. *See also* cimetidine
  for peptic ulcer, 77
human plasma protein fraction (Plasmanate)
  for burns, 107
  practice test for, 298
hydatidiform mole, 171
hydration, for cerebrovascular accident, 57
hydrocephalus, 197–198
  practice test for, 368–369

hydrogen peroxide mouthwash, 118
hyperbilirubinemia, neonatal, 186–187
hyperemesis gravidarum, 170
    practice test for, 342
hyperglycemia
    practice test for, 372
    signs of, 231
hypertension, 62–64
    practice test for, 292
    pregnancy-induced, 170–171
hyperthyroidism, 96–97
hypertropia, 200
hypnotics, 250–251, 252t, 253t
    abuse of, 262–263
hypochondriasis, 272, 273
hypoglycemia
    diabetes and, 94t
    signs of, 231
hypoglycemic agents, for diabetes mellitus, 95
hypothyroidism, 97–99
hypoxia, in congestive heart failure, 43
hysterectomy, 134, 137
    for cervical and uterine cancer, 141
    practice test for, 312
hysterosalpingogram, 135

imipramine hydrochloride (Tofranil), 248t, 271. *See also* antidepressant agents
immunization, for infants and children, 196t
    practice test for, 364, 365
immunoglobulin, for hepatitis, 92
implementation, in nursing process, 14t, 18
independent nursing interventions, definition of, 14t, 18
infant, 193–211
    accidents and, 220
    care of, 181–182
    developmental assessment for, 193, 194t
    family relationships and, 193, 196
    health assessment for, 193
    health problems of, 196–211
        abuse and neglect, 208–209
        acute respiratory infections, 202–203
        allergies, 207–208
        cleft lip and cleft palate, 198–199, 367
        congenital heart disease, 200–201
        congenital hip dysplasia, 199–200
        diarrhea and dehydration, 204–205, 367–369
        failure to thrive, 210–211
        Hirschsprung's disease, 206–207
        hydrocephalus, 197–198, 368–369
        intussusception, 206
        iron deficiency anemia, 205–206, 370
        myelomeningocele, 196–197, 368–369
        phenylketonuria, 209–210
        pyloric stenosis, 203–204
        strabismus, 200, 367
        sudden infant death syndrome, 209, 350
        tracheoesophageal fistula, 201–202
    high risk, 183
    hospitalization and, 196
        practice test for, 366–367
    immunization for, 196t
    nutritional requirements of, 193
infant respiratory distress syndrome, 178
    practice test for, 350
infection(s)
    chemotherapy and, 102–103
    ear, 214–215
    helminthic, 223–224
    maternal, neonate and, 189
    neonatal, 187
    postpartal, 183
    pregnancy and, 171
    respiratory, acute, 202–203
    of tonsils and pharynx, 213–214
infertility, 169
    practice test for, 340
inguinal hernia, 228
insulin therapy
    for diabetes mellitus, 95
    for pancreatitis, 93
    practice test for, 296
    pregnancy and, 170
interdependent nursing interventions, definition of, 14t, 18
interpersonal control, definition of, 32
interpersonal skills. *See* communication, nurse-client interviewing
    definition of, 32–33
    skills for, 28–30
intramuscular injections of antipsychotic/neuroleptic agents, 245
intussusception, 206
involvement, definition of, 33
IRDS. *See* infant respiratory distress syndrome
iron deficiency anemia, 100–101, 205–206
    practice test for, 370
    pregnancy and, 170
iron supplements
    for mitral stenosis, 47
    for nutritional anemia, 100
    for pernicious anemia, 99
Ismelin (guanethidine), for hypertension, 63
isocarboxazid (Marplan), 248t. *See also* antidepressant agents
isoimmunization, 186–187
isoniazid, for tuberculosis, 68–69

isoproterenol (Isuprel)
   practice test for, 289
   for second degree heart block, 50, 51
Isuprel (isoproterenol), 50, 51, 289

jaundice
   cirrhosis of liver and, 88
   hepatitis and, 91
   neonatal, 186–187
   pernicious anemia and, 99
   practice test for, 350
joint dysfunction, 129–132
   gout as, 130–131
   osteoarthritis as, 129–130
   practice test for, 301–302
Jones' criteria, for acute rheumatic fever, 229, 229t

ketoacidosis
   diabetes and, 94t
   pregnancy and, 170
kidney, cancer of, 154–155
King, I., 24
Korsakoff's syndrome, 259

labor, 169, 173–178. *See also* delivery
   analgesia during, 175
   anesthesia during, 175–176
   complications of, 177–178
   definitions for, 174t, 175t
   fetal response to, 174–175
   induction of, oxytocin and, 176, 177–178
   practice test for, 343–345
   premature, 178
   signs of, 169
   stages of, 173–174, 174t
   true vs. false, 169
   vital signs and, 174
lactation, 179–181
lactulose
   for cirrhosis of liver, 90
   for hepatic coma, 89
language development, 194–195t
   practice test for, 363, 364
Lanoxin (digitalis), 44, 47, 56, 201, 289, 290, 369–370
laparoscopy, 136
laparotomy, 136
large-for-gestational-age infant, 188
laryngectomy, 118–119
   practice test for, 302
larynx impairment, 118–119
Lasix (furosemide), for congenital heart disease, 201
L-dopa (levodopa), for Parkinson's disease, 117

leiomyomas, uterine, 133–134
leukemia, 102–103. *See also* acute lymphocytic leukemia
leukorrhea, pregnancy and, 166
levodopa (L-dopa), for Parkinson's disease, 117
LGA infant. *See* large-for-gestational-age infant
Librium (chlordiazepoxide), 250, 252t, 261, 399–400
life events, 278
linea nigra, pregnancy and, 166
listening skills, 27–28, 30, 32
lithium carbonate, 248–250, 251t
   practice test for, 399
lithotripsy, 154
liver and pancreas dysfunction, 88–93
   cancer of liver as, 91
   cirrhosis of liver as, 88–91
   hepatitis as, 91–92
   pancreatitis as, 92–93
liver biopsy, 89
   practice test for, 295–296
liver cancer, 91
lobectomy, 67
lochia, 179
   practice test for, 347
lorazepam (Ativan), 250, 252t. *See also* benzodiazepines
Love, B. H., 23–24
loxapine (Loxitane), 246t. *See also* antipsychotic/neuroleptic agents
Loxitane (loxapine), 246t
Ludiomil (maprotiline hydrochloride), 248t
lumbar sympathectomy, for Buerger's disease, 59
Luminal (phenobarbital), 80, 237, 252t
lumpectomy, 140
lung cancer, 66–68
   practice test for, 286

malabsorption disorder, 217
manic-depressive disorder. *See also* bipolar disorders
MAO inhibitors. *See* monoamine oxidase inhibitors
maprotiline hydrochloride (Ludiomil), 248t. *See also* antidepressant agents
Marplan (isocarboxazid), 248t
masochism, sexual, 274
mastectomy, 140
   practice test for, 313
mastitis, 183
   practice test for, 348
McBurney's point, appendicitis and, 228
mebendazole (Vermox), for helminthic infections, 224
meconium-stained amniotic fluid, 175
Mellaril (thioridazine), 246t
Meniere's syndrome, 120–121
   practice test for, 306
meningitis, 112–113
   practice test for, 303

mental health problems
    adjustment disorder as, 277–279
    organic, 256–266
        alcohol intoxication, 259–262
        amphetamine abuse, 264–265
        barbiturate and sedative abuse, 262–263
        cocaine abuse, 265–266
        delirium, 256–257
        mental retardation, 256–257
        opioid abuse, 263–264
    in postpartum client, 183
    practice test for, 390–404
    from psychological causes, 267–279
        anorexia nervosa, 275
        anxiety disorders, 271–272
        bipolar disorders, 269–270
        bulimia, 275–276
        depressive disorders, 270–271
        obsessive–compulsive disorders, 272
        physical diseases and, 274–275
        schizophrenia, 267–269
        sexual disorders, 273–274
        somatoform disorders, 272–273
    treatment modalities for, 243–255. *See also names of specific treatment modalities;* psychotropic medications
mental retardation, 224, 266
    practice test for, 375
meperidine hydrochloride (Demerol)
    for pancreatitis, 93
    practice test for, 371–372
meprobamate (Equanil; Miltown), 252*t*. *See also* antianxiety agents
mesoridazine (Serentil), 246*t*. *See also* antipsychotic/neuroleptic agents
metabolic acidosis, diabetes and, 94*t*
metabolic dysfunction
    Addison's disease as, 98–99
    diabetes mellitus and, 93, 94*t*, 95–96
    hyperthyroidism as, 96–97
    hypothyroidism as, 97–99
methylxanthine derivative bronchodilators, for chronic obstructive pulmonary disease, 65
methyprylon (Noludar), 252*t*. *See also* antianxiety agents
metoclopramide (Reglan), for hiatal hernia, 76
milieu therapy, 254
Miltown (meprobamate), 252*t*
miotics
    for cataracts, 123
    for glaucoma, 122
mitral stenosis, 47–49, 48*f*
Moban (molindone), 246*t*
Mobitz I, 48*f*, 50. *See also* heart block
Mobitz II, 49*f*, 50. *See also* heart block

molindone (Moban), 246*t*. *See also* antipsychotic/neuroleptic agents
moniliasis, 171–172
    practice test for, 341, 350
    pregnancy and, 189
monoamine oxidase inhibitors, 248*t*, 249*t*. *See also* antidepressant agents
morning sickness, during pregnancy, 165
morphine sulfate, for myocardial infarction, 42
motor development, 194–195*t*
mouthwash, hydrogen peroxide, 118
mucolytics, for chronic obstructive pulmonary disease, 65
mucous plug, pregnancy and, 169
multiple sclerosis, 113–114
    practice test for, 304
muscle relaxants, for multiple sclerosis, 114
myasthenia gravis, 114–115
    practice test for, 304
Mycobacterium tuberculosis, 68–69
    practice test for, 289
mydriatics
    for cataracts, 123
    for detached retina, 124
myelomeningocele, 196–197
    practice test for, 368–369
myocardial infarction, 40, 41*t*, 42
myomectomy, 134
myringotomy tube insertion, 215
myxedema, 97–99

NANDA. *See* North American Nursing Diagnosis Association
narcotics
    for burns, 107
    for detached retina, 124
    for leukemia, 103
    for ovarian cancer, 138
    for renal calculi, 154
    for sickle cell anemia, 101
Nardil (phenelzine sulfate), 248*t*
nasoseptoplasty, 125
National League for Nursing Mobility Profile II Examinations, 3–4
Navane (thiothixene), 246*t*
Nembutal (pentobarbital), 252*t*
neomycin
    for cirrhosis of liver, 90
    for diverticulitis, 88
neonate, 184–189
    complications in, 185–188
        congenital anomalies, 187
        hyperbilirubinemia, 186–187
        jaundice, 186

neonate, complications in (*continued*)
   respiratory problems, 185–186
   gestational age and, 188
   high risk, 187–188
   immediate care of, 177
   maternal problems and, 188–189
   nutritional needs of, 185
   physical asessment of, 184–185
   physiological changes in, 184
   in postpartal period, 181–182
   post-term, 188
   practice test for, 349–350
   preterm, 187
nephrectomy, 155
nephrolithiasis, 153–154
nephrosis, 218–219
   practice test for, 367
nerve blocks
   for labor and delivery, 175–176
   practice test for, 345
neuroleptic agents. *See* antipsychotic/neuroleptic agents
niacin, for arteriosclerosis, 62
nitrogen mustard, Hodgkin's disease and, 104
nitroglycerin
   for angina pectoris, 39
   for myocardial infarction, 42
   practice test for, 287
Noctec Somnos (chloral hydrate), 252*t*
Noludar (methyprylon), 252*t*. *See also* antianxiety agents
noncompliance, 244–245
nonsteroidal anti-inflammatory drugs
   for gout, 131
   for osteoarthritis, 130
   for rheumatoid arthritis, 132
nonsystemic antacids, for peptic ulcer, 77
Norpramin (desipramine hydrochloride), 248*t*
North American Nursing Diagnosis Association, 15, 16*t*
nortriptyline hydrochloride (Aventyl), 248*t*. *See also* antidepressant agents
nose impairment, 124–125
NSAIDs. *See* nonsteroidal anti-inflammatory drugs
nurse-client relationship, phases of, 244. *See also* communication, nurse-client
nursing diagnosis
   components of, 14*t*, 15, 15*t*
   example of, 19*f*
   medical diagnosis vs., 15
   NANDA-approved, 16*t*
   steps involved in planning phase of, 17*t*
nursing intervention, definition of, 14*t*, 18
nursing process, 13–20, 14*t*
   assessment in, 13, 14*t*—17*t*, 15
   components of, 14*t*
   evaluation in, 14*t*, 18, 20

   implementation in, 14*t*, 18
   planning in, 14*t*, 15, 17–18, 19*f*
nutritional anemia, 100–101

obesity, adolescent and, 235–236
objective data, definition of, 13
obsessive–compulsive disorder, 272
oophorectomy, 137
open-ended questions, definition of, 33
ophthalmia neonatorum, 176
   practice test for, 349
opioid abuse, 263–264
oral hygiene, 118
orchiectomy, 145
Ortolani's sign, 199
osteoarthritis, 129–130
osteogenic sarcoma, 236
ostomy care, 83, 85*t*
otitis media, 214–215
otosclerosis, 119–120
outcome criteria, definition of, 17
ovarian cancer, 138–139
ovum, 165
oxygen, deficiency of delivery of. *See* cardiac dysfunction; pulmonary dysfunction; vascular dysfunction
oxygen therapy
   for angina pectoris, 39
   for myocardial infarction, 42
   practice test for, 288–289
oxytocin (Pitocin), 175–178
   practice test for, 344, 345

pacemaker, for second degree heart block, 50, 51
pain
   abdominal
      appendicitis and, 228
      ovarian cancer and, 138
      ruptured spleen and, 104
   burns and, 106
   chest, 37, 40, 287
      practice test for, 287
   chlamydia and, 148
   endometriosis and, 136
   fractures and, 125
   gallbladder disease and, 78
   genital herpes and, 147
   herpes zoster and, 105
   laryngeal tumors and, 118, 119
   leukemia and, 102
   pancreatitis and, 93
   peptic ulcer and, 76
   renal calculi and, 153

rheumatoid arthritis and, 132
  sickle cell anemia and, 101
  uterine, 133
pancreas and liver dysfunction, 88–93. *See also* liver and pancreas dysfunction
pancreatic enzyme supplements
  for cystic fibrosis, 216, 228
  practice test for, 366–367
pancreatitis, 92–93
  practice test for, 298
panic disorder, 271
  practice test for, 399
paracentesis, 89
  practice test for, 296
paranoid delusions, 267–268
  practice test for, 391–392, 394, 398
paraphilias, 273–274
parity, 166
Parkinson's disease, 116–118
  practice test for, 304
pedophilia, 274
pelvic inflammatory disease, 135–136
  chlamydia and, 148
  practice test for, 313–314
pentobarbital (Nembutal), 252*t*. *See also* barbiturates
pentoxifylline (Trental), for arteriosclerosis, 62
peptic ulcer, 76–78
percutaneous transluminal coronary angioplasty, 38–39
perforation, with peptic ulcer, 77
peritoneal dialysis, 157–158
pernicious anemia, 99–100
  practice test for, 297
Pertofrane (desipramine hydrochloride), 248*t*
phenelzine sulfate (Nardil), 248*t*. *See also* antidepressant agents
phenobarbital (Luminal), 252*t*. *See also* barbiturates
  for gallbladder disease, 80
  for seizures, 237
phenothiazines, 246*t*
  practice test for, 391
phenozapyridine hydrochloride (Pyridium), 159
  practice test for, 308
phenylketonuria, 209–210
phenytoin (Dilantin), for epilepsy and seizures, 112, 237
phlebography, for thrombophlebitis, 53
phosphates, for renal calculi, 154
phototherapy, for neonate, 186
PID. *See* pelvic inflammatory disease
PIH. *See* pregnancy-induced hypertension
pilocarpine, 122
  practice test for, 300
pilonidal cyst, 86
pinworms, 223–224
Pitocin (oxytocin), 176–178, 344, 345

pituitary adenoma, 109–111
  practice test for, 303
placenta previa, 171
  practice test for, 343
Placidyl (ethchlorvynol), 252*t*
plan of care, development of, 14*t*, 15, 17–18, 19*f*
  format for, 18, 19*f*
  goals in, 17, 17*t*
  nursing interventions in, 14*t*, 18
Plasmanate (human plasma protein fraction), 107, 298
plethysmography, for thrombophlebitis, 53
pneumonia, 70–71
poisonous substances, ingestion of, 216–217
  practice test for, 366
positive regard, 24
postpartal period, 179–183
  complications of, 182–183
  educational needs during, 181–182
  physiological adaptation during, 179–180
  practice test for, 347
  psychosocial problems during, 183
post-term infant, 188
preeclampsia, 170
  practice test for, 342
pregnancy, 165–172. *See also* delivery; labor; postpartal period
  childbirth education during, 168
  complications of, 170–172
    bleeding disorders, 171
    hypertension, 170–171
    infections, 171–172
    TORCH, 172
  developmental tasks of family during, 168
  diagnosis of, 166
  discomforts of, 165–166
  drug use during, 167
  fetal assessment during, 167–168
  insulin therapy and, 170
  iron-deficiency anemia and, 170
  leg cramps and, 167
  multiple, 169
  nutritional care during, 167
  objective changes and diagnosis of, 166–167
  physiological adaptations to, 165–167
  practice test for, 338–343
  preexisting medical conditions as factors in, 169–170
  prenatal care for, 167
  rest and activity during, 167
pregnancy-induced hypertension, 170–171
  practice test for, 342
pregnancy tests, 166
preschooler, 212–220
  dental health for, 212
  family relationships and, 212–213
  growth and development of, 195*t*, 212

preschooler (*continued*)
  health problems of, 213–220
    accidents, 220
    appendicitis, 218, 368, 376
    celiac disease, 217
    cystic fibrosis, 215–216, 374
    hemophilia, 219–220
    ingested poisons, 216–217, 366
    nephrosis, 218–219, 367
    otitis media, 214–215
    tonsillitis and tonsillectomy, 213–214, 369
  hospitalization and, 213
  nutritional requirements of, 212
preterm infant, care of, 187
  practice test for, 348, 350
probenecid (Benemid)
  for gout, 131
  for pelvic inflammatory disease, 136
probe questions, definition of, 33
procainamide hydrochloride (Pronestyl), for mitral stenosis, 48
prolapsed cord, 177
Prolixin (fluphenazine hydrochloride), 246*t*
Prolixin Decanoate (fluphenazine decanoate), 246*t*
Pronestyl (procainamide hydrochloride), for mitral stenosis, 48
propanediol, 252*t*, 253*t*. *See also* antianxiety agents
prostatectomy, 142
  practice test for, 310–311
prostatic cancer, 143–144
  practice test for, 311
psychiatric nursing, general considerations for, 243
psychological factors, physical diseases and, 274–275
psychosocial therapies, 254–255
psychotropic medications, 244–253. *See also names of specific psychotropic medications*
  antianxiety agents as, 250–251, 252*t*, 253*t*
  antidepressant agents as, 246, 248, 248*t*
  antihistamine agents as, 251, 253
  antimania agents as, 248–250, 251*t*
  antiparkinsonian agents as, 251, 253
  antipsychotic/neuroleptic agents as, 245–246, 246*t*, 247*t*
  general considerations for, 244
  noncompliance and, 244–245
PTCA. *See* percutaneous transluminal coronary angioplasty
pulmonary dysfunction, 64–73
  acute respiratory infection as, 70–71
  adult respiratory distress syndrome as, 71–73
  asthma as, 69–70
  cancer of lung as, 66–68
  chronic obstructive pulmonary disease as, 64–66
  in congestive heart failure, 43
  tuberculosis as, 68–69

pulmonary embolism, 55–56
  practice test for, 291
pyloric stenosis, 203
Pyridium (phenozapyridine hydrochloride), 159, 208

question analysis procedure, for test-taking, 9–10
Questran (cholestyramine), 62, 295
quickening, 166
Quinidine, for mitral stenosis, 48

radiation therapy
  for bladder tumors and neoplasms, 160
  for breast cancer, 140
  for cervical and uterine cancer, 141
  implants for, 140–141
  practice test for, 309–310
  for testicular cancer, 144–145
radioactive iodine, for hyperthyroidism, 96–97
Raynaud's phenomenon, 60
  practice test for, 291–292
regional enteritis, 80–81
Reglan (metoclopramide), for hiatal hernia, 76
relaxation exercises, as test-taking strategy, 11
renal calculi, 153–154
  practice test for, 308
renal dysfunction, 152–161. *See also* renal failure
  bladder tumors and neoplasms as, 160–161
  cystitis as, 159
  glomerulonephritis as, 152–153
  renal calculi as, 153–154
  renal tumor as, 154–155
renal failure
  acute, 155–157
  chronic, 157–158
  practice test for, 307–308
renal transplantation, 158
reproductive problems. *See also* sexually transmitted diseases
  female, 133–141
    breast cancer, 139–140
    endometriosis, 136–138
    ovarian cancer, 138–139
    pelvic inflammatory disease, 135–136
    uterine and cervical cancer, 140–141
    uterine fibroids and leiomyomas, 133–134
    uterine prolapse, 134–135
  male
    benign prostatic hypertrophy, 141–142
    prostatic cancer, 143–144
    testicular cancer, 144–145
respiratory dysfunction, in preterm infant, 187–188
respiratory infections, acute, 70–71, 202–203
Restoril (temazepam), 250, 252*t*

rheumatic fever
    acute, 229t, 229–230
        practice test for, 342, 371, 374–375
rheumatic heart disease, 45–47
    mitral stenosis and, 47
    practice test for, 291
rheumatoid arthritis, 131–132
    practice test for, 301
Rh-negative blood factor, 186–187
    practice test for, 341
RhoGAM, 186–187
    practice test for, 341
ritodrine, premature labor and, 178
RN mobility programs, 3–5
Rogers, C., 24
ROM. *See* rupture of membranes
rubella, pregnancy and, 172
Rubin's test, 135
ruptured spleen, 104–105
    practice test for, 297
rupture of membranes, pregnancy and, 169

sadism, sexual, 274
safe sexual practices, 151
salicylates
    for rheumatic heart disease, 46
    for rheumatoid arthritis, 132
salmonella, 204
salpingectomy, 137, 141
salpingitis, 135–136
    chlamydia and, 148
salt-poor albumin, for cirrhosis of liver, 90
schizophrenia, 267–269
    medication for, 245–246, 246t
    practice test for, 390–391, 400
school-age child, 221–233
    growth and development of, 221–222
    health problems of, 223–233
        accidents, 223
        acute glomerulonephritis, 226, 371
        acute lymphocytic leukemia, 224–225, 373
        acute rheumatic fever, 229t, 229–230, 342, 371, 374–375
        appendicitis, 228–229, 368, 376
        asthma, 226–227, 370, 393–394
        brain tumors, 225–226, 303, 372
        burns, 231–232, 342, 371, 374–375
        cystic fibrosis, 227, 374
        diabetes mellitus, 231. *See also* diabetes
        fractures, 125–127, 232–233
        helminthic infections, 223–224
        inguinal hernia, 228
        mental retardation, 224, 375
        sickle cell anemia, 230, 299, 374

    health promotion for, 222
    hospitalization and, 222–223
sclerotherapy, 90
scoliosis, 236–237
    practice test for, 373
secobarbital (Seconal), 252t. *See also* barbiturates
Seconal (secobarbital), 252t
sedatives, 250–251, 252t, 253t. *See also* names of specific sedatives
    abuse of, 262–263
    for ulcerative colitis, 82
seizures
    adolescent and, 237
    brain tumors and, 109, 110
    epilepsy and, 111–112
    head injury and, 108, 109
    meningitis and, 112–113
    practice test for, 300–301, 303–304, 370–371
self-disclosure, definition of, 33
sensorimotor impairment, 108–132
    central nervous system impairment as, 108–111
    convulsive disorders as, 111–118. *See also* convulsive disorders
    ear impairment as, 119–121
    eye impairment as, 121–124
    joint dysfunction as, 129–132, 301–302
    larynx impairment as, 118–119
    nose impairment as, 124–125
    skeletal dysfunction as, 125–129
separation anxiety, children and, 196
Serentil (mesoridazine), 246t
sexual abuse, of children, 208–209
sexual disorders, 273–274
sexuality
    adolescent and, 235
    school-age child and, 222
sexually transmitted diseases, 145–152, 171–172
    adolescent and, 237–238
    AIDS as, 149–152
    chlamydia as, 148–149, 172, 238
    genital herpes as, 147–148, 172, 189, 309
    gonorrhea as, 146–147, 172, 238, 308–309, 372
    syphilis as, 145–146, 172
SGA infant. *See* small-for-gestational-age infant
shigellosis, practice test for, 367
shingles, 105
sibling rivalry
    newborn and, 181
    preschooler and, 213
sickle cell anemia, 101–102, 230
    practice test for, 299, 374
SIDS. *See* sudden infant death syndrome
silver nitrate, for newborn, 176
Sinemet (carbidopa), for Parkinson's disease, 117
Sinequan (doxepin hydrochloride), 248t

skeletal dysfunction, 125–129
   amputations as, 128–129
   fractures as, 125–127
   spinal cord injuries as, 127–128
skin breakdown, prevention of, 197
   diarrhea and, 205
small-for-gestational-age infant, 188
smoking. *See* cigarette smoking
sodium bicarbonate, for sickle cell anemia, 101
sodium levothyroxine (Synthroid), for hyperthyroidism, 97
sodium luminal, for alcohol intoxication, 261
somatization disorder, 272, 273
somatoform disorders, 272–273
spinal cord injury, 127–128
   practice test for, 305
splenectomy, 104
   practice test for, 297
sponge, for birth control, 182
stapedectomy, 120
station, definition of, 174
Stelazine (trifluoperazine), 246*t*, 399
steroid therapy. *See also* cortisone
   for contact dermatitis, 106
   for detached retina, 124
   for multiple sclerosis, 114
   practice test for, 367
   for rheumatoid arthritis, 132
stoma care, 119
stool softeners, for spinal cord injuries, 128
strabismus, 200
   practice test for, 367
stress, physical diseases and, 274–275
striae gravidarum, pregnancy and, 166
stroke, practice test for, 292
study skills, 6–9, 7*f*
subjective data, definition of, 13
submucosal resection, 125
substance abuse. *See* drug abuse
Sucralfate (carafate), for peptic ulcer, 77–78
sudden infant death syndrome, 209
suicide
   adolescent and, 238–239
   intervention for, 255
   practice test for, 391–392
sulfinpyrazone (Anturane), for gout, 131
sympathomimetic bronchodilators, for chronic obstructive pulmonary disease, 65
sympathomimetic organic mental disorders, 264–265
syphilis, 145–146
   pregnancy and, 172

TAH-BSO. *See* total hysterectomy and bilateral salpingo-oophorectomy

Taractan (chlorprothixene), 246*t*
Tegretol (carbamazepine), for epilepsy and seizures, 112
temazepam (Restoril), 250, 252*t*. *See also* benzodiazepines
testicular cancer, 144–145
   practice test for, 311
test-taking strategies, 9–12
   for anxiety, 10–11
   for content questions, 283
   for process questions, 283–284
   for validation examination, 4–5
tetanus prophylaxis, for burns, 107
tetracyclic antidepressants, 248*t*, 249*t*. *See also* antidepressant agents
tetracycline, for chlamydia, 149
theophylline, for asthma, 226, 227
therapeutic communication. *See* communication, nurse-client
therapeutic relationship
   phases of, 244
   practice test for, 402–403
thiamine, for alcohol intoxication, 261
thiazide, for hypertension, 63
thioridazine (Mellaril), 246*t*. *See also* antipsychotic/neuroleptic agents
thiothixene (Navane), 246*t*. *See also* antipsychotic/neuroleptic agents
thioxanthenes, 246*t*. *See also* antipsychotic/neuroleptic agents
Thorazine (chlorpromazine), 246*t*, 399
thromboangiitis obliterans, 59–60
thrombolytic agents
   for myocardial infarction, 42
   for pulmonary embolism, 56
thrombophlebitis, 53–55
   postpartal, 183
thrombosis, 53–55
   practice test for, 293
thyroidectomy, practice test for, 298
thyroid replacement, for hypothyroidism, 98
toddler, 212–220. *See also* preschooler
   growth and development of, 195*t*
Tofranil (imipramine hydrochloride), 248*t*, 271
toilet training, 212–213
   practice test for, 364
tonsillitis and tonsillectomy, 213–214
   practice test for, 369
TORCH, 172
total hip replacement, 126–127
   practice test for, 298–299
total hysterectomy and bilateral salpingo-oophorectomy, 137
toxoplasmosis, pregnancy and, 172

tracheoesophageal fistula, 201–202
tranquilizers
  for epilepsy and seizures, 112
  for ulcerative colitis, 82
Transactional Analysis, 24–28, 27f, 33
transition, definition of, 33
transplantation, renal, 158
transvestic fetishism, 274
Traxene (chlorazepate dipotassium), 250, 252t
trazodone (Desyrel), 248t. *See also* antidepressant
    agents
Trendelenberg's sign, 199
Trental (pentoxifylline), for arteriosclerosis, 62
tricyclic antidepressants, 248t, 249t. *See also*
    antidepressant agents
trifluoperazine (Stelazine), 246t. *See also* antipsychotic/
    neuroleptic agents
  practice test for, 399
triflupromazine (Vesprin), 246t. *See also* antipsychotic/
    neuroleptic agents
trust, definition of, 33
tubal ligation, 182
  practice test for, 345
tuberculosis, 68–69
  practice test for, 289

ulcer, peptic, 76–78
ulcerative colitis, 81–82
ultrasound, for fetal assessment, 168
uremic frost, 157
urinary dysfunction
  benign prostatic hypertrophy and, 141–142
  cancer of prostate and, 143–144
  cancer of testes and, 144–145
urinary tract infection, 159
  postpartal, 183
  practice test for, 368–369
  pregnancy and, 171
uterine and cervical cancer, 140–141
  practice test for, 309–310
uterine fibroids and leiomyomas, 133–134
uterus
  inversion of, 178
  prolapse of, 134–135
  rupture of, 178

vagotomy, for peptic ulcer, 77
validation
  definition of, 3
  preparation for, 4–5

validation examination
  administration and scoring of, 4
  material covered in, 4
  study skills in preparation for, 6–9, 7f
  test-taking strategies for, 10–12
  types of, 3
Valium (diazepam), 42, 112, 250, 252t, 261
value systems, in nurse-client communication, 21–23
valve replacement, 46
  for mitral stenosis, 47
varicose veins, 58–59
  practice test for, 293
vascular dysfunction, 51–64
  aneurysm as, 51–53
  arteriosclerosis as, 61–62
  Buerger's disease as, 59–60
  cerebrovascular accident as, 56–58
  hypertension as, 62–64
  pulmonary embolism as, 55–56
  Raynaud's phenomenom as, 60
  thrombophlebitis as, 53–55
  varicose veins as, 58–59
vasectomy, 182
vasodilator agents
  for congestive heart failure, 44
  for hypertension, 63
  for Raynaud's phenomenon, 60
vasopressor drugs, for pulmonary embolism, 56
vein ligation and stripping, 58
  practice test for, 293
venereal diseases. *See* sexually transmitted diseases
venous congestion, in congestive heart failure, 43
venous thrombosis, 53–55
  practice test for, 293
ventilatory therapy, for head injury, 109
Vermox (mebendazole), for helminthic infections, 224
Vesprin (triflupromazine), 246t
vincristine, practice test for, 373
viral pharyngitis, practice test for, 369
visualization, as test-taking strategy, 11
vital signs, postpartal, 180
vitamin B_{12}, for pernicious anemia, 99
vitamin K
  for cirrhosis of liver, 90
  for hepatitis, 92
  for newborn, 176
  practice test for, 346
vitamin supplements
  for cirrhosis of liver, 90
  for nutritional anemia, 100
vomiting
  pyloric stenosis and, 203
  self-induced, 275–276
voyeurism, 274

warfarin sodium crystalline (Coumadin)
　　for pulmonary embolism, 55
　　for thrombophlebitis, 54
weight gain, pregnancy and, 166
Wenckebach, 48f, 50. *See also* heart block

Xanax (alprazolam), 252t

Zarontin (ethosuximide), for seizures, 237